D1413716

The Jossey-Bass Health Series brings together the most current information and ideas in health care from the leaders in the field. Titles from the Jossey-Bass Health Series include these essential health care resources:

FUNDAMENTALS OF HEALTH CARE FINANCIAL MANAGEMENT

A Practical Guide to Financial Issues and Activities

SECOND EDITION

Steven Berger

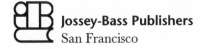
Jossey-Bass Publishers
San Francisco

Published by

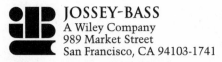

JOSSEY-BASS
A Wiley Company
989 Market Street
San Francisco, CA 94103-1741

www.josseybass.com

Jossey-Bass books and products are available through most bookstores. To contact Jossey-Bass directly, call (888) 378-2537, fax to (800) 605-2665, or visit our website at www.josseybass.com.

Substantial discounts on bulk quantities of Jossey-Bass books are available to corporations, professional associations, and other organizations. For details and discount information, contact the special sales department at Jossey-Bass.

We at Jossey-Bass strive to use the most environmentally sensitive paper stocks available to us. Our publications are printed on acid-free recycled stock whenever possible, and our paper always meets or exceeds minimum GPO and EPA requirements.

Library of Congress Cataloging-in-Publication Data

Berger, Steven H.
    Fundamentals of health care financial management : a practical guide to fiscal issues and activities / Steven Berger. — 2nd ed.
        p.   cm. — (The Jossey-Bass health series)
    Previously published under the title: Fundamentals of healthcare financial management : a systematic approach to fiscal issues and activities.
    Includes bibliographical references and index.
    ISBN 0-7879-5980-4
    1. Health facilities—Business management.   2. Health facilities—Finance.   I. Berger, Steven H. Fundamentals of healthcare financial management.   II. Title.
    RA971.3 .B465 2002
    362.1′068′1—dc21
    2001038582

SECOND EDITION
HB Printing   10 9 8 7 6 5 4 3 2 1

CONTENTS

TABLES, FIGURES, AND EXHIBITS

Tables

Figures

Exhibits

PREFACE

Starting right now, we are embarking on a journey into the interesting and compelling world of the health care financial manager. Though not on the front line of the patient's care, the health care financial manager needs to be involved in or apprised of all decisions related to operating or planning the facility. Because of this, the financial manager develops a unique understanding of the business of health care.

Whether in a hospital, a skilled nursing facility, a physician office, a home health agency, a psychiatric facility, or any of the other operations doing business in this industry, the basic concepts are essentially the same. Health care and how it is financed have several characteristics unique to this industry alone:

- The health insurance system separates the consumer from the buying decision. Because of this, the consumer seldom has to make a rational choice in the amount or level of product consumption. This is the number one reason the cost of health care is so high in the United States.
- The health care system is pluralistic, a mixture of government and non-government providers and payors.
- The payment system is very technical and complex. Every payor has its own set of benefits, and often they are not spelled out clearly. The consumer (patient) may believe she has a certain set of benefits, but when she finally needs care she may find out that she is in fact not covered for a particular

set of illnesses or therapies. This often puts the provider in the difficult situation of denying or postponing care until these coverage issues are settled.

• Ultimately, health care is personal. It affects everyone. No other industry encounters the intensity of emotion engendered in health care. The patient, whose illness may lead to death (or in the case of maternity care, life) is always at personal risk. So, too, are the loved ones who congregate around the patient and the provider, often with great anxiety and trepidation.

This, then, is why health care, and how it is financed, is so important. Knowing this helps to explain why the role of the finance manager takes on great importance within the industry. The financial manager is responsible for financial reporting and the budget, both of which summarize financial results of the organization, actual and projected. These summaries are a direct reflection of the decisions made before the fiscal year begins and day to day as the year moves along. The astute financial manager, who needs to learn as much as possible about every aspect of the organization's operation, is often in a better position than any other manager to assess the operation in an objective and nonpartisan manner.

At the same time, the health care financial manager needs to learn, understand, and absorb myriad rules, regulations, policies, and procedures that reflect the highly unique world of American health care practices and its finances. This book is dedicated to the proposition that you the reader can learn much about the unique financial underpinnings of your industry. There is so much to know and so little time. The challenge is how to make these complex ideas presentable in a basic text.

Imagine, if you will, an industry in which the billing rules for only one of its many payors, Medicare, are forty-five thousand pages long. Then imagine that in 1997, Medicare's enforcement division claimed that a billing mistake constitutes fraud, not an honest error.

Or imagine an industry in which the largest group of nongovernmental payors, known as health maintenance organizations (HMOs) or preferred provider organizations (PPOs), together commonly referred to as managed care, creates incentives for its contracted providers of care (the hospitals, doctors, and other caregivers) to limit the care given. This is done in the name of saving money for the premium payor, who is usually the employer. Yet these same insurers generally do not offer coverage for screening tests that could either rule out or determine illness that, if caught early, would cost those self-same insurers less money through less intensive treatment.

OK, you get the idea. Crazy policies. Not always in the best interest of the patient. More than likely in the best interest of the insurer. But ask yourself: *When was the last time I reached into my own pocket to pay the full list price for my health care?* Most probably never. Very few employed, elderly, or poor people in America have. They seldom ask the question, which we will do, "Why does health care cost so much?" The biggest part of the answer is that if one of your loved ones gets sick, you will spare no expense (primarily the insurance company's money) to make sure he or she gets well. The providers of care in America have therefore built their industry to respond to the needs and desires of the market.

The problem here is what the market desires is in conflict. Because very few patients (customers) pay out of pocket, the patient's desires are often at odds with the desires of the payors and employers who pay the premiums. Caught in the middle, then, are the providers, attempting to be cost-efficient, produce quality outcomes, and create a high level of patient satisfaction while earning a positive financial return on their investment.

How all this came to happen and how a particular fictional provider contributes to overall industry expenditures is a case study for learning. This book covers the basic health care financial management issues, but from a distinct perspective. You, the reader, get to act like a health care financial manager for the most common financial reporting period, one calendar year. Starting on January 1, you will experience the highs and lows of a health care finance officer as he (in this case, a man) weaves his way through busy times and slow times—mostly busy!—and through the conflicting issues that populate the health care financing landscape.

This particular book is written from the perspective of a finance officer for a hospital. However, many of the other primary industry providers are also profiled because the organization in this case study also operates a hospital-based skilled nursing facility, a home health agency, and a psychiatric unit, and it employs a dozen physicians in office practices.

Finally, this text is not intended as an academic treatise. Rather, it is a practical guide to how an integrated health care finance division operates in this era, day to day. It is an attempt to meld practice with theory. As we go through the year, various concepts are highlighted and highlighted again, just as often really happens. This helps to clarify those issues that are of overriding importance to sound financial management.

November 2001   Steven Berger
Libertyville, Illinois   stevenberger@aol.com
                                                  http://www.healthcareinsightsllc.com

To my wife Barbara,
who provides a great sense of joy
and stability for me and our family.

ACKNOWLEDGMENTS

I would like to thank a number of people for bringing me to the point in my life where the opportunity to write this book coincided with reality. On the professional side, I would like to thank two of the best bosses anyone could possibly be lucky enough to have had—Ken Knieser and Jack Gilbert—for never telling me to stop doing what I thought was right. Thanks also to John Dalton, for encouraging me to become a writer and editor of health care finance material more than ten years ago. Finally, my thanks to Jim Curcuruto, who, more than two decades ago, was the first professional I worked with who took the time to stop what he was doing and give me my first taste of understanding the concepts of health care finance.

I would also like to thank those people with the experience and knowledge to help me improve this book. They took the time and effort to read the entire first-edition manuscript in draft and offer terrific suggestions for refinement and embellishment. They are my good friends, who continue to offer constructive advice, Bob Carlisle and the aforementioned Jack Gilbert and Ken Knieser. The fourth reader of the original book, Mary Grace Wilkus, has subsequently become my business partner. Her insightfulness has helped to make the contents of this book more cogent.

In addition, several people with expertise in some specific areas of health care financial management contributed their time and effort to review those sections and offer insightful comments that helped to improve this book. They are Jane

Bachmann on Medicare step-down advice, Robert Alcaro for contributing his review of the HIPAA section, Julie Micheletti for her astute knowledge of Ambulatory Payment Classifications (APCs), and Keri Wulf for her review of financial statements. I would also like to give special mention to the editor of the first edition of this book, Kristine Rynne, who has helped to guide me through some murky publishing waters.

I continue to thank my former staff at Highland Park Hospital for doing their jobs so well that I felt comfortable taking the time to write a book. My particular thanks to Keri Wulf again; Guy Sanchez; Diana Wright (without whom I would not have been so effective on the job); and my former assistant, Patty Holland, who always kept me heading in the direction I needed to be going.

On the personal side, I am indebted to my family, who made the biggest sacrifice involved in creating this book. The nights and weekends I labored on it often took me away from them. My wife, Barbara, kept the household together, holding a menagerie of active children in a relative state of equilibrium. I am blessed to have four kids who keep me younger in spirit than in body. Ben, Arlie, and Emmalee make me smile all the time. But how would I have ever been able to finish this book without Sam, who looked over my shoulder every day to check my progress and whisper encouragement in my ear, like, "Come on, Dad, what do you mean you only did one page since yesterday? Let's move it, move it, move it!"

ABOUT THE AUTHOR

Steven Berger is president of Healthcare Insights (http://www.healthcarein sightsllc.com), which specializes in teaching and consulting on general and financial management issues in health care. In addition, Healthcare Insights has developed dynamic decision support software solutions for the health care industry.

Prior to assuming his role at Healthcare Insights, he was vice president, finance, for seven years at the two hundred and fifty–bed Highland Park Hospital in suburban Chicago. Before that and since 1978, he was a hospital or health system finance officer in New York, New Jersey, and Missouri at diverse organizations including urban and suburban facilities, both academic and nonteaching, ranging in size from one hundred to four hundred beds. He began his career as a Medicare auditor for the Blue Cross Blue Shield Plan of Greater New York and has also worked for a small CPA firm in New York City.

Berger has twenty-six years of health care financial management experience. He holds a bachelor of science degree in history and a master of science in accounting from the State University of New York at Binghamton. He is a certified public accountant (CPA) and a fellow (FHFMA) of the Healthcare Financial Management Association, where he currently serves as immediate past president of the First Illinois chapter. He has recently completed a three-year term on the HFMA's National Board of Examiners. He is also a diplomate of the American College of Healthcare Executives (CHE).

In addition, over the past several years he has presented many health care finance-related seminars throughout the United States and Canada, including three two-day classes on Fundamentals of Health Care Financial Management (which is the basis for this book); Turning Data into Useful Information (how to effectively collect, analyze, and report financial and clinical data to enhance decision making in health care), which trains both data users and data crunchers in understanding each other's needs and practical ways in which to meet those needs; and Hospital Financial Management for the Nonfinancial Manager, which teaches clinical and operating managers how to use financial tools and techniques to improve the financial results in their own departments. He has also cowritten articles on health care information systems that were published in *Healthcare Financial Management* and a February 2000 commentary in *Modern Healthcare* on the lack of training in the industry.

CHAPTER ONE

JANUARY

"Daddy, what do you do all day at work?" the seven-year-old asks plaintively.

"What do you mean?" blinks Samuel Barnes, the daddy.

"You know, like when you go out so early in the morning and then don't come back until after other daddies are already home. What are you doing? Why does it take so long?" asks the curly-haired tot.

Sam has to think for a moment. "Well, honey, that's a good question. I guess I'm out there trying to make the hospital I work for as successful as it can be."

"But what do you do?"

"Susie, I'm in charge of all the money that comes into the hospital. I'm also respon-sible for all the money paid out to the people who work there. I also make sure that all the other people who send us stuff that we use to make the sick people better, like food and medicine, get paid."

"Daddy, do you ever have any money left over after you pay these people?"

"Well, Susie, that's the whole point. To be successful, you want to have as much left over as you can."

"But what do you do with all that leftover money? Do you put it in the bank like I do with my allowance?"

"Well, sort of. But instead of putting it into the bank, we put it into a kind of bank that lends it out to other people who need money in their businesses. They then pay us back with a little extra money to thank us for letting them use our money for a while. It's called interest."

"So the hospital has all this leftover money and then you have even more money from these other people paying you interest. I'm glad that you work at a company that's making money because I heard on the news that some people were losing their jobs. I guess you or any of the people you work with won't lose their jobs."

"Actually, Susie, I wish I could tell you it was that clear-cut, but it's not. Part of my job is to make sure that the hospital makes as much money as we decided we wanted to make before the year starts. Sometimes that means we believe we will need less people working for us if we think less people will come to the hospital to be taken care of."

"But," Susie asks quizzically, "how can you know about all these things?"

"Ah, honey," he says, "that's a long story."

It is one minute past midnight on January 1. Outside, the New Year's revelers are just beginning their celebrations. Inside the bowels of the powerful computers

1

of Ridgeland Heights Medical Center (RHMC), a fictional health care system, a different kind of ritual is taking place. At this moment, the automated pricing mechanism is executing its programming, effectively increasing the ten thousand or so charges related to individual services or supplies provided to patients. These increases, so carefully planned, are meant to help the organization improve its bottom line.

How these charges came to be, and why they are important, is only a small part of the story that constitutes the art of health care financial management. Financial management in practically any industry has its own policies, procedures, and practices. In most cases, generally accepted accounting principles (GAAP) and financial procedures require estimates and approximations based on the company's, and the estimator's, previous experience within the industry. This experience is often timeworn. Financial statements are produced month after month, year after year. Over time, most companies doing business within any industry report financial results in conformance with industry standards.

A standard is "something considered by an authority or by general consent to be an approved or acceptable model." In the health care industry, standards represent the ability to properly report operating results for any particular period of time requested as well as the net assets of an organization.

For RHMC, the price increase, although not entirely desired by the organization's administration because of its possible negative public relations, is vital to its continued financial success. The size of the price increase is a function of change in volume, severity, and expense, all forecast and budgeted by the medical center. These changes are the result of strategic planning initiatives, newly planned services, shifts in the payor mix, and demographic fluctuations. They are also related to expense increases or decreases projected as a result of the change in volume.

This book examines these issues and many more. To begin to understand health care financial management and many of its key components, we must build a framework from which to operate. This framework takes the form of a diary and a primer. It chronicles a year in the life of one health care institution and one health care financial administrator. It explores how this organization, the board of directors, and the clinical and financial executives go about making decisions and how these decisions are then implemented. It further explores the organization through the natural life cycle of the institution, day by day and month by month, just as a real institution operates.

This book offers practical and informative points on health care decision making, usually from the financial point of view. In the end, the objective is to create greater understanding of *how* the industry operates on a detailed financial level, and *why*. Our fictional medical center, Ridgeland Heights, was chosen because its bed complement of 256 falls in the range of a great many hospitals in the United States today. According to *Health, United States, 2000* (one edition of an annual compilation of health care statistics across the United States published since 1993 by the National Center for Health Statistics of the Department of Health and Human Services), of the 33.8 million admissions to all hospitals in 1998, 6.2 million were made to hospitals in the range of 200 to 299 beds. When you add up the admissions of hospitals in the range from 100 to 399 beds, the result is 17.9 million, 53 percent of all admissions (*Health, United States, 2000, with Adolescent Health Chartbook*). Consequently, this book is representative of more than half of the typical hospitals in the country.

Before we begin to explore health care financial management systems and techniques, it is necessary to first define some terms.

What Is Health Care?

What is health care? It is "the field concerned with the maintenance or restoration of the health of the body or mind." This may seem obvious, but maybe not. The health care industry at the current time encompasses much more than just hospitals and doctors. Although together they are associated with the majority of industry expenditures, there is a considerable number of other reputable health care providers that make up the remainder. Figure 1.1 shows the current breakdown of expenditures within the health care industry.

Remarkably, one of the largest segments of the industry is in the "other" category. "Complementary" or "alternative" medicine (CAM) currently dominates this category. CAM is generally categorized as non-Western medicine and therapies, which are not currently accepted as a standard of care by most U.S. doctors. Some therapies included in this grouping are chiropractic, massage therapy, acupuncture, Chinese herbal medicine, aromatherapy, meditation, and yoga. According to a study published in the *New England Journal of Medicine* (*NEJM*) in 1993, consumers spent about $13.7 billion on alternative care in 1990 (Eisenberg and others, 1993). Of that amount, $10.3 billion was out-of-pocket, not paid for by any insurance. The *NEJM* study further indicated that 34 percent of the respondents in the national survey said they had used at least one alternative therapy in the preceding year.

Interestingly, it is probable that over the last decade, through 2001, even more Americans embraced CAM as a fundamental treatment option. Yet in the 2000 AHA Annual Survey of Hospitals, it was found that only an estimated 10.2 percent of all hospitals in the United States and 11.2 percent of all community hospitals offered CAM services in 1999. This was a sharp jump from 1998, when

FIGURE 1.1. NATIONAL HEALTH EXPENDITURES, 1960–1999.

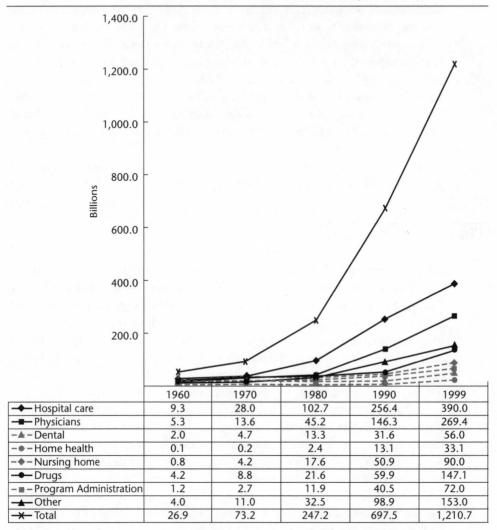

	1960	1970	1980	1990	1999
◆ Hospital care	9.3	28.0	102.7	256.4	390.0
■ Physicians	5.3	13.6	45.2	146.3	269.4
▲ Dental	2.0	4.7	13.3	31.6	56.0
● Home health	0.1	0.2	2.4	13.1	33.1
◆ Nursing home	0.8	4.2	17.6	50.9	90.0
● Drugs	4.2	8.8	21.6	59.9	147.1
■ Program Administration	1.2	2.7	11.9	40.5	72.0
▲ Other	4.0	11.0	32.5	98.9	153.0
✕ Total	26.9	73.2	247.2	697.5	1,210.7

Source: Office of the Actuary, National Health Statistics Group, Health Care Financing Administration (HCFA). January 2001. (http://www.hcfa.gov)

7.7 percent of all hospitals and 8.6 percent of community hospitals gave CAM care. Furthermore, the study indicates that the likelihood of offering CAM services varies sharply according to the number of beds in the institution, with just 3.4 percent of hospitals having six to twenty-four beds offering CAM but 33 percent of hospitals with five hundred or more beds providing it. In itself, this indicates a significant expansion opportunity for a variety of hospitals.

Still, the important principle here is to recognize the breadth of a $1.2 trillion industry. The health care industry is huge and has grown that way in the most dramatic fashion over the past thirty-five years, really starting its climb in 1966 with the advent of the Medicare and Medicaid programs. These programs are explored in greater detail in Chapter Four. However, suffice it to say that they opened the floodgates of money to the industry. At the time the programs began, the industry absorbed 5.7 percent of the gross domestic product (GDP) in the country (*Health, United States, 2000*). The GDP is the market value of goods and services produced by labor and property located in the United States. In the intervening thirty-three years, through 1999, health care's percentage of GDP has grown to 13.0 percent, a 228 percent increase (*Health, United States, 2000*). This means that as a country we have decided, either by intent or accident, to expend a considerable amount of additional national resources and wealth in the pursuit of our health.

It is important to note that the 13.0 percent of U.S. GDP absorbed for health care leads the industrialized world by a large margin. The next five highest GDPs by country are Canada at 9.8 percent, Austria and France at 9.7 percent, Switzerland at 9.6 percent, and Germany at 9.5 percent (*Health, United States, 2000*). So significantly more is spent on health care in the United States than any place else in the world. There are many reasons for this. First, Americans have more discretionary income than anyone else and have chosen to spend some of it on health care. Second, Americans have been trained since the end of World War II to expect unlimited treatment for illness. This training has come from organized medicine—defined as the American Medical Association, the American Hospital Association, the American College of Surgeons, and many more groups. Health care is big business, and major administrative services have sprung up to handle the load.

Figure 1.1 highlights the financial scope of the health care industry. It is over one point two trillion dollars. $1,200,000,000,000. That's a lot of zeros. It is also the total amount of money spent on health care services in 1999. This means that there are tremendous resources available to the companies that service patients—and tremendous opportunities. Health care is now one of the largest industries in the country. This money should be consumed in pursuit of the best possible outcomes, offered in the most consumer-friendly way, and at the least possible cost. This is the role and objective of health care. The financial manager plays a large role in trying to achieve these outcomes through his or her involvement and leadership in budget planning and reporting, charge setting, contract negotiations, and general financial consulting to the organization's department managers.

What Is Management?

Before looking for a definition of financial management, it is first important to define general management. In most for-profit firms, management's overarching objective is to maximize the owners' or shareholders' wealth. To accomplish this goal, management has been assigned certain roles and responsibilities:

Leading

Planning

Organizing

Coordinating

Motivating

Controlling

In the case of the health care industry, an overwhelming majority of hospitals and skilled nursing facilities are classified as not-for-profit through section 501(c)(3) of the Internal Revenue Code. Still, though their employers are not-for-profit, health care industry managers are required to produce the best possible bottom line. They simply need to do so in the context of providing optimal patient care in the most efficient manner.

In the for-profit world, "management must administer the assets of the enterprise in order to obtain the greatest wealth for the owner" (Berman, Weeks, and Kukla, 1986, p. 4). Therefore, management's goal is to find the combination of earnings and risk associated with producing those earnings that yields the highest possible value.

In the not-for-profit world, earnings or profits are called margin. In the case of both for-profit and not-for profit health care firms, the profit or margin is what remains after expenses, or costs, are subtracted from revenues. To reiterate, the role of management is to produce the best possible financial outcomes while minimizing risk to the organization. Not-for-profit health care providers place a somewhat greater emphasis on social goals than for-profit providers, but in the end management's success or failure—as defined by each organization's board of directors—is primarily related to the quality of its bottom line.

What Is Financial Management?

Financial management can now be defined as strategizing the organization's financial direction as well as the performance of its day-to-day financial operation.

Therefore financial management has a twofold purpose. The first is to point the strategic financial direction of the organization. This function is usually performed at the executive level of the financial ladder by the chief financial officer (CFO). The primary job is to prepare and present the organization's strategic financial plan to the board for endorsement and approval. In many organizations, this job may also include the treasury function, which is charged with investing the organization's financial assets in the most prudent manner as set down in board-approved investment policies.

The second purpose is management of day-to-day financial operations. The organization's second-in-command finance officer, often called the controller, usually carries this out. This function means making sure that the payroll and the suppliers are paid, and that the revenues generated by the operation are billed out in an accurate and timely manner and collected efficiently with a minimum of write-offs.

Financial management has a role within the overall context of general management. Sound financial management aids the general managers in carrying out the six management concepts expressed previously. According to Berman, Weeks, and Kukla (1986), "Financial management tools and techniques can aid management in providing the community with quality services at least cost by furnishing the data that are necessary for making intelligent capital investment decisions, by guiding the operations of certain hospital subsystems, and by providing the systems and data needed to monitor and control operations" (p. 4).

Thus making data available and helping to analyze the financial implications of the data across the health care organization's setting is a primary role of financial management. Financial management involves the finance staff in a number of highly visible and important matters:

- Setting prices for the services provided (often called gross charges)
- Producing and analyzing the discounts (often called contractual allowances) taken by a third-party payor—defined as anyone other than the patient who pays for the patient's services (the large third-party payors are Medicare, Medicaid, and hundreds of managed care organizations or MCOs, often called health maintenance organizations or HMOs, preferred provider organizations or PPOs, or point of service organizations or POSs, all across the country)

- Recording and analyzing cost information across the organization and at the department level (this involves comparing actual costs to budgeted costs and determining variance analysis; it may also involve a detailed cost accounting program)
- Preparing and reporting financial projections to help successfully guide the organization in its future endeavors (a short-term projection of up to a year into the future is called a budget, and a long-term projection of one to five years into the future is called a strategic financial plan)

Why Is Financial Management Important?

Financial management has a primary and a secondary role in the financial health of the health care organization. Its secondary role is reporting financial results periodically, usually monthly. Its primary role, however, is as a broker of information. Those who control the information usually have quite a bit of power in any organization. The finance division of most organizations, and in most industries, has generally been the storer and reporter of information.

Remember, an organization can have little success without the proper financial information on which to base its decisions. The whole purpose of having and using information is to make the most appropriate decision. Making a decision is any manager's number one priority. Making the proper decision is a function of experience and appropriate information.

Keep in mind that there is a significant difference between information and raw data. Data streams inundate most managers all day long. Raw data are often useless, and sometimes harmful, in the process of making the best decision. The value of information is that it brings context to the data, presenting them in a format that enhances a manager's ability to understand what is happening and to make a good decision.

Management has been described as the art of making decisions, usually under uncertain and difficult conditions. Thus financial management can be said to be important because, if applied properly, it maximizes the operating manager's ability to make difficult yet good decisions, under uncertainty, by presenting information in the best possible format. In addition, it allows the finance division to maximize reimbursement (net revenue) for the health care organization. (This is covered in Chapter Four.)

Ridgeland Heights Medical Center: The Primary Statistics

Ridgeland Heights Medical Center is a (fictional) medium-sized medical center in a northern Chicago suburb. For IRS purposes, it was classified as a community, not-for-profit hospital under Internal Revenue Code Section 501(c)(3) because of its charitable mission, dating back to 1925. In addition to its current complement of 180 acute care medical and surgical beds, it also has a 20-bed maternity unit, a 22-bed Medicare PPS-exempt psychiatric unit, a Medicare-certified home health agency (HHA) and hospice, and a 30-bed hospital-based skilled nursing facility (SNF).

Ridgeland Heights also owns ten primary care physician practice sites, which employ thirteen full-time physicians. This practice is managed through a corporate affiliated management service organization (MSO), which also manages six nonowned primary care physician practices.

In addition, RHMC is half owner of a physician hospital organization (PHO), the other half owned by an independent practice association (IPA), a group of physicians legally organized to negotiate contracts with MCOs. The PHO negotiates contracts on behalf of both the medical center and the IPA. In many instances, this is well received by the managed care companies because of its time-saving and cost-reducing principles.

Volume indicators are critical to understanding any institution. A volume indicator generally defines the level of financial viability. RHMC provides both inpatient and outpatient services. Table 1.1 highlights the inpatient volumes for the year just ended as well as the current budgeted year.

Although the medical center always received a majority of its gross revenues from its inpatient services, the 11,000 or so inpatient admissions are now dwarfed by more than 180,000 outpatient services each year. (See Table 1.2 for the analysis.)

This development brought a series of unexpected consequences to the medical center. Although the administration had for several years talked about redefining its service lines to be somewhat more aligned with the outpatient business, it had not yet done so. The continuing decline in the inpatient census coupled with outpatient increases drove the powers-that-be to complete plans for a renovation and expansion, primarily for improved and updated outpatient and physician services. At the same time, the medical center decided to take some dramatic action with regard to its dwindling inpatient census.

TABLE 1.1. RIDGELAND HEIGHTS MEDICAL CENTER 2000 ACTUAL AND 2001 BUDGETED INPATIENT VOLUMES.

		Admissions		
	Number of Beds	2000 Actual	2001 Budget	Percentage Variance
Medical, surgical	120	2,700	2,800	3.7
Intensive care	24	1,800	1,900	5.6
Pediatrics	10	600	660	10.0
Maternity	24	2,000	2,200	10.0
Births	26	1,950	2,145	10.0
Psychiatric	20	1,000	1,200	20.0
Skilled nursing facility	30	800	840	5.0
Totals	254	10,850	11,745	8.2

TABLE 1.2. RHMC 2000 ACTUAL AND 2001 BUDGETED OUTPATIENT VISITS.

	Visits		
	2000 Actual	2001 Budget	Percentage Variance
Emergency department	19,000	20,000	5.3
Outpatient surgery	4,500	5,000	11.1
Same-day surgery	3,700	4,000	8.1
Observation patients	1,950	2,000	2.6
Home health services	26,000	30,000	15.4
Other outpatients	112,000	120,000	7.1
Totals	167,150	181,000	8.29

Managed Care Inroads

Over the past few years, managed care companies have made significant inroads into RHMC's primary and secondary service areas. In doing so, these companies have brought with them a utilization review philosophy that generally reduces access to care to those beneficiaries covered by insurance. This is not by accident. Employers, who usually foot the bills for employee medical insurance, grew tired of the seemingly never-ending round of double-digit premium increases each year throughout the 1980s. When old-style indemnity insurance, which generally

	Patient Days			Length of Stay	
2000 Actual	2001 Budget	Percentage Variance	2000 Actual	2001 Budget	Percentage Variance
13,000	14,000	7.7	4.81	5.00	3.8
6,500	7,220	11.1	3.61	3.80	5.2
1,500	1,716	14.4	2.50	2.60	4.0
4,000	4,400	10.0	2.00	2.00	0.0
3,900	4,290	10.0	2.00	2.00	0.0
6,500	8,160	25.5	6.50	6.80	4.6
8,800	8,400	−4.5	11.00	10.00	−9.1
44,200	48,186	9.0	4.07	4.10	0.7

paid the health care providers (hospitals, physicians, SNFs, home health agencies, and so on) failed to reign in these increases, employers turned to managed care companies.

These companies claimed they could control the rate of premium increases using a series of strategies that would reduce both the number of health care provider contacts as well as the intensity of the services received. Here is a summary of the cost control strategies used by managed care companies:

Utilization Controls

- Preauthorization of necessity (before approval for service)
- Second opinion, to determine need for service or alternatives
- Concurrent review and case management of continuing service necessity during a hospital stay
- Quality management programs, monitoring treatment type and duration for outpatient services
- Patient outcome research, to determine the efficacy of new clinical services

Reimbursement and Payment Controls

- Minimizing level of payment to service providers through tough negotiation
- Approval of payment methodologies that minimize provider incentives to continue treatment
- Imposition of patient copayment to discourage utilization of services

RHMC's Actions to Counter Dwindling Inpatient Census

The rate of decline in the inpatient census was alarming to the RHMC administration. They recognized that the decline in the inpatient census was partially causing an increase in lower-paying outpatient services. Still, to maintain viability as a full-service, stand-alone medical center, the administration knew that admissions had to be increased. There were only a few ways to do it:

1. Steal market share from other service providers (always an option in any business in any industry; the secret is not in the trying but in the succeeding). This could be attempted in a number of ways:

   Improved consumer marketing or more of it. Historically, this is not the most effective means. Health care is an industry that has always resisted consumer marketing because referral is generally through a physician, or more recently through managed care contractual coverage.

   Improved physician marketing or more of it.

   A better mix of clinical services. This would be a much more effective strategy given the reasons that previous marketing strategies have not worked. A health care organization that can meet the demands of physicians and payors is likely to survive and thrive in the current climate of downsized institutions.

2. Grow market share by providing services that are not being offered in the service area. This could mean being on the leading edge of technology (a potentially expensive place to be) or assessing the local market through focus groups and surveys to determine the current needs, wants, and desires of the community. An example is complementary or alternative care services, as mentioned earlier in this chapter.

3. Grow market share by recruiting additional physicians at RHMC and encouraging physicians who practice at more than one hospital to practice exclusively at RHMC.

RHMC Decision Time

Through its administration, RHMC decided to try a mix of solutions. It would perform more targeted marketing and advertising to highlight those services where it already had a substantial clinical advantage as well as those services that it wanted to build on. Yet the RHMC administration understood that the concept of target marketing and advertising in health care is complex because it is difficult to identify the decision makers who ultimately purchase the service. For instance, is it the patient, patient's family, physician, insurer, or someone else? The answer is, it depends on the particular health care service. Thus the administration intended to proceed carefully.

In addition, the Medical Center planned to build new services, particularly outpatient surgeries and services, that appear to be where the heaviest industry growth is headed. Finally, it would put some of its limited financial and intellectual resources into developing more advanced clinical services (often called tertiary services) to differentiate itself from some of its other community-based, nonacademic teaching facility competitors.

Financial Management Implications

Almost every decision made by the health care organization's administration has implications for financial management. There should be intended consequences that were expected and in fact desired when the decision is made. There are also unintended consequences, those results that are unforeseen (and that have a 100 percent likelihood of happening). In any event, the finance division is counted on (no pun intended) to present the most appropriate and conservative estimate of the likely projected financial results. This usually means producing what is called a *pro forma*, a projected income statement incorporating all known assumptions. This should be done using assumptions that represent best-case, worst-case, and most-likely scenarios.

Pro Forma Development

Developing pro formas is extremely important to the financial well being of the organization. A pro forma is usually performed when the organization is planning to develop a new service or acquire any type of equipment, the capitalized cost of which exceeds some internally generated amount of money. It is also usually performed in conjunction with the organization's strategic plan. This book goes into some detail on the concepts of strategic plan, strategic financial plan, capital goods, and capital budgeting in Chapter Three, but for now let's assume that RHMC always performs pro forma analysis for all capital acquisitions costing more than $500,000.

Net Present Value and Internal Rate of Return

The art of pro forma development is best described as the ability to assemble a series of assumptions that lead to a go or no-go decision with respect to capital acquisition. This is generally accomplished by having the final result of the pro forma produce either a net present value (NPV) or internal rate of return (IRR) for the project.

NPV is defined as the present value of the future cash inflow of an investment less the investment's cash outflow. Whereas NPV measures a project's dollar profitability, IRR measures a project's percentage profitability, or its expected rate of return (Gapenski, 1996). The computation summarizes quite a number of assumptions into a single percentage that has value for the decision maker. The organization may well have a "hurdle rate," established for its IRR for a new project. This is defined as the minimum percentage return that the organization expects to achieve through funding the project. The hurdle rate reflects the percentage return on its investment that the organization wants to realize. It is a function of the amount of interest income it could earn if it were to invest in the stock or bond market and the additional risk associated with the volume and rate projections used in the pro forma. By concluding a pro forma with an IRR, it is easy, at a glance, to determine whether the hurdle rate has been exceeded, thus giving the decision maker the appropriate information with which to make the go or no-go decision.

The reason for establishing a hurdle rate and internal rate of return involves money (that is, the capital resources used to pay for all purchases, whether operating expenses or capital expenses). Money, or the organization's capital, is scarce. There is always a list of conflicting priorities to be funded. Therefore, it is imperative that any health care organization establish its own hurdle rate, know why it is doing so, and adhere to it to stay financially viable into the future.

Volume Assumptions

The most important feature of pro forma development is the "validity" or best-guess nature of the assumptions. The most sensitive assumption in any pro forma is that of volume. Absolutely no other assumption drives the bottom line result as much as volume, because volumes drive three of the four essential elements of the income statement (gross revenue, net revenues, and variable expenses). The only element that it does not primarily control is fixed expenses. The age-old question is always how to verify, how to validate, or simply to believe that the volumes being proposed are achievable in the future for a service that has never been performed at the organization in the past.

Various methods can be used to construct a best-guess for volume. But again, because it is in the future, there is no guarantee that it will be achieved.

A good example of volume uncertainty and its potential validity can be seen in a pro forma that was developed at RHMC three years prior to the January of our discussion. The medical center decided it would make good clinical sense to install a magnetic resonance imaging (MRI) device, a highly sophisticated diagnostic radiology tool costing $1.75 million for the machine and another $250,000 for construction of the MRI suite. Up to that time, whenever physicians ordered MRI tests for patients, RHMC staff had to load the patients into an ambulance (at a cost of $60,000 a year) to be taken to an MRI provider twenty minutes away. An in-house unit would give better patient satisfaction and better physician satisfaction as a result of faster turnaround time on results. But it was the responsibility of the finance division to determine whether or not it would be a good financial investment.

Working with the radiology department manager, RHMC's finance manager developed a series of assumptions (see Table 1.3). The radiology manager contributed the all-important verifiable volumes, while the finance manager developed the information on gross and net revenue. Volume is the most important number on the page because both revenues and expenses are driven by it. In this case, the volumes were developed from two sources, one internal and one external.

The internal source was the number of MRI scans that RHMC was already sending to the outside provider annually. This number had great validity since it was historical. The external source was vendor-generated (usually suspect because the vendor is trying to sell its product). It consisted of the average number of MRI scans that should be needed at the medical center based on the number of current diagnostic radiology tests being performed. The vendor backed up the figures with a number of years of research. It is usually difficult to validate this type of claim, but it is important to try, particularly if the health care organization is considering spending $2 million. A survey of RHMC physicians most likely to order MRI scans can be used to validate the reasonableness of the vendor projection. In addition, external benchmarks of user rate per existing radiological procedure are available to help validate the projections.

Revenue and Expense Assumptions

Other aspects of the pro forma become almost as critical to ultimate success or failure of the venture. In this case, the published price per scan (the gross charge) needed to be set at a prevailing market rate, so various individuals performed "secret shopper" phone calls to other MRI providers within a thirty-mile radius. This helped the finance manager set prices for the types of scan performed by the MRI machine that should maximize the return to RHMC and be acceptable to the community.

Maximization of net revenue is a function of the number of Medicare, Medicaid, and managed care patients expected and in what percentages to the total. This is important because none of these payors reimburses the organization by its

TABLE 1.3. RHMC PRO FORMA OF PROPOSED MRI SERVICE FINANCIAL AND VOLUME ASSUMPTIONS, JULY 1998.

Capital Costs		Useful Life
Equipment (MRI)	$1,750,000	5 years
Construction, renovation	250,000	5 years
Total	$2,000,000	

	1999	2000
Volumes		
Inpatient	350	371
Outpatient	1,610	1,707
Total volumes	1,960	2,078
Total per day	8	8.48
Charge per test	$680	$714
Revenues		
Inpatient	238,000	264,894
Outpatient	1,094,800	1,218,798
Total revenues	$1,332,800	$1,483,692
Payor mix		
Medicare	34.20%	35.00%
Medicaid	3.80%	4.00%
Managed care	26.80%	30.00%
All other	35.20%	31.00%
Total payor mix	100.00%	100.00%
Contractual allowances		
Inpatient		
Medicare	100.00%	100.00%
Medicaid	100.00%	100.00%
Managed care	20.00%	20.00%
All other	5.00%	5.00%
Outpatient		
Medicare	53.00%	53.00%
Medicaid	80.00%	80.00%
Managed care	15.00%	15.00%
All other	5.00%	5.00%
Free care		
All other		
Inpatient	0	0
Outpatient	10.00%	12.00%

set price. Instead, Medicare and Medicaid mandate what they pay (no negotiations, thank you very much), while each managed care payor attempts to negotiate the lowest price that the provider is willing to accept.

Direct variable expenses for this new service are purely a function of volume. The number of employees, also known as full-time equivalents (FTEs), who must be hired is a function of the number of scans expected to be performed and the

2001	2002	2003	Total
393	417	442	1,973
1,809	1,918	2,033	9,076
2,202	2,335	2,475	11,049
8.99	9.53	10.1	
$750	$787	$827	
294,632	328,256	365,333	$1,491,115
1,356,207	1,509,821	1,680,364	$6,859,991
$1,650,839	$1,838,077	$2,045,697	$8,351,105
35.50%	36.00%	37.00%	
4.20%	4.40%	4.60%	
33.00%	36.00%	39.00%	
27.30%	23.60%	19.40%	
100.00%	100.00%	100.00%	
100.00%	100.00%	100.00%	
100.00%	100.00%	100.00%	
20.00%	20.00%	20.00%	
5.00%	5.00%	5.00%	
53.00%	53.00%	53.00%	
80.00%	80.00%	80.00%	
15.00%	15.00%	15.00%	
5.00%	5.00%	5.00%	
0	0	0	
14.00%	16.00%	18.00%	

amount of time it takes to perform the tests. Because staffing costs generally account for a majority of service costs, it is useful to project conservatively (that is, lower volume).

Fringe benefits are always a significant expense within any pro forma that has staffing expenses. There are two ways to reflect fringe benefits. One is to determine the exact cost. Fringe benefits are commonly represented by these items:

EXHIBIT 1.1. RHMC ANALYSIS OF FRINGE BENEFIT PERCENTAGE.

1A. OASDI at 6.2% of gross salary (up to a maximum of $76,200)		6.20%
1B. Medicare Part A trust fund at 1.45% of gross salary (no cap)		1.45%
2. Non-FICA fringe benefits:		
Total non-FICA fringe benefit costs	$4,600,000	
Total gross salaries	$36,000,000	
Non-FICA fringe benefit percentage	12.78%	12.78%
3. Staffing replacement fringe benefits— average allowable days off:		
Sick	8	
Holiday	6	
Vacation	10	
Total allowable days off per year	24	
Total paid days per year	260	
Staffing replacement fringe benefit percentage	9.23%	9.23%
Total fringe benefits as a percentage of gross salaries		29.66%

- Old age survivor and disability insurance (OASDI) withholding, which is also known as Social Security
- Medicare Part A trust fund withholding
- Medical, dental, and life insurance
- Short- and long-term disability
- Pension expense
- Tuition reimbursement
- The value of sick, vacation, and holiday time off

The only amounts easily quantifiable are these:

- OASDI, which the federal government has set at 6.2 percent of an employee's gross wages, with a cap ($76,200 in 2001)
- Medicare Part A trust fund, set by the federal government at 1.45 percent of an employee's gross wage, without a cap

All other fringe benefits are much harder to quantify, if only because none of them are paid for as a percentage. Instead, they are all employee-specific, with criteria such as sex, age, family size, and employment longevity as factors.

Therefore, a second method to reflect fringe benefit cost on a pro forma is generally preferred and used. This is as a percentage of gross salary. Health care organizations differ in the percentage used to represent their particular institution. RHMC has settled on a 30 percent rate, which is reflective of its experience over a period of several years. Exhibit 1.1 shows an analysis of the fringe benefit rate.

The results, as shown in Table 1.4, are presented in financial statement format with an IRR calculated over a five-year period. IRRs are easily calculated by any popular brand of electronic spreadsheet—a real time saver because the assumptions change constantly throughout the process. The 14.32 percent IRR seen in Table 1.4 is above RHMC's hurdle rate of 14.0 percent. Thus this project was accepted because it exceeded the hurdle rate and was going to improve customer satisfaction and make testing more efficient for the onsite clinical staff.

Convinced that this was a worthwhile project, the medical center administration recommended it for approval to the finance committee of the board of directors, which approved it. But as with all major projects, the finance committee wanted to track the investment over time. It required that projects costing more than $1 million be brought back to the committee annually for review.

So the finance manager, through finance staff, prepared an actual profit and loss statement for this program on an annual basis. The report was prepared in January 2001 so that at the February finance committee meeting the CFO could present this second annual report on the MRI program that went live two years earlier, in January 1999. The results are presented in Table 1.5. As can be seen, this new clinical program is performing acceptably on the basis of financial return, doing better than budget on the bottom line in its first two years.

Living with the Finance Committee and Board of Directors' Calendar

An important aspect of proper health care financial management is understanding the information needs of the ultimate decision makers in any organization, the board of directors. This is true whether the organization is set up as a taxable or a nontaxable entity. The board sets the policy direction for the organization, which is then carried out by the administration through its management team.

The board and its standing committees expect and require certain information, in a certain format, at specified intervals (committee meetings). It is essential that delivery of the information expected by the board be accurate and timely. Many health care organizations have a calendar, published before the year begins, specifying which topics are discussed throughout the year. The finance committee of the board of directors is one such committee. It has specific authority in and responsibility to the organization, enumerated in the bylaws of the organization:

- Present to the board for approval an annual budget consistent with the medical center's plan for providing care to meet patient needs
- Present a long-term capital expenditure plan to the board for approval

TABLE 1.4. RHMC PROPOSED MRI SERVICE PRO FORMA, STATEMENT OF REVENUES AND EXPENSES, JULY 1998.

	1999	2000
Revenues		
Gross revenues	$1,332,800	$1,483,692
Less contractual allowances	402,390	415,143
Less free care allowances	38,537	45,339
Net revenues	891,873	1,023,209
Expenses		
Variable expenses		
Salaries		
2.0 technicians	70,000	73,500
1.0 clerical	18,000	18,900
Total salaries	88,000	92,400
Fringes @ 30%	26,400	27,720
Medical supplies	82,320	91,622
Reduction of ambulance cost	(60,000)	(60,000)
Total variable expense	136,720	151,742
Fixed expenses		
Cryogens	23,000	35,000
Equipment maintenance contracts	0	115,000
Utilities	40,000	42,000
Legal and accounting (incl. billing)	20,000	21,000
Insurance	30,000	31,500
Office supplies	5,000	5,250
Marketing	50,000	52,500
Facility lease	96,665	101,498
Interest	0	0
Miscellaneous	10,000	10,500
Total fixed expense	274,665	414,248
Total cash outflows	411,385	565,990
Net cash inflows/(outflows)	480,488	457,219
Less depreciation expense	400,000	400,000
Net operating profit/(loss)	80,488	57,219
Internal rate of return		

- Review monthly and quarterly reports on financial matters
- Review and approve the budget of any special project or committee, when appropriate
- Annually, review the sources of funding for the corporation in conjunction with preparation of the budget
- Recommend independent auditors for the medical center

2001	2002	2003	Total
$1,650,839	$1,838,077	$2,045,697	$8,351,105
425,351	435,559	449,525	2,127,969
51,834	57,011	58,678	251,400
1,173,654	1,345,507	1,537,494	5,971,737
77,175	81,034	85,085	386,794
19,845	20,837	21,879	99,461
97,020	101,871	106,965	486,256
29,106	30,561	32,089	145,877
101,975	113,499	126,324	515,740
(60,000)	(60,000)	(60,000)	(300,000)
168,101	185,931	205,378	847,873
36,750	38,588	40,517	173,854
120,750	126,788	133,127	495,664
44,100	46,305	48,620	221,025
22,050	23,153	24,310	110,513
33,075	34,729	36,465	165,769
5,513	5,788	6,078	27,628
55,125	57,881	60,775	276,282
106,573	111,902	117,497	534,135
0	0	0	0
11,025	11,576	12,155	55,256
434,961	456,709	479,544	2,060,127
603,062	642,640	684,922	2,907,999
570,592	702,867	852,572	3,063,737
400,000	400,000	400,000	2,000,000
170,592	302,867	452,572	1,063,737
			14.32%

RHMC's finance committee meets periodically to carry out its responsibilities. Table 1.6 is the finance committee calendar for the center. In addition to the routine matters that are brought forth at every meeting, the calendar clearly defines those topics to be formally reviewed in a defined time frame. As can be seen, the RHMC finance committee meets every other month except March, which is special because of an additional meeting dedicated solely to the

TABLE 1.5. RHMC MRI SERVICE, ANNUAL STATEMENT OF REVENUES AND EXPENSES, JANUARY 2001.

	1999 Budget	1999 Actual	Percentage Variance	2000 Budget	2000 Actual	Percentage Variance
Revenues						
Gross revenues	$1,332,800	$1,264,800	−5.1%	$1,483,692	$1,591,200	7.2%
Less contractual allowances	402,390	379,440	−5.7%	415,143	561,111	35.2%
Less free care allowances	38,537	24,034	−37.6%	45,339	24,034	−47.0%
Net revenues	$891,873	861,326	−3.4%	1,023,209	1,006,055	−1.7%
Expenses						
Variable expenses						
Salaries						
2.0 technicians	$70,000	72,000	−2.9%	73,500	76,000	−3.4%
1.0 clerical	18,000	17,000	5.6%	18,900	18,500	2.1%
Total salaries	88,000	89,000	−1.1%	92,400	94,500	−2.3%
Fringes @ 30%	26,400	26,700	−1.1%	27,720	28,350	−2.3%
Medical supplies	82,320	74,500	9.5%	91,622	88,900	3.0%
Reduction of ambulance costs	(60,000)	(60,000)	0.0%	(60,000)	(60,000)	0.0%
Total variable expense	136,720	130,200	4.8%	151,742	151,750	0.0%
Fixed expenses						
Cryogens	23,000	20,000	13.0%	35,000	34,550	1.3%
Equipment maintenance contracts	—	—	n/a	115,000	115,000	0.0%
Utilities	40,000	34,000	15.0%	42,000	45,000	−7.1%
Legal and accounting (incl. billing)	20,000	—	100.0%	21,000	—	100.0%
Insurance	30,000	—	100.0%	31,500	25,000	20.6%
Office supplies	5,000	4,500	10.0%	5,250	4,900	6.7%
Marketing	50,000	60,900	−21.8%	52,500	64,000	−21.9%
Facility lease	96,665	96,665	0.0%	101,498	101,498	0.0%
Interest	—	—	n/a	—	—	n/a
Miscellaneous	10,000	—	100.0%	10,500	—	100.0%
Total fixed expense	274,665	216,065	21.3%	414,248	389,948	5.9%
Total cash outflows	411,385	346,265	15.8%	565,990	541,698	4.3%
Net cash inflows/(outflows)	480,488	515,061	7.2%	457,219	464,357	1.6%
Less depreciation expense	400,000	400,000	0.0%	400,000	400,000	0.0%
Net operating profit/(loss)	$80,488	$115,061	43.0%	$ 57,219	$ 64,357	12.5%

organization's strategic financial plan. Every organization determines its own preferred timing between meetings. Common intervals are monthly, bimonthly, and in some cases, quarterly.

Each item the finance committee requires to be reviewed is important, if only because they are on the governing board and this information aids in conducting their fiduciary responsibility.

TABLE 1.6. RHMC ANNUAL FINANCE COMMITTEE AGENDA.

	Routine Agenda Items, Every Meeting	(Chapter Number in This Book)
	(1) Approval of minutes	
	(2) Financial statement review, including review of financial ratios	2
	(3) Accounts receivable update	5
Bimonthly Standing Agenda Items		
February	(1) Bond debt status	2
	(2) Health insurance annual review	2
March	(3) Strategic financial plan	3
April	(4) Results of annual audit and management letter review	4
June	(5) Human resource report, salary budget decisions	6
	(6) Pension status and actuaries report review	6
August	(7) Review next year's budget assumptions	8
	(8) Annual materials management, inventory level review	8
October	(9) Finalize and approve operating and capital budgets	10
	(10) Review progress toward management letter comments	10
December	(11) Review malpractice insurance coverage	12
	(12) Review and approve auditors and fees	12
As-Needed Items		
	(1) Information system plans	10
	(2) Investment opportunities	

Routine Matters

There are several items that the RHMC finance committee reviews at each meeting. The most important are the monthly financial statements. Although the committee meets every other month, it still receives individual monthly financial statements for review. At the meeting, the most recent financial statement is reviewed, while the prior statement is mentioned only if there was some event that warrants discussion. Preparation and review of the financial statements by the finance division are discussed in Chapter Two.

The other routine item presented at every meeting is an analysis of the organization's accounts receivable. Accounts receivable is often the largest current asset in a health care organization and has the most significant impact on daily cash flow. Smaller is considered better because any organization would much rather have cash assets to invest instead of non-interest-bearing receivables. Accounts receivable practices are discussed in Chapter Five, while the all-important accounts receivable ratio, which is the number of days of revenue represented by the receivables, is discussed in Chapter Three.

The finance committee is primarily interested in the calculation of number of days of receivables, how it compares to recent months, and how it compares to the budget to judge the performance of management. The committee is also interested in the amount of bad-debt write-off and whether or not they judge it to be excessive. Finally, with respect to receivables, the committee is interested in the aging of the various open balances to judge whether management is allowing accounts to grow too old to collect.

Periodic Review Matters

As can be seen from Table 1.6, there are a number of areas under periodic review by the finance committee. Each item, its importance, and implications for financial management are discussed elsewhere in this book. For the moment, though, the real importance to financial managers is that they are expected to produce reports and information that allow the members of the governing board to pursue their duties. The periodic review calendar allows the financial managers to set up their upcoming year, knowing the schedule they are required to keep.

Year-End Closing

At the same time the finance managers are preparing for the next finance committee meeting in February, they are engaged in one of the two most onerous tasks they are required to perform each year: the year-end closing. (The other is the budget process.) Although the regular monthly closing becomes routine, the year-end closing always requires an extraordinary amount of effort. This is because an outside accounting firm audits the financial books and records of the organization and so the year-end balance takes on added importance.

Preparing for the auditors is an arduous and time-consuming task, particularly if the organization has not performed ongoing account analysis throughout the year. The auditor's job is to validate the transactions that are reflected in the client's financial statements—in this case, Ridgeland Heights Medical Center. Because it is the auditor's role to determine that the financial statements "present fairly, in all material respects, the financial position (balance sheet) of [its client], as well as the results of the operations, changes in net assets and cash flows for the years then ended, in conformity with generally accepted accounting principles

(GAAP)," the auditors need to examine the underlying transactions (AICPA, 1996, p. 117).

Therefore, the finance staff of RHMC needs to give the auditors a series of analyses for every balance sheet account, listing by category and date the transactions made as well as the other side of each entry. If the staff performed this throughout the year, the task would be less onerous. However, many organizations have trouble maintaining and updating these analyses monthly and thus are required to recreate their annual transactions in a short time frame (say, within thirty days). This is necessary because most administrators and boards require the audit to be complete and the auditor's report to be presented to the board within a short time period (two to four months) after the close of the fiscal year.

The staff and accounting director at RHMC do a better job than some of their peers and therefore do not face so great an obstacle in finishing their task. Still, the accounting director has created a list enumerating the tasks that the department faces in January and part of February (see Table 1.7). This consumes most of the staff time during these two months.

TABLE 1.7. RHMC YEAR-END ACCOUNTING PROCEDURES, DEC. 31, 2000.

Account Number and Person Responsible	Account Name	Procedure	Due Date
Cash	Petty cash accounts	Verify balances are correct	1/16/01
	Accounts payable, checking	Complete December and all prior-month reconciliation; adjust G/L balance accordingly	1/16/01
Payroll		Complete December and all prior-month reconciliation; adjust G/L balance accordingly	1/16/01
Investment	Money market sweep	Tie out to bank statement	1/16/01
	Unrestricted investments	Tie out to month-end investment schedule; adjust valuation allowance so all investments are stated at market value; verify that balance in unrealized gain/loss account is proper	1/19/01
	Trusteed investments	Tie out to investment manager statement; verify that balance in unrealized gain/loss account is proper	1/16/01
	Endowment fund	Tie out balance to statement; adjust for interest if necessary; verify that balance in unrealized gain/loss account is proper	1/16/01
Patient accounts receivable	Patient posted cash	Reconcile G/L balance to cash summary from patient accounts; adjust if necessary	1/20/01
	Accounts receivable	Complete December reconciliation of accounts receivable trial balance to the general ledger; adjust if necessary	1/12/01
	Refund clearing	Determine validity of balances; verify refunds issued in January; reclassify to liability section	1/16/01
	Contra A/R, in-house and discharged, not final billed	Record adequate contra accounts receivable reserve to reflect accounts receivable at net realizable value	1/16/01
	Allowance for doubtful accounts (bad-debt reserve)	Test reserve by applying approved percentage allowances against appropriate aging category of receivables; recommend adjustment for excess/shortage of reserve requirement	1/12/01
Other accounts receivable	Credit card clearing	Verify that the G/L balance represents December charges not yet reimbursed	1/16/01
	Collection agency clearing	Reconcile balances to collection agency statements; follow up on outstanding items	1/16/01
Inventory, prepaid, deferred costs	Pharmacy inventory	Adjust balance to physical inventory	1/16/01
	Dietary inventory	Verify G/L balance per inventory schedule	1/16/01
	Central supply inventory	Verify G/L balance per inventory schedule	1/16/01

Category	Account/Item	Procedure	Date
	Prepaid insurance	Review schedule of all policies for completeness and accuracy; determine prepaid amount remaining at year end; adjust G/L if necessary; tie out amortized amount in 2000 per schedule to insurance expense on the income statement	1/14/01
	Bond issues	Verify balances to amortized schedules; analyze actual bond issue costs paid and compare to estimate of bond issue costs used for amortization schedule; investigate differences; adjust if necessary	1/14/01
	Annual financing costs	Verify zero balances—all 2000 costs should be expensed; balance only if amount prepaid for 2001	1/14/01
Fixed assets, depreciation	Fixed assets	Reconcile December plant ledger reports to G/L, both by fixed asset category and in total; recommend adjustments and/or reclassification, if necessary; make all necessary adjustments for disposal of fixed assets; tie out net of all disposal adjustments to gain/loss in disposal on the income statement	1/26/01
	Construction in progress	Verify that all completed projects have been included in fixed assets at year end; validate balances in CIP as ongoing projects that have not been completed at year end	1/20/01
	Depreciation reserve	Reconcile plant ledger reports to G/L, both by fixed asset category and in total; recommend adjustments and/or reclassification, if necessary	1/26/01
Accounts payable, accrued expenses	Accounts payable	Reconcile subsidiary ledger to general ledger	1/16/01
	Accrued accounts payable	Update schedule identifying balance in detail; determine propriety of accruals at year end; recommend adjustment if necessary	1/16/01
	Security deposits	Agree to schedule maintained by Facilities Department	1/16/01
	Accrued payroll	Determine if any adjustments are necessary due to void or any other reason	1/16/01
	Interest payable	Verify payable balance includes current year expense for all bond issues not paid as of year end; tie out annual expense to debt schedules	1/20/01
	Accrued pension	Verify balance against actuarial report; adjust if necessary	1/16/01
	Accrued malpractice	Test against 12/31/00 malpractice insurer report; round balances due to estimate	1/20/01
	Unemployment compensation	Adjust balance to estimated liability at year end based on historical claims; prepare schedule supporting calculation	1/16/01
	Workers' compensation	Determine necessary accrual based on WC agent's estimate of future claims and estimate of future liability based on unreported claims	1/16/01
	Third-party reserves	Determine adequacy of reserves and realizability of receivables; adjust if necessary	1/16/01
	Current retirement of long-term debt	Agree current portion for all bond issues to debt schedules; adjust, if necessary	1/16/01
Long-term debt	Bonds payable	Agree amounts payable for all bond issues to debt schedules	1/16/01
	Unamortized bond discount	Agree unamortized discount for all applicable bond issues to amortization schedules	1/16/01

CHAPTER TWO

FEBRUARY

"Honey, you sure have been working some late nights the last few weeks," says Becky Barnes to her nearly exhausted husband, Samuel.

"Yeah, you know how it is," says Sam. *"We have the finance committee meeting in two weeks, and there's some extra stuff to prepare for this month. In addition to the usual material, like the financial statements and accounts receivable report, we're in the middle of the year-end closing and audit that follows. So it's been a tough month."*

"I'm confused. I know you've been doing this health care financial management thing for a long time. But how can you, with only your finance background, know enough to deal with and understand all the things that are required in a clinical program like an MRI?"

"Well, you know, that's a question I've been asked before," Sam says to his long-suffering wife. *"You've heard me say that I believe no finance person, no matter what level of responsibility they have, can be truly effective unless they intimately know the operations of the business they're in. This is true for manufacturing, banking, airlines, any industry. The only way to be sure the financial statements accurately reflect the results of operations is to know those operations. It's imperative that the finance person learn how those operations work, whether through formal study, continuing education, or on-the-job training."*

"Yeah, I've heard you say that before. But MRIs are just one clinical program. Being an ICU nurse, I'm deeply involved in some complicated clinical programs myself, and I know you've been involved in preparing the financial analyses for them. How can you be sure you're being given enough, or all, the information you need to put together the proper analysis?"

"Actually, the truth of the matter is there's never enough information. That's because we're dealing with the future and no one can accurately predict the future. So we get as much information as we can about an entire program by asking questions developed over years of asking the same kinds of questions, and then hope we haven't missed anything big."

"Sam, I know you haven't missed much over the past few years, but it seems like it's getting tougher and tougher lately, with you working on shorter and shorter time frames with fewer and fewer staff people to help with the analysis."

"Yeah. It's the nature of this beast."

It is a cold, clear, and crisp day in northern Illinois in early February. Although the ice and snow of the previous week cling to the narrow branches of dormant trees, creating a beautiful frozen tableau, the accountants of Ridgeland Heights Medical Center are busy at work. Their priority assignment is to finish preparing analyses required for presentation to the auditors by the third week of February. The auditors, from one of the Big Five international accounting and auditing firms, scheduled their usual three-week audit to be ready to present their findings at the April finance committee meeting.

Preparation and attestation of the year-end financial statement are a critical aspect of health care financial management. These statements are the backbone of the financial reporting and analysis of this $1.2 trillion industry. Because health care as an industry does not stand in isolation in this country, it is important that the reporting be accurate and timely so that industry statistics can be combined for aggregate national data.

Accounting Principles and Practices

As with other industries, health care has a set of principles and practices established through authoritative pronouncement, regulation, and historical precedent. All the books and records that are audited, whether a for-profit or a not-for-profit organization, are required to follow generally accepted accounting principles. For the health care industry, GAAP is formally presented in the *Audit and Accounting Guide for Health Care Organizations* (or *AAG-HCO*), published by the American Institute of Certified Public Accounting (AICPA) (1996).

The hierarchy of GAAP for not-for-profit organizations starts at paragraph 1.23 of the *AAG-HCO*. It states that "not-for-profit organizations should follow the guidance in effective provisions of ARBs (Accounting Research Board), APB Opinions (Accounting Principles Board) and FASB Statements and Interpretations (Financial Accounting Standards Board), unless the specific pronouncement explicitly exempts not-for-profit organizations or their subject matter precludes such applicability." The *AAG-HCO* also defines the GAAP hierarchy for government organizations as well as all other health care organizations that do not qualify as not-for-profit or government entities (these exceptions being generally for-profit organizations).

Here is the general definition of the three major types of health care organization, as listed in the *AAG-HCO* on page 1:

- Not-for-profit, business-oriented organizations, which are characterized by no ownership interests and essentially are self-sustaining from fees charged for goods and services. The fees charged by such organizations generally are intended to help the organization maintain its self-sustaining status rather than to maximize profits for the owner's benefit. Such organizations are exempt from federal and state income taxes and may receive tax deductible contributions from corporations or individuals that support their mission.

- Investor-owned health care enterprises, which are owned by investors or others with a private equity interest and provide goods or services with the objective of making a profit.
- Government health care organizations, which are public corporations and bodies corporate and politic. Also organizations are presumed to be governmental if they have the ability to issue directly (rather than through a state or municipal authority) debt that pays interest exempt from federal taxation.

All of the accountants at RHMC have formal accounting training and thus understand the background of these pronouncements. In addition, they are aware that interpretation of accounting rules for their industry is often covered in the *AAG-HCO*; as such, each accountant keeps a copy within reach at all times.

As we saw in Chapter One, RHMC is a not-for-profit corporation; therefore it follows the rules for such an organization. They are essentially the same whether the organization is a hospital, skilled nursing facility, psychiatric facility, or home health agency. Physician office practices are generally some form of for-profit partnership or corporation and as such follow for-profit accounting rules.

Objectives of Financial Reporting

Because RHMC has a hospital-based skilled nursing facility, home health agency, and psychiatric unit, it employs these basic not-for-profit accounting rules across the various financial statements. It also follows the objectives of financial reporting that were set down and are summarized in the FASB's Statement of Financial Accounting Concepts Number 1, which states that financial reporting should give information of the following types:

- Useful to current and potential investors, creditors, and other users in making rational investment, credit, and similar decisions
- Concerning the economic resources of an enterprise, the claims to those resources, and the effects of transactions, events, and circumstances that change resources

- Regarding an enterprise's financial performance during a period
- Describing how an enterprise obtains and spends cash, about its borrowing and repayment of borrowing, about capital transactions, and about other factors that may affect liquidity or solvency
- Describing how management of an enterprise has discharged its stewardship responsibility for the use of enterprise resources
- Useful to managers and directors in making decisions in the interest of owners

Ultimately, the whole point of preparing, auditing, and disseminating the financial reports for an enterprise is to allow the stakeholders to determine the financial performance of the organization. Some of the stakeholders include the following:

- For-profit equity shareholders
- Not-for-profit community board members and community members themselves
- Politicians who charge governmental agencies with spending budgeted dollars

Basic Accounting Concepts

At RHMC, the accountants are well aware of the importance of their work. They are in fact extremely diligent in the care they give to preparing the financial statements. In addition, because of their accounting training, they are aware of the basic accounting concepts that have been developed over the years, and they follow them along with their peers. There are six basic accounting concepts of which they are particularly aware:

1. *Entity.* This concept expresses that the corporate structure, or entity, is capable of taking economic actions apart from the individuals running the entity. Accounts are kept for the business entity and reflect events that affect the business. This concept is further expanded by the "going concern" theory, which suggests that the entity will live on indefinitely, regardless of the individuals in control. This is important because it allows accountants to use a continuity assumption in valuing assets, rather than "fire sale" liquidation value at the end of each accounting period.

2. *Transactions.* This simple concept requires all financial transactions that affect an organization to be included in the accounting records and reports. This

is necessary to ensure that accounting data and reports are dependable and valid. If all transactions are not included, then the financial records could be inaccurate, creating the possibility that the accounting numbers are massaged or finessed undesirably and inappropriately.

3. *Cost valuation.* This is a corollary to the transaction concept. It requires that all financial transactions be recorded at "cost," that is, the price paid to acquire any item or good. Cost is preferable to any other valuation because it is determinable, definite, objective, and verifiable. Other valuation methods such as sale price and replacement cost are not always definite and may be a matter of conjecture or opinion. Although the cost method of valuation is not perfect, primarily because it does not properly value inflationary or deflationary trends in times of highly fluctuating prices, its merits outweigh the demerits.

4. *Double entry.* This is the granddaddy of all accounting concepts. Developed in 1492, it requires that accounting records be constructed in such a manner as to reflect two aspects of each transaction, that is, the change in assets, and the change in the source of financing (liabilities). Thus for accounting records to reflect fully the effect of any transaction, two entries must be made.

5. *Accrual.* This concept acts as a guide in accounting for revenues and expenses. The accrual concept requires that revenues be recorded in the accounts when they are realized and that expenses be recorded in the period in which they contribute to operations. In practice this means, for example, that supplies purchased and used at the end of a month should be recorded as expenses for that month. But if the supply distributor has not sent out an invoice for the goods, the accrual concept requires the organization's accountants to estimate the value of the supplies and record it in that month's financial records. This concept permits proper allocation of income and expenses to the appropriate fiscal period.

6. *Matching.* This concept requires that all associated revenues and expenses be matched in the financial records in any given month to properly determine net income. If it were not necessary to match related items, revenues, and expenses, then it would be possible to manipulate income from various types of activity to produce whatever operating picture is desired (adapted from Berman, Weeks, and Kukla, 1986).

As the accountants prepare their entries, these concepts are second nature to them and used in all their work. They know it is critical that their work be accurate and timely. Accuracy is a function of properly applying the basic concepts. Timeliness is a function of management's will and persistence. As the accountants prepare their automated and manual journal entries, they are repeatedly reminded of the lessons learned along the way.

TABLE 2.1. BASIC FINANCIAL STATEMENTS OF A HEALTH CARE ORGANIZATION.

Financial Statement	Primary Purpose
Balance sheet	Presents a snapshot of the financial condition of the health care organization at a single point in time.
Statement of operations	Presents summarized revenues and expenses of an organization, resulting in a profit or loss, for a given period of time.
Statement of changes in net assets (or equity, if for-profit)	Presents a summary of the financial elements that caused a change in net assets, or equity, during a given period of time.
Statement of cash flows	Presents a summary of the assets and liabilities that caused a change in the main cash balances, during a given period of time.
Notes to the financial statement	Presents disclosure and discussion of the information underlying the numbers reported on the financial statements.

Basic Financial Statements of a Health Care Organization

What the RHMC accountants are preparing are financial statements.* The basic financial statements of a health care organization consist of a balance sheet, a statement of operations, a statement of changes in net assets, a statement of cash flows, and footnotes (notes) to the financial statement (see Table 2.1).

It is important to note that every one of these five items must be present, or else the financial statement is not complete. Each item is only a part of the whole, a whole that can tell the knowledgeable reader a great deal about the organization whose financial statement he or she is reviewing.

Uses of Financial Information

As we said earlier in this chapter, the reason for preparing, auditing, and disseminating enterprise financial reports is to allow the stakeholders to determine the

*Part of the analysis for this section is derived from the Healthcare Financial Management Association's (HFMA) Certification Examination Preparation—CORE manual, 1998, Chapter 11, as authored by Phyllis Cowling, chief financial officer at Baptist St. Anthony's Health System in Amarillo, Texas.

financial performance of the organization. Additionally, financial reporting is important because it enhances the ability of many stakeholders to make decisions about the organization. According to William Cleverly (1997), a professor of health care financial management, five uses of financial information may be important in decision making:

1. Evaluating the financial condition of an entity
2. Evaluating stewardship within an entity
3. Assessing the efficiency of operations
4. Assessing the effectiveness of operations
5. Determining the compliance of operations with directives

A number of stakeholders would want to be able to make appropriate decisions about the organization using financial information:

• *Governing board.* The board reviews the financial performance (the bottom line results and the level of assets and liabilities—that is, the financial condition) as well as the organization's actual financial ratios compared to budget and industry benchmarks. The governing board is also interested in the auditor's review of the organization's internal financial controls during the attestation process, sometimes called the "management letter" (stewardship).

• *Senior management.* The same criteria apply here as with the governing board. In addition, senior management wants to review operating ratios such as departmental productivity (efficiency) and departmental budget variances (effectiveness).

• *Department management.* Managers review the results during the period to determine their efficiency (did they make their budget numbers?) and to prepare analysis for any budget variances.

• *Investment bankers, rating agencies, and bondholders.* These people determine whether the value of any outstanding bonds has deteriorated or increased during the reviewed period (financial condition). Millions of dollars could be at stake in the secondary market for individuals or mutual fund holders.

• *Community.* Community members must determine if their resource is functioning appropriately. This may mean different things to different communities. For example, the standard in one community may mean that a not-for-profit's board of directors prescribes that the organization should not earn a "profit" greater than 2 percent because if it does the community may think it is "gouging" community members. Another community's standard, however, may lead the not-for-profit organization to budget and achieve a much higher net margin.

• *Benefactors.* These people are a subset of the community, inasmuch as most organizations or individuals who give charitable donations reside in or around the community. These donors want to know whether or not their donations are being used appropriately for an organization that will remain self-sustaining (financial condition).

  • *Equity investors.* These are individuals and investment fund managers who are concerned with their investment and may require either stock price appreciation or dividends to maintain their participation with the stock.

The Financial Statements

So we have theories, concepts, and practices of accounting that both the preparers and the users of financial statement information have been trained to analyze and understand. It is time to review the financial statements and the value they bring to users in understanding the financial health of the organization.

Balance Sheet

The order of financial statement presentation is always the same, as was indicated in Table 2.1. This has been established over time. The balance sheet has always been first because of the age-old concept that places the organization's assets, liabilities, and net assets or equity balance in a primary position ahead of periodic profit or loss (the income statement). The rationale is that an organization with a strong balance sheet can withstand a short run of losses or reduced profits, while an organization with a weak balance sheet will not be able to do so easily. An investor's eye quite naturally looks first to the balance sheet and then the income statement.

Table 2.2 is the RHMC balance sheet at December 31, 1998. A significant amount of financial information can be extracted from the balance sheet alone. Yet it is also used in conjunction with the other parts of the financial statements, along with additional financial and volume-related information, to form a complete picture of the medical center's financial resources.

Though it is just one part of a complete financial statement, the balance sheet by itself can yield some interesting information applicable to internal or external users. Quick perusal of RHMC's balance sheet highlights several matters of import. First, it can be noted that RHMC has $213.9 million in total assets, a considerable amount.

Next, it can be noted that RHMC has three large groupings of assets: cash (in several forms), accounts receivable, and fixed assets. The large percentage of assets tied up in fixed assets (characterized as property, plant, and equipment, or PP&E) indicates that RHMC, illustrative of the industry as a whole, is capital-intensive.

TABLE 2.2. RHMC BALANCE SHEET (IN THOUSANDS OF DOLLARS).

	December 2000	December 1999
Current assets		
Cash	$ 1,200	$ 2,000
Investments, short-term	6,500	5,400
Total cash and cash equivalents	7,700	7,400
Accounts receivable	22,000	22,800
Less allowance for doubtful accounts	(5,800)	(5,600)
Net patient receivables	16,200	17,200
Inventory	500	400
Prepaid expenses	400	300
Other current assets	900	700
Total current assets	24,800	25,300
Long-term investments, unrestricted	95,500	87,000
Trusteed investments	22,000	30,000
Endowment fund investments	300	300
Deferred financing costs	3,300	3,400
Other noncurrent assets	121,100	120,700
Property, plant, and equipment (PP&E)		
Land and land improvements	8,000	7,000
Buildings	70,000	60,000
Leasehold improvements	3,000	2,800
Equipment and fixtures	56,000	51,600
Construction in progress	3,000	4,000
Total PP&E	140,000	125,400
Less accumulated depreciation	(72,000)	(61,000)
Net PP&E	68,000	64,400
Total assets	$213,900	$210,400
Current liabilities		
Accounts payable and accrued liabilities	$12,000	$10,000
Third-party liabilities	4,000	4,500
Current portion on long-term debt	3,500	3,400
Total current liabilities	19,500	17,900
Long-term debt	120,000	123,400
Other long-term liabilities	4,000	4,100
Total long-term liabilities	124,000	127,500
Long-term liabilities	143,500	145,400
Net assets		
Unrealized gain/(loss) on investments	2,000	3,000
Other unrestricted	67,900	61,500
Temporarily restricted	200	200
Permanently restricted	300	300
Total Net Assets	70,400	65,000
Total Liabilities and Net Assets	$213,900	$210,400

We will see later when we review the income statement (or statement of operations) that it is also labor-intensive.

Third, it is reported that there is $125.2 million in cash and investments on the asset side of the balance sheet (which is made up of cash of $1.2 million, short-term investments of $6.5 million, plus unrestricted long-term investments of $95.5 million and trusteed investments of $22 million). There is also $123.5 million of debt on the liability side ($120 million in long-term debt and $3.5 million as the current portion on long-term debt), which may indicate a highly leveraged financial position. The organization is able to determine its leverage position during ratio analysis (see Chapter Three).

Finally, it can be seen that RHMC has net assets of $70.4 million. Net assets in a not-for-profit organization are the equivalent of equity in a for-profit business. There are some technical aspects to net assets, particularly the concepts surrounding classification of unrestricted, temporarily restricted, and permanently restricted. In general, though, unrestricted net assets in most organizations constitute a large majority of the total net assets. At first glance, RHMC looks to be financially stable.

A word of interest is in order here. You can see that RHMC has only $400,000 in inventory on its balance sheet, a low dollar amount compared to the $213.9 million in total assets. This is one area where health care as a service industry differs considerably from most manufacturing and other industries, which have a considerably larger percentage of their total assets tied up in inventory.

Statement of Operations

The statement of operations (known as the income statement before publication of the AICPA's updated health care audit guide in 1992) can give a knowledgeable reader both summary and some detailed information as to the periodic financial results of an organization. Depending on how many line items are shown in the statement of operations and the amount of trending information conveyed, a reader could glean a wealth of intelligence.

For example, initial review of the RHMC income statement in Table 2.3 indicates that for the year ending December 31, 1998, the organization had an operating margin of $5.2 million and a net margin of $6.4 million. Without additional trending information or ratio analysis, this appears to be a good set of bottom lines for the organization. These margins were the result of $145 million in gross patient revenues less discounts, and charity care given of $51.6 million. Gross patient revenues are a manifestation of charging list price for all services rendered by the health care facility. The majority of the discounts were a consequence of contracting with managed care companies and accepting a variety of discounts through negotiation.

TABLE 2.3. RHMC STATEMENT OF OPERATIONS FOR THE YEAR-TO-DATE ENDING DECEMBER 31, 1999 AND 2000 (IN THOUSANDS OF DOLLARS).

	2000	1999	Percentage Change
Revenues			
Inpatient revenue	$ 73,000	$74,000	−1.35
Outpatient revenue	72,000	69,000	4.35
Total patient revenue	145,000	143,000	1.40
Less			
Contractual and other adjustments	(49,000)	(48,000)	2.08
Charity care	(2,600)	(2,200)	18.18
Net patient service revenue	93,400	92,800	0.65
Add			
Premium revenue	2,100	1,300	61.54
Investment income	6,400	5,500	16.36
Other operating income	1,200	1,200	0.00
Total revenue	103,100	100,800	2.28
Expenses			
Salaries	36,000	34,000	5.88
Contract labor	1,000	1,500	−33.33
Fringe benefits	7,000	6,800	2.94
Total salaries and benefits	44,000	42,300	4.02
Bad debts	4,600	4,400	4.55
Patient care supplies	15,500	15,000	3.33
Professional and management fees	3,600	3,600	0.00
Purchased services	5,400	5,600	−3.57
Operation of plant (including utilities)	2,600	2,500	4.00
Depreciation	11,000	10,500	4.76
Interest and financing expenses	7,400	7,600	−2.63
Other	3,800	5,200	−26.92
Total expenses	97,900	96,700	1.24
Operation margin	5,200	4,100	26.83
Nonoperating income			
Gain/(loss) on investments	1,200	600	100.00
Total nonoperating income	1,200	600	100.00
Net income	$ 6,400	$ 4,700	36.17

It should be noted that the 1992 edition of the *AAG-HCO* mentioned earlier in this chapter took a position that gross patient revenue and contractual adjustments and charity care should no longer be reported on an audited financial statement. The industry has had to adopt this for annual external reporting (as with the audited financial statement); however, in practice monthly financial statements prepared for the administrators and the board continue to include this information. Health care facilities administrators know that gross patient service revenue can be an indicator of business growth or decline and is important in relation to variances between this year's budgeted and the prior year's revenue. The increase or decrease in contractual adjustments is likewise important to budgeted and prior year's results. Large variance causes the reviewer to raise pertinent questions, such as what caused the change, is it part of a trend, and what can be done to improve it?

Premium revenues indicate that the health care facility has contracted with insurance-type organizations (usually managed care companies) to accept capitation payment for treating members of the managed care company. This concept of capitation is reviewed in Chapter Three. For purposes of the financial statement, however, suffice it to say that premium revenue on the statement of operations means that the health care organization has decided to take the risk of a financial gain or loss for providing health care services. It does so by agreeing to provide all contracted health care for insurance members, with no additional payment beyond the insurance premiums. In other words, a health care organization that takes capitation has effectively, for at least part of its services, become an insurance company.

Interest income is the revenue earned on investment of excess funds made by the organization. RHMC has more than $120 million in excess funds; its investment policies determine the most appropriate mix of equities (stocks), bonds, and other financial instruments. As you can see, RHMC earned $6.4 million on investment of its money. That is a return of 5.33 percent. By itself, this return may not look substantial (although not bad for a down market in 2000). Yet this represents only the interest paid out by its holdings in bonds and other fixed instruments and the dividends paid out by its stock holdings. It does not include the unrealized appreciation (or depreciation) in the price of stocks and bonds. The cumulative amount of these unrealized gains or losses is available on the balance sheet in the net assets section. For purposes of analysis, total investment return, which is reported internally, includes appreciation or depreciation of assets as a percentage.

Placing interest income in the "other operating income" of the statement of operations is somewhat controversial. GAAP appears to allow this placement, which is "above the line" and therefore included in the operating margin. The more common and traditional treatment is "below the line," in the nonoperating income section of the statement of operations and therefore not part of the operating margin. A review of financial statements around the country reveals that one or the other method is used and certified by the CPA firms that issue audit opinions. In fact, an article in *Modern Healthcare* states that "much like medicine, auditing is not an exact science. One set of numbers can be interpreted many ways, each of which may be correct. Finance experts say health care accounting rules allow a great deal of leeway in accounting for investment income, for example. Some systems may classify those earnings as 'nonoperating income.' Other systems lump investment income with 'other revenue'" (Pallarito, 1998, p. 2). Interestingly, because of this lack of consistency, operating margin is no longer considered a good benchmark. Many investment and commercial bankers, bond rating agencies, investment managers, and consultants use only the net margin ratio as a consistent indicator for comparison.

"Other operating income" is an aggregation of disparate types of miscellaneous income not directly related to patient care. The most common type includes cafeteria revenue, revenue from drugs sold to patients, sale of the silver in old X-ray film, and rebates for volume discount from vendors. It should be noted that some of these items of other operating income are subject to income tax even though the health care organization is tax-exempt. A tax-exempt organization must file an IRS 990-T form along with its IRS 990 form for all appropriate items of other operating income that qualify as taxable.

Salaries is the most significant expense item on the statement of operations. This line includes only wages paid to its employees by the organization that are subject to employment taxes.

Any work being carried out in the organization by individuals who are not subject to employment taxes is reported on the statement of operations as either *contract labor* or *purchased services*.

Contract labor represents laborers employed by an outside organization. The health care organization contracts with an outside entity to have its employees perform work. Contract labor often mounts if there is a shortage of certain types of skilled labor within the industry. For example, RHMC spent $1 million in 2000 on contract labor. Some of these funds were spent on physical therapists, while another significant amount was spent on registered nurses. In both cases, the funds were expended because there was a shortage of these specific personnel types in the region. The budget had assumed that the hospital could hire more of its own therapists and nurses, but it was not successful in doing so and hence needed to resort to these outside agencies, at twice the price.

Purchased services often represent engagement of outside help in a larger context. The organization's administration may decide that it wants to outsource management of a department or departments to companies that specialize in certain skilled or unskilled areas rather than recruit and retain its own management staff. Therefore RHMC purchases services for these areas (environmental, previously called housekeeping; laundry; operation of the physical plant; dietary; and information systems).

The *fringe benefits* line is an aggregation of several types of expense paid for by the organization to enhance the quality of life for its employees or to comply with federal, state, and local laws. Development and magnitude of fringe benefit expenses was previously explored in Chapter One.

Bad debts represent the amount of gross charges that the provider of health care services will not collect from the financial guarantor of the individual who receives the health services. The financial guarantor could be the patient, the patient's relative, or the third-party payor (an insurance company). Usually, it is not the insurance company but the patient or family member who has to pay out of pocket, either for the entire scope of services or just a deductible or coinsurance amount. Here is a useful distinction between bad-debt expense and charity care write-off:

- Charity care: patients are *unable* to pay for the health care services received
- Bad debt: patients are *unwilling* to pay for the health care services received

Chapter Five discusses how the health care organization knows whether the patient is unwilling or unable to pay.

"Patient care" and other supplies, "professional and management fees," "operation of plant," and "other" expenses represent the normal costs of doing business in health care. For example, the line for patient care supplies includes medical supplies and drugs used in the patient's care as well as mundane office supplies needed to run the operation. Professional and management fees include the cost of external auditors, attorneys, and consultants. Operation-of-plant costs represent the expenses of running the physical facility, such as the nuts, bolts, and screws used in minor repairs as well as the heat, light, and power bills needed to keep the facility operating.

Depreciation expense is the periodic portion of the cost of building the physical plant and purchasing all the capital equipment used within it. Depreciation expense is determined by dividing the original cost of a building project or capital equipment purchase by the estimated useful life of the asset. A review of RHMC's statement of operations reveals that depreciation is the second largest expense. This is in keeping with the capital-intensive nature of the health care industry. Depreciation therefore has a large impact on the organization's bottom line. Because of its size and the nature of the calculation, depreciation is subject to being finessed. There are three major ways an organization could attempt to manipulate its bottom line through the use (or misuse) of depreciation expense:

- Nonstandard estimated useful life
- An accelerated method of depreciation rather than a straight-line method
- Capitalization policy inconsistent with reasonable industry standards

Nonstandard Estimated Useful Life. In theory, an organization could pick any useful life, which allows altering the bottom line of the statement of operations to suit its needs. In practice, however, the industry has adopted a generally accepted source for establishing asset lives: a pamphlet from the American Hospital Association titled *Estimated Useful Lives of Depreciable Hospital Assets* (1988). It was developed for two reasons:

1. GAAP would not permit a range of options for useful life. If allowed, there would be no "general acceptance." So external auditors wanted to be sure that an authoritative source was available.

2. Medicare was established in 1966 as a third-party payor that reimbursed providers for service based on cost. It did not want to pay more than reasonable cost, and so it also needed an authoritative source for the denominator of the calculation. Medicare has stated that employing useful life as presented in the AHA booklet is deemed acceptable for cost-reporting purposes.

Accelerated Methods of Depreciation. The second major way for any organization to manage depreciation expense is through using any method that accelerates it. The most common method of depreciation is called *straight line*. It is simple to use; you simply divide the cost of the asset by the number of years of estimated useful life. Table 2.4 shows a comparison of the straight line method of depreciation with two *accelerated* methods: *double declining balance* and *sum of the years digits*.

The main point is that the method used can have a big impact on the total depreciation expense recorded in each accounting period. As you can see, the straight line method literally smoothes the depreciation expense of each asset for each year of its estimated useful life. The two accelerated methods place a greater proportion of the expense in the early years and a smaller portion in the later years.

One reason to use an accelerated depreciation methodology is that a financial advantage can be gained from doing so. It needs to be done thoughtfully because, as we have seen, accelerating depreciation puts extra expense on the statement of operation, which makes the bottom line worse than perhaps it should be. But this is an established practice in the for-profit world because the income tax code gives favorable treatment. Specifically, because the tax code allows accelerated depreciation to be used for tax-reporting purposes, the extra expense that decreases the bottom line means that the for-profit organization pays less tax. Further, the organization is not harmed financially for doing so because depreciation is a non-cash expense. The organization is, in fact, helped financially.

As stated earlier, most health care organizations in this country are not-for-profit. Therefore there is no tax advantage to using accelerated depreciation. Although there is no tax advantage, there may still have been an advantage because

TABLE 2.4. COMPARISON OF STRAIGHT LINE AND ACCELERATED DEPRECIATION METHODS.

	Straight Line	Accelerated Depreciation Method				
		Double Declining Balance with Optimum Switch*	Actual Declining Balance	Optimum Switch, Double Declining Balance	Sum of the Years Digits	SYD Years
Cost of asset (radiology fluoroscope)	$300,000	$300,000			$300,000	
Estimated useful life	5	5			5	
Annual depreciation						15
Year 1	60,000	120,000	180,000		100,000	5
Year 2	60,000	72,000	108,000		80,000	4
Year 3	60,000	43,200	64,800		60,000	3
Year 4	60,000	32,400	38,880	25,920	40,000	2
Year 5	60,000	32,400	23,328	15,552	20,000	1
Total depreciation	$300,000	$300,000		$41,472	$300,000	15

*Optimum switch method allows the organization to switch to straight line depreciation after the straight line method exceeds the double declining balance method. On a five-year life, the switch would occur in the fourth year. On a ten-year life, the switch would occur in the seventh year. Without optimum switch, the declining balance extends many years past the original useful life determination.

of the cost reimbursement nature of the Medicare program. Although we explore Medicare in greater detail in Chapter Four, it is important to note here that at least through 1998 all Medicare costs except those for acute inpatient services were reimbursed at cost. However, because Medicare was aware of this potential advantage, it specifically forbade use of any type of accelerated depreciation for cost-reporting purposes. Therefore, with no tax advantage and no Medicare advantage, most not-for-profit organizations chose to stick with the easy and familiar straight-line method.

It turns out, as a result, that the only real advantage to using accelerated depreciation is operational. It makes sense to charge new capital acquisition a higher depreciation in the early years, when it needs little maintenance. Then in later years, it is financially responsible to charge the asset a lower level of depreciation when it needs and receives service and maintenance charges.

Capitalization Policy Inconsistent with Industry Standards. Once again, Medicare has had a large impact in the area of capitalization policy. The question is, at what dollar level should a purchase be capitalized? When Medicare came into existence in 1966, it established a rule that defined a capital asset as having a useful life greater than one year and a cost over $500. Therefore, anything bought under $500 was, by definition, an operating expense. At that time, it was important to the Medicare program to use as small a dollar figure as possible because it wanted to limit its cost reimbursement. Although a Medicare provider could conceivably have set capital policy at a higher level, there was no incentive to do so because it still had to report to Medicare at the $500 level.

Although Medicare changed its method of reimbursing for the capital related to acute inpatient care in 1990, thereby rendering some of the rationale no longer applicable, it was not until 1998 that Medicare revised its 1966 practice. Since 1998, Medicare has allowed providers to consider a purchase with a useful life of more than one year and cost of $5,000 and above to be considered capital (Health Care Financing Administration transmittal no. 402, June 1998). This allows providers to more properly classify many purchases as operating expenses, bringing more reality to operations and hence decreasing depreciation expense in the future.

Over the course of the last thirty years, RHMC has always followed the prescribed guideline, recognizing that it was in the best interest to use the AHA's pamphlet along with the straight line method and the $500 capitalization policy. However, it is pleased that the $500 level has at last been revised. RHMC has in fact decided to revise its capitalization to $2,500 next year. RHMC further recognizes that in doing so, it must allow additional operational budget dollars for those purchases that in prior years would have fallen into the $500 to $2,499 range.

Interest and financing expenses are a result of $123.4 million of prior-year tax-exempt bond debt on the liability side of the balance sheet. At the time the bonds were issued, the tax-exempt interest rate RHMC was able to obtain for 2000 was 5.5 percent (0.055 × $123.4 million = $6,787,000 plus $600,000 in bond insurance fees, or a total of $7.4 million). This rate was 85 basis points less than the thirty-year taxable rate at the time the bond was issued. This amounted to savings of several million dollars that RHMC will not have to pay over the life of the bonds. The entire topic of interest and financing falls under the rubric of treasury management and is the subject of several books; we touch on the topic briefly in Chapter Three in reviewing strategic financial planning.

Finally, the next to last line on the RHMC statement of operations is realized *gain or loss on investments.* This is the profit or loss made when the organization or its investment managers sell any financial instrument held for investment. These instruments are usually bonds or stocks, and the difference between the purchase price and the selling price is always reported in the nonoperating section (see Table 2.3).

TABLE 2.5. RHMC STATEMENT OF CHANGES IN UNRESTRICTED NET ASSETS FOR THE YEARS-TO-DATE ENDED DEC. 31, 1999 AND 2000.

	2000	1999
Unrestricted net assets		
Excess of revenues over expenses	$ 6,400	$ 4,700
Change in net unrealized gains and losses on investments other than trading securities	(1,000)	(2,000)
Increase (decrease) in net assets	5,400	2,700
Net assets, beginning of year	65,000	62,300
Net assets, end of year	$70,400	$65,000

Statement of Changes in Unrestricted Net Assets (or Equity)

The statement of changes in unrestricted net assets (or equity; see Table 2.5) is the least used part of the financial statement. Its primary purpose is to roll forward the net assets from the end of the prior period to the current period. In many cases, the most common change in the unrestricted net assets from one period to the next is one of these:

• Excess of revenue over expense
• Any unrealized gain or loss on other than trading securities
• Net assets released from restriction used to purchase property and equipment

All positive results in any of these areas increase the organization's net worth, while negative results decrease it.

Complex organizations such as RHMC may require separate statements to segregate the net assets into the three categories of unrestricted, temporarily restricted, and permanently restricted.

Statement of Cash Flows

The statement of cash flows (see Table 2.6) is generally the most useful section of a typical financial statement. Although many readers of financial statements turn first to the income statement and then to the balance sheet in an attempt to understand an organization's financial results and financial position, they often overlook the cash flow statement. At a glance, it gives the knowledgeable reader an interesting set of information regarding the organization's sources and uses of cash.

The statement of cash flows has one purpose: to allow the reader to understand the financial statement elements that make up the change in cash in the

TABLE 2.6. RHMC STATEMENT OF CASH FLOWS FOR THE YEARS-TO-DATE ENDED DEC. 31, 1999 AND 2000.

	2000	1999
Cash flows from operating activities		
Increase (decrease) in net assets	$ 6,400	$ 4,700
Change in net unrealized gains and losses on investments other than trading securities	(1,000)	(2,000)
Changes in net assets		
Adjustments to reconcile changes in net assets		
Depreciation and amortization	11,100	10,500
Net accounts receivable (increase) decrease	1,000	(700)
Other current assets (increase) decrease	(200)	(1,500)
A/P and accrued liabilities (decrease) increase	2,000	(1,000)
Other long-term liabilities (decrease) increase	(100)	200
Third-party settlement (decrease) increase	(500)	1,200
Current portion of long-term debt (decrease)	100	100
Net cash provided by (used in) operating activities	18,800	11,500
Cash flows from investing activities (increase) decrease		
Net investments	(500)	0
Other noncurrent assets	0	(200)
Capital expenditures	(14,600)	(6,200)
Net cash provided by (used in) investing activities	(15,100)	(6,400)
Cash flows from financing activities		
Proceeds from the issuance of long-term debt	0	0
Payments on long-term debts	(3,400)	(2,500)
Net cash provided by (used in) financing activities	(3,400)	(2,500)
Net increase (decrease) in cash and cash equivalents	300	2,600
Cash and cash equivalents, beginning of year	7,400	4,800
Cash and cash equivalents, end of year	$ 7,700	$ 7,400

Note: Supplemental disclosure of cash flow information: cash paid for interest (net of amount capitalized) in 2000 and 1999 was $7,700,000 and $7,500,000, respectively.

organization's operating checkbook. The statement begins by recording the organization's change in net assets (which primarily consists of the bottom line). After that, all noncash items included in the bottom line, such as depreciation and amortization, are added back because the purpose of this statement is to recognize cash transactions only. Finally, the statement is designed to show the balance sheet items that increase and decrease an organization's checkbook balance.

In the not-for-profit industry, the statement of cash flows is divided into cash flow from operations, investing activity, and financing activity. These designations represent cash flows from the organization's principal activity (operations), investment and capital expenditure (investing), and proceeds of debt activity (financing). Although a for-profit organization does not use the same categorizations, the end result is the same, which is to describe net increase or decrease in cash and cash equivalent.

Some interesting and useful line items on the statement of cash flows:

- *Capital expenditures.* This line shows the total change in capital expenditures during the reporting period. The changes involve acquisition of any new capital as well as any capital items that are discarded.
- *Proceeds from issuance of long-term debt.* This line exhibits any long-term debt issued by the organization during the reporting period. At a glance, the reader can determine the amount of debt taken on by the organization.
- *Payments on long-term debt.* This line represents all principle payments made during the reporting period. It quickly isolates the amounts in question.

Notes to the Financial Statements

The notes have considerable importance for the overall quality of a full-scope financial statement. GAAP requires notes to be included in an audited statement. They add a level of understanding to the other four statements by describing various accounting concepts used by the reporting organization. In addition, the notes allow the organization to present any message it wants to illustrate to the reader of the statements. The notes give supporting detail that cannot easily be placed on the face of the financial statements themselves. Internal monthly financial statements often exclude a formal set of notes because it is assumed that the readers of these internal statements are already familiar with the information that may be included in the notes.

Preparing for the Auditors

As stated earlier in this chapter, the RHMC accounting director and her accountants spent several weeks just prior to the end of the fiscal year as well as several weeks into the new calendar year employing once-a-year actions to get ready for the arrival of the auditors. They are paying special attention to preparing analysis to be given to the auditors for both balance sheet and income statement accounts. This is, in fact the biggest difference between regular month-end and end-of-year closings.

During a regular month-end closing, the accountants are generally more concerned with getting the books closed, publishing the financial statement, and getting ready for the next month's close. There is usually not enough time during a regular month-end closing to be concerned with the accuracy involved in a year-end closing. This is because the senior administration and the board want to know the results of operations as soon as possible after the close of the month.

For the year-end closing, extra time is allotted for the close of the month and hence the year's end. This is allowed because finance administration is aware that there will be extra scrutiny in the audit, and from a political viewpoint it is much better to make sure that the accounting staff make all required accounting entries rather than have them proposed by the auditors. This extra time is always used for additional analysis, which, owing to time constraints, is not always performed during the rest of the year.

In the previous chapter, the tasks involved in a year-end closing were enumerated in Table 1.7. This is the baseline for the work paper analysis that is prepared by the RHMC accounting staff and given to the external auditors. The work paper is referred to as "prepared by client" (PBC); it allows the auditors to begin their audit already armed with the details behind the financial statement accounts. The extra closing time, coupled with the PBC, permits a clean year-end financial statement and practically ensures that the auditors will not find any financial transactions that should have been recorded but were not, were recorded in error and need to be eliminated, or were recorded in error and must be changed.

A couple of items are worthy of note. First, a health care facility is better served if it maintains good account analysis month to month. This simply follows good management practices. Not maintaining monthly account analysis means that the administration and the accounting staff can be absolutely sure the published financial statements are not as accurate as possible. Because of this, they do not know if a major adjustment will be required, which can make the already published statements misleading and get the accountants, the accounting director, or the chief financial officer fired.

Second, the six most sensitive accounts (that is, those most likely to receive audit adjustments in the financial statements) are the following:

1. Contractual adjustments (income statement)
2. Accounts receivable (balance sheet)
3. Allowance for doubtful accounts (ADA, in the balance sheet)
4. Bad-debt expenses (income statement)
5. Allowance for contractual adjustments (ACA, in the balance sheet)
6. Due to or from third-party settlements (balance sheet)

These accounts are sensitive because determining the balance involves a great deal of *estimation*. There are, of course, accounting rules that set down proper estimation techniques. These are, in fact, the rules that the auditors use when they do their analysis. But amazingly, many health care organizations want to follow these techniques but have trouble because of time or talent, or they decide they have a better way and thus choose to follow their own methodology. This often causes significant audit adjustments after the health care facility has closed its books for the year.

There is some good advice to follow in this regard: always ask your auditors to share the exact methodology *they* use to analyze these accounts. Ask them to explain their methodology. Then, after it becomes understandable, adopt it. If the health care organization is using the same methodology as the auditors, so long as there is no problem with the numerical input there is no potential for audit adjustment. In other words, unless the facility has some reason not to adopt the auditor's method (perhaps it is only a long-standing tradition), just do it! It significantly minimizes the risk of adjustments, which is the name of the game in year-end preparation for the auditors.

Analysis of Sensitive Accounts

This chapter explains the financial statements and their elements, so this is a good opportunity to further discuss the six sensitive accounts just mentioned.

1. *Contractual adjustments.* These have become the second largest line item on the income statement of many a health care organization, after gross revenue. This is because many organizations have chosen not to limit any increase to their gross charges (price list) while at the same time absorbing extraordinary increases in discount (contractual adjustments) that they agree to give to third parties. Because of its size on the income statement, even a small discrepancy can have big consequences for earnings. The timing of the contractual adjustment on the patient's account as well as the accuracy of the adjustment are crucial items that affect potential audit adjustments. Development of contractual adjustments is given detailed review in Chapter Four, along with the concept of net revenue generation.

2. *Accounts receivable.* The concept of accounts receivable management is discussed in Chapter Five. It is a detailed analysis of methods to minimize the dollar level and aging of the amount owed to the health care facility for the services it has provided to patients (customers). The reason for this importance and sensitivity lies in size and the percentage of assets that it represents. In most other industries, accounts receivable is usually the third largest current asset, behind inventories and cash. In health care, however, accounts receivable is often the largest asset. In addition, accounts receivable involves a high degree of detailed analysis to verify that the gross and net receivables on the books are, in fact, valid.

3. *ADA.* One of the oldest, most time-honored concepts in accounting has its own special rules in the health care industry. Allowance for doubtful accounts represents the dollars subtracted from gross accounts receivable to help arrive at the net amount expected to be collected from all patients. It is always an estimate, because it is impossible to know, with certainty, how many accounts receivable dollars will not be collected. Because of the high dollar value of ADA (which is often 10 to 30 percent of the gross accounts receivable, depending on each organization's payor mix), there are significant implications for a bottom line adjustment if not done appropriately. We review, in detail and with examples, how to prepare a monthly ADA analysis in Chapter Five.

4. *Bad-debt expense.* This is sometimes called provision for bad debts. The finance committee keeps a close eye on this income statement line. This expense is called a provision because, like the ADA, it is also an estimate. Indeed, it is specifically related to ADA; the higher the ADA in any accounting period, the higher the bad-debt expense, and vice versa. Bad-debt expenses have a direct effect on the bottom line. Minimizing this expense depends on the kind of accounts receivable management practiced; in many cases it also depends on the socioeconomic neighborhood in which the organization is located. Still, in those aspects that are controllable, the finance committee requires that these expenses not vary greatly from year to year without good reason. In addition, it is important that bad-debt expense be properly estimated throughout the year so that no large negative entry is made to the income statement in December or as an audit adjustment.

5. *ACA.* Like ADA, allowance for contractual adjustments is used to reduce the gross accounts receivable down to its net collectible value. ACA is an estimate of contractual adjustments that should be taken when the health care organization receives payment for services from the many third-party payors with which it has contracted. These third-party payors are usually categorized into Medicare, Medicaid, or managed care. Also like ADA, this allowance, or estimate, can have a meaningful impact on earnings. If the organization does not properly prepare its estimate, the audit adjustment can cause havoc with the year-end closing numbers. Detailed explanation of ACA is in Chapter Five.

6. *Due to or from third parties.* This is an accounting concept that has been used in most health care organizations since 1966, at the inception of Medicare. This balance sheet account represents the amount of money either owed to a third-party payor by the provider (liability) or additional reimbursement owed by the payor to the provider (asset). This balance sheet account is necessary only if the type of reimbursement agreed to by provider and payor is cost-based and retrospective, which means that all payments throughout the year are only interim (temporary) and would be finalized (or finally settled) after a year-end cost report

is filed. This was how Medicare originally reimbursed providers (who were then mostly hospitals). Since 1983, inpatient hospital reimbursement has changed and is no longer retrospective; all such rates are set before the year begins (called prospective). Still, since passage of the Balanced Budget Act of 1997, most other industry types that Medicare reimburses have changed from retrospective to prospective (skilled nursing facility, home health agency, outpatient hospitalization, rehabilitation). Consequently, this line item will be considerably less sensitive in the future and continue to diminish as previous years not yet resolved by the Medicare intermediary are taken care of and no additional settlements are required.

February Finance Committee Special Reports

As reported earlier, RHMC's board finance committee meets bimonthly to review routine matters such as the operating results of the organization, as represented by the statement of operations (income statement), balance sheet, and statement of cash flows. Other routine items of interest are review of the accounts receivable balance and capital expenditures, budgeted and unbudgeted.

In addition, at every meeting, certain items are formally reviewed on a specific and periodic schedule. This is done so that these items, which have been deemed important but not requiring review at every meeting, are not forgotten. In February, two of these items are on the agenda.

Bond Debt Status

RHMC has issued $150 million of bond debt over the last several years. This is a substantial amount of money, particularly to the individuals and corporations that bought the debt. In fact, both the purchasers and the issuers of the debt (the latter represented by the RHMC board) have the same concerns. Namely, is the organization that issued the bond still financially viable and able to continue to repay principal and interest on the outstanding bond issue?

A good way to determine financial viability and ability to repay principal and interest on a bond issue is to use financial statement ratios. The capital structure ratio analysis given here was adapted from *The Almanac of Hospital Financial and Operating Indicators* (Ingenix, 2001). Three ratios are particularly important for this analysis:

1. *Long-term debt to capitalization.* This is defined as the proportion of long-term debt divided by the sum of long-term debt plus unrestricted net assets or

EXHIBIT 2.1. SELECTED BOND REPAYMENT RATIOS.

1. Long-term debt to capitalization ratio:

$$\frac{\text{long-term liabilities}}{\text{long-term liabilities} + \text{unrestricted net assets}}$$

2. Debt service coverage ratio:

$$\frac{\text{cash flow (total margin} + \text{depreciation expense)} + \text{interest expense}}{\text{principal payment} + \text{interest expense}}$$

3. Cash flow to total debt:

$$\frac{\text{revenues and gains in excess of expenses and losses} + \text{depreciation}}{\text{current liabilities} + \text{long-term debt}}$$

equity. A high value for this ratio implies reliance on debt financing and may signal reduced ability to carry additional debt.

2. *Debt-service coverage.* This measures total debt-service coverage (interest plus principal) from the organization's cash flow. A high value for this ratio indicates good ability to repay debt.

3. *Cash flow to total debt.* This is defined as the proportion of cash flow to total liabilities, current and long-term. It has been found to be an important indicator of future financial problems or insolvency.

These ratios are the ones most commonly used throughout the health care industry to measure bond repayment capability. Actual calculations for these ratios are presented in Exhibit 2.1.

We explore ratios further in the next chapter.

Because of their importance, these ratios are computed and presented on the financial statement each month for review and discussion by the finance committee. Still, once a year, the administration deems it important to prepare an in-depth review of the organization's debt status for the finance committee. The review includes

1. A summary of the bond debt expense for the past ten years
2. A discussion of any changes in the organization's bond debt rating by the three major rating agencies (Moody's, Fitch, and Standard & Poor's).

Table 2.7 shows the analysis and review.

TABLE 2.7. RHMC ANALYSIS OF THIRTY-YEAR BOND DEBT, 1988–2000 (IN THOUSANDS OF DOLLARS).

	Interest Rate	Principal	Interest Expense	Total Annual Payments	Debt Balance	Additional Expenses*
1988					150,000,000	
1989	4.4%	1,740,000	6,600,000	8,340,000	148,260,000	600,000
1990	4.7%	1,900,000	6,968,220	8,868,220	146,360,000	600,000
1991	4.9%	2,000,000	7,171,640	9,171,640	144,360,000	600,000
1992	5.0%	2,100,000	7,218,000	9,318,000	142,260,000	600,000
1993	5.2%	2,220,000	7,397,520	9,617,520	140,040,000	600,000
1994	5.3%	2,320,000	7,422,120	9,742,120	137,720,000	600,000
1995	5.3%	2,440,000	7,299,160	9,739,160	135,280,000	600,000
1996	5.3%	2,660,000	7,169,840	9,829,840	132,620,000	600,000
1997	5.4%	2,820,000	7,161,480	9,981,480	129,800,000	600,000
1998	5.4%	3,100,000	7,009,200	10,109,200	126,700,000	600,000
1999	5.5%	3,300,000	6,968,500	10,268,500	123,400,000	600,000
2000	5.5%	3,400,000	6,787,000	10,187,000	120,000,000	600,000

*Additional expenses include (1) the cost of bond insurance at 40 basis points, or 0.4 percent (to receive a AAA rating from the bond rating agencies); (2) related consulting fees; and (3) related legal fees, all of which are being amortized over the life of the bond.

Note: Based on the ratio analysis of RHMC's current financial statement, there has been no upgrade or downgrade of RHMC's bond ratings by Moody's, Fitch, or Standard & Poor's.

Health Insurance Annual Review

As in many towns around the country, the health care organization is the largest employer. There are several interesting twists here. Because RHMC is an employer as well as a health care provider, it knows better than most the costs associated with providing care for its employees. This is the *cost* of care, not the price of the care.

Therefore, when negotiating with a health insurer to cover its employees, RHMC is at an advantage and a disadvantage simultaneously. The advantage is knowing its own costs for providing care, which affords a measuring stick when the prospective health insurer makes a bid to insure the medical center's employees. The disadvantage is that RHMC must negotiate with these self-same insurers for managed care contracts over other employers. It cannot reveal too much of the underlying cost structure without risking loss of some negotiating leverage on its other contracts.

The other interesting twist is that RHMC has learned that employee use of health services greatly exceeds that of employees in any other industry. This is no fluke and no accident. It is, in fact, extremely logical. Because health care workers are exposed to these services every day as service providers, there is no mys-

EXHIBIT 2.2. RHMC 2000 HEALTH INSURANCE INFORMATION.

During 2000, RHMC offered a single health insurance plan through ABC Healthcare, a midwestern regional-based health maintenance organization. We offered a preferred provider organization (PPO) plan that featured managed care benefits for the employee staying in the ABC network and indemnity-type benefits for going outside the ABC network.

The budget for health insurance for 2000 was $2.4 million. Actual premiums paid during 2000 were $2 million. The savings resulted from lower participation levels following staff reductions and a different mix of single/couple/family employee participation than what was budgeted.

Dental insurance continued to be offered through XYZ Dental Program. Two programs were offered: a dental maintenance organization (DMO) plan and an indemnity plan. These plans, which were fully paid for by the participating employees, had four hundred participants in 2000. The 2000 premiums paid by the employees were $960,000.

tery and no fear in using health care. These workers, in general, are the greatest users of health care services in the country. But because of this, the health care insurer wants and needs to charge health care providers a higher monthly premium rate, owing to high usage, than it would for workers in other industries.

Each year, the administration presents a wrap-up of the previous year's health insurance information for the finance committee so that it can assess variance from budget and determine any potential variances in the coming year. This is particularly important if the organization is self-insuring its employees' medical coverage. Because RHMC self-insured its medical coverage in past years, this report to the finance committee has become a habit. Thus, although RHMC currently offers regular insurance coverage in the current year, it continues to present this report. A summary is presented in Exhibit 2.2.

CHAPTER THREE

MARCH

Sam is restless. He has just begun to prepare information for his organization's annual update of its strategic financial plan. But he is having a rare moment of doubt. At such times, he always does the right thing: he calls his ex-boss for some advice.

"Jim, I've got a problem and I need your help," says Sam to his ever-understanding and patient colleague and friend.

"Yeah? What's up today?" asks Jim Jordan, who just happens to be the chief financial officer of a six-hundred-bed academic medical center in the glorious state of Florida. Jim is always available to take a call from his former protégé.

"I'm about to start gathering information for the upcoming five-year strategic plan, and it seems like we just finished the work from last year. I'm having trouble redoing this again year after year. I've forgotten what value we get from this exercise."

Now, Jim—who is not only his facility's CFO but also the senior vice president for strategic planning—is a patient man. He has to be, listening untiringly to Sam's stream-of-consciousness, free-association ramblings. So he says, "Come on. Buck up. You've gotten into these funks before. It will pass; it always does.

"Let me remind you of something you told me just last year, Sam. You called me and you were very excited. You were preparing last year's plan and you realized you'd made an assumption that Medicare reimbursement wouldn't go down as much as had been predicted by one of those consultants that your hospital retains. Your reading of the literature led you to a better prediction. And since your administration listened to you last year instead of the other guy, the hospital didn't have to cut an additional ten employees."

"What? Oh my gosh, that's right. I forgot about that. Actually, that was important for a number of reasons, particularly because the administration put more credence in my work for the first time. You are so right. As usual, you've been fabulous, Jim. Thanks a lot. How do you always do that?"

"Sam, Sam, Sam, I've told you this before. It's not a matter of talking—you just need to listen."

The month of March opened in a very promising fashion in Chicago. The weather was unusually warm, allowing people to shake off their winter blues. Unfortunately, the blue period lingered in the health care industry. As in the previous few years, events further diminished both the reputation and the finances of industry participants. The federal government was continuing its two-pronged attack on the industry's financial and billing practices.

On the billing front, the feds decided that they had probable cause to conclude that a great deal of the industry was filing erroneous Medicare and Medicaid claims; this determination was made within the statutes of the 1863 Civil War law dubbed the False Claims Act. In addition to believing that these erroneous billings constituted fraud, the Office of Inspector General of the United States and many state attorneys general felt they could raise their own revenues using the fining powers granted under the False Claims Act.

On the financial front, passage of the federal Balanced Budget Act (BBA) in August 1997 (which became effective in October of that year) exacerbated a decline in hospital reimbursement that had begun a few years earlier, concurrently with the increase in power and strength of the managed care industry. The BBA, which primarily affected Medicare reimbursements and to a lesser degree Medicaid, immediately began to have an impact on the financial bottom line of every segment of the health care industry. Hospitals were the first to feel the brunt of the $116 billion, five-year payment reduction act. Home health agencies were also immediately affected and felt the impact from the Interim Payment System segment of the BBA, with 752 agencies shutting their doors in the first nine months after the October 1, 1997, implementation (Ngeo, 1998). Other segments of the industry, such as skilled nursing facilities and physician office practices, took their share of the legislation a year later. Further, hospital outpatient services were affected on August 1, 2000, upon implementation of the Hospital Outpatient Prospective Payment System (HOPPS), which used the Ambulatory Payment Classification (APC) system for reimbursement of services. (We explore the BBA and its many industry implications in the next chapter.)

Strategic Financial Planning: Five-Year Projections

Meanwhile, back at Ridgeland, the accounting and finance staff were gearing up to present the implications of any new 2001 BBA or managed care issues and several other significant operational changes to the administration. They do this through annual preparation and presentation of a five-year strategic financial plan.

A health care organization's strategic financial plan can be defined as quantification of a series of strategic planning policy decisions. The strategic financial plan is meant to quantify the tactics surrounding the organization's strategic plan. To be successful, it is important that any organization wanting to be financially competitive possess a number of critical attributes:

- The chief executive has conceived a financial vision.
- Management follows the simple rule that "What gets measured gets done."
- Management understands and applies principles of corporate finance.
- Management has a sophisticated financial plan.
- The organization favors a quantitative capital allocation process.
- Management consistently applies quantitative decision-support tools.
- Management sets annual financial goals and objectives, welcoming organizationwide input.
- The organization has a visible operating plan and disseminates its financial goals.
- The organization has a strategic plan that takes into account the requirements of the capital market.
- Management reduces expenses while improving service and quality (Kaufman and Hall, 1994)

Ridgeland Heights Medical Center believes in these attributes and attempts to follow them as closely as possible. In particular, the center updates its five-year strategic plan every year to remain current with contemporary strategic and financial changes within the industry. Doing so helps it manifest a number of the attributes just listed.

Strategic Planning

To begin a successful strategic financial plan, management must finalize its own strategic plan. This is updated every two or three years and presented for approval to the planning committee of the board of directors, and then finally to the full board. The strategic plan can be defined as a statement of missions or goals (or both) required to offer guidance to the organization; it incorporates a set of programs or activities to which the organization commits resources during the plan period (Cleverly, 1997).

A strategic plan is imperative to proper functioning of any successful organization. Yet in many places, the strategic plan is looked on as an added inconvenience. Department heads, as well as administrators, may want to just "manage" (that is, simply operate their department or division without taking the time to determine where they are headed). The strategic plan focuses the organization on the important changes in demographics, payor mix, payor reimbursement methodology, physician recruitment and retention policy, new programs or other initiatives, strategic market share practices, and any other area pertinent to maintaining or improving the organization's financial position.

It is important to note that both strategic planning and financial planning are the primary responsibility of the board of directors. To be sure, although senior administration has a role in carrying out the plans, the future vision of the organization begins with the board. The vision of the organization's CEO is also highly relevant. The CEO serves as a link between the board (usually as a member) and management. The final link between the board and administration involves the board setting key financial policy targets. These targets should include debt policy and profitability objectives (for instance, operating margin percentage and return on net assets) as well as a capital plan.

The purposes of the strategic plan are as follows:

- Identify key future issues and priorities.
- Allow managers an opportunity to understand and contribute to the organization's direction.
- Identify resource needs and guides on how they can be allocated.
- Ensure that the strategic plan supports board policy.

To determine these strategies, it is necessary to carry out this procedure:

1. Assess external environmental conditions.
2. Assess internal environmental conditions, such as current organization issues.
3. Describe the strategic gap from the desired position to the current one with respect to organizational and environmental variables.
4. Identify competencies and resources needed to close the gap.
5. Determine strategic initiatives that can move the organization forward toward successful completion of the plan.
6. Allocate capital or operating dollars to each initiative.

After the strategic initiatives are determined, the organization needs to identify the tactics it will use to activate the strategies. The tactics are the actual steps the various departments take to implement those changes developed within the strategic plan. It is imperative that management be given (and understand its) accountability in carrying out the tactics. Without accountability the tactics have a great chance of not being implemented, thereby causing the strategic plan to fail.

Converting Vision (Strategic Plan) into Financial Reality: Market Share, New Services, and the Medical Staff

According to Cleverly (1997), there are four steps involved in developing a strategic financial plan: the organization needs to analyze its financial position and prior growth patterns, determine the growth in total assets needed for the planning period, define an acceptable level of debt for both current and long-term categories, and assess the reasonableness of the required growth rate in equity (net assets). RHMC generally follows these steps. After approval of the strategic plan, the finance department goes to work on the strategic financial plan. There are a number of specific steps taken to translate the organization's vision into financial reality. Some of them may be performed concurrently, while others need to await completion of previous steps.

At RHMC, the first step is for the finance officer to call a meeting of senior administration. The objective of the meeting is to determine volume changes over the next five years. This is often a result of market share analysis and the organization's current and proposed market share position. For example, suppose that the organization's current share across all markets (the primary one and all secondary markets) is 12 percent. Also let us suppose that the organization has determined that for it to enjoy continued success, it must increase market share to 18 percent, an increase of 50 percent. This is not the kind of change that happens easily. The quickest way to increase market share in the short term is to buy it. This, of course, presumes that there is a willing seller in the market. Numerous scenarios can play out if acquisition is the desired method of choice.

The next likely method for increasing market share is to determine the services that are most desired by the local market. A good way for the organization to make this determination is through surveys, focused and general. They help to determine the demand for any new or expanded services that are already being met, the alternative being to create demand for services that the market may not yet know it really wants.

Medical Staff Issues

There are many examples of what a demand analysis may uncover. For example, let's say that an organization is in an area where a majority of its residents favor alternative medicine such as chiropractic, acupuncture, and massage therapy. Let's say the survey reveals 43 percent of the population has already used at least one of these therapies in the past twelve months. In this case, the organization can surmise that a lot of health care is being administered to local residents who are prospective patients, but without its input. Although this might be an interesting finding, it may not allow the organization to do anything about it.

A logical action plan might be to research these services and begin to offer them upon completion of an implementation plan. But in the health care industry, nothing is quite so simple. This is particularly true because of the hospital's interdependence with its affiliated medical staff. All community-oriented hospitals and academic medical centers have bylaws that grant their medical staff a series of privileges to practice medicine in the facility, based on their academic and professional credentials.

Members of the medical staff are charged with checking the credentials of physicians new to the staff as well as periodically reviewing existing credentials. This periodic review is usually at intervals of two or three years, depending on the organization. A medical executive committee (MEC), sometimes called the medical board, represents the organization's medical staff. The MEC is made up of elected and appointed physician representatives. Initial approval by the MEC is required for a physician to practice at the hospital, but because of the interdependence just mentioned, final approval is required by the full board of directors of the health care organization.

One other privilege granted to the MEC is its ability to decide and determine the kinds of medicine practiced in the organization. The MEC is made up of long-serving members of the medical staff who understand the community they serve and the general needs and desires of its resident population. They have specific roles and responsibilities with regard to medical practice performed in the facility. Specifically, the bylaws of health care organizations such as RHMC might have language saying "subject to the authority of the board, the MEC shall determine all policy and shall have the authority to make final decisions on all questions relating to the practice of medicine within the institution."

Thus it is quite possible that there could be a major conflict between the organization's administration and its medical staff, as represented by the MEC. The administration is eager to add what it perceives to be needed services (as well as increase its market share), while the MEC may reject this addition because it does not perceive alternative medicine as being in the best interest of the community—or the medical staff. The MEC may reason that there has not been enough academic peer review in regard to alternative medicine—meaning, the efficacy of the treatments has not been proven. In addition, it may reject any treatments not approved by the state's medical professional licensing board. Any of these considerations may stymie the desire of the organization in question to use alternative medicine as a way to increase its market share.

RHMC Strategic Financial Planning

With the foregoing discussion of strategic financial planning as a backdrop, it is now possible to develop a plan for RHMC.

Volume Assumptions

RHMC's senior officers responsible for planning and implementation need to take the lead in determining the increase or decrease in volume over the upcoming five years. Although the crystal ball may be somewhat snowy, it is an essential part of an administrator's job responsibility to do this prognostication with appropriate inputs. Several types of volume must be reviewed for both current and proposed programs:

Inpatient Volume

- Admissions
- Average length of stay
- Patient days

Outpatient Volumes

- Emergency department
- Same-day surgery
- Observation days
- Home health services
- Other outpatient (defined as all other revenue-producing services rendered to outpatients:
    Laboratory services
    Radiology services (general, ultrasound, CT scanning, MRI)
    Physical therapy, occupational therapy, speech therapy
    Pharmaceutical (drug) sales
    Renal dialysis
    Other outpatient ancillary services

Physician Office Visit Volume

- Fee-for-service visits
- Capitated lives (or members)
- Relative value units (RVUs)

The volumes should be arrayed to show the trends over the past two to four years. This enables the administrators to make an informed decision on future volume as they review their market share assumptions. The future volumes are generally described as a percentage increase or decrease from current volume, by year. RHMC has conducted an analysis of its current market to determine the various volume assumptions and reviewed certain areas:

- The demographics of the organization's service area (particularly the age trend)
- The projected population growth rate of the area
- The current age of the physician staff
- The shifting criteria for inpatient admissions as dictated by various insurance companies
- The continuing shift from inpatient to outpatient care

    Thus RHMC's summarized volume assumptions looks like this:

- We expect a moderate decline in acute care volume each year:
    Discharges decline 2 percent per year
    Lengths of stay decline 4 percent per year
    Thus patient days decline 6 percent per year
- Emergency department volume is expected to increase 4 percent per year
- Other outpatient and physician volumes are projected to increase 8 percent per year

Payor Mix

Another major set of assumptions project the percentage mix of third-party insurance companies making payments on behalf of clients (employers, employees, and individual subscribers). It is important to determine the potential mix of payors simply because each payor is likely to be paying a different amount to RHMC for the same services. This is usually based on each insurance company's ability to negotiate its best rate with RHMC (referred to as the provider of services). The insurer's ability to negotiate a better or worse rate with the provider is generally a function of unique market conditions and the provider's need to capture the volume offered up by the insurer.

Payors vary dramatically:

- The dominating nature of the Medicare and Medicaid programs
- Control of HMO providers of managed care
- Laissez-faire PPOs of managed care
- Lack of control among POS providers of managed care

In addition, there is the unique reimbursement associated with worker's compensation and motor vehicle accidents, and the diminishing role of commercial

TABLE 3.1. CURRENT AND PROJECTED PAYOR MIX.

	Current Year	Annual Change, Next Five Years
Medicare	38%	−0.5%
Medicaid	6%	0.0%
HMO, managed care	16%	+0.5%
PPO, managed care	14%	+1.0%
Workers compensation	4%	0.0%
Commercial insurers	8%	−0.5%
Other	12%	−1.0%
Capitation, Medicare	2%	+0.5%
Capitation, commercial	0%	0.0%

insurers. Finally, the industry constantly redefines the concepts inherent to patient-pay or self-pay patients, which often depends on the socioeconomic conditions of the community around the health care organization. In some communities, *self-pay* means "pay," while in other areas it really means "no-pay."

In this year's strategic financial plan, RHMC has once again performed a review, based on actual data from the current year. It has examined current trends within various health insurance companies and employer fringe benefit areas. From this review, RHMC administration has adopted the payor mix assumptions seen in Table 3.1.

Rates and Reimbursements

The next major set of assumptions involve reimbursement rates, which represent the net revenue the health care organization expects from the various payors throughout the industry. In this industry, there is one dominant payor: the federal government. The two primary programs covered by the government are Medicare and Medicaid. The federal government pays 100 percent of its agreed-upon rates (not the organization's charges) for services rendered to Medicare recipients. In addition, the federal government pays at least 50 percent of the rate for services rendered to Medicaid recipients while each state government pays a varying percentage that makes up the 100 percent.

Between Medicare and Medicaid, the government pays more than 50 percent of every health care dollar directed to providers. (We review the Medicare and Medicaid programs in more depth in the next chapter.) Still, it is important to note that for purposes of the strategic financial plan, making one's best guess on the direction of the Medicare and Medicaid programs in the near future—say, the next five years—is essential to a quality outcome.

TABLE 3.2. RHMC MANAGED CARE SUMMARY OF PERCENTAGE OF DISCOUNT FOR GROSS CHARGES.

	Year 1	Year 2	Year 3	Year 4	Year 5
HMOs	30	32	35	38	42
PPOs	18	21	25	29	34
Medicare	46	48	50	52	54
Medicaid	68	69	70	71	72

After the Medicare and Medicaid programs, the next largest payor group is categorized as managed care. The term *managed care* is a catch-all for a variety of health insurance that is designed to limit the cost of health care through a range of utilization and reimbursement techniques. The various managed care companies attempt to reduce costs by focusing on lowering the price paid to the provider, limiting the volume of care rendered to subscribers, and reducing the intensity of services used.

Managed care concepts are reviewed in Chapter Four. For purposes of the strategic financial plan, it is important to recognize the implications of the reduction strategies used by these companies. Managed care methodology favors reduction in admissions and length of stay, thereby further reducing the number of days that the subscriber spends as an inpatient in a health care facility. The chosen methodology also cuts outpatient visits wherever possible. In addition, managed care companies negotiate aggressively with providers to secure the best (that is, lowest) prices possible.

There are more than a dozen reimbursement methodologies that managed care companies may attempt to negotiate and impose. The easiest way to express the discount taken off of the provider's list price of services (usually called gross charges) is as an overall percentage. This allows the provider to summarize a list of various managed care contracts into one consistent number for calculation, analysis, and trending. The summary for rate payors is usually expressed as shown in Table 3.2.

Keep in mind that the percentages in Table 3.2 are fully blended between inpatient and outpatient rates. They are usually determined and reported separately between inpatient and outpatient categories.

Capitation: Implications for Revenue

There is one other concept that should be explored at this time, which began to have an effect on the revenue and rate structures of many health care organizations in the 1990s. This is the insurance concept known as capitation. Capitation shifts the risk of coverage from the insurer to the provider of care. It is defined as "a flat periodic payment per enrollee to a health care provider that is the sole reimbursement for providing defined services to a defined population. These defined services are specific to the contract between the provider and the insurer but may include coverage for the enrollee's entire assortment of health care needs. The word *capitation* is derived from the term *per capita,* which means per person. Generally, capitation payments are expressed as some dollar amount per member per month (PMPM), in which the word *member* typically means enrollee in a managed care plan, usually a health maintenance organization (HMO)" (Gapenski, 1996, p. 378).

Capitation can be paid to providers of services at various rates. Providers that typically accept capitation include primary care physicians (PCPs), specialist physicians, hospitals, and home health agencies. Again, the rates vary depending on the provider and the age and sex of the enrollee. For example, a primary care physician may accept capitation from an insurance company on a large or small set of enrollees. The PCP may receive $10–14 PMPM for accepting the contract. Assume that the contract calls for the insurance company to supply one thousand members. The PCP, if paid $12 PMPM, would receive $12,000 per month, or $144,000 per year in reimbursements. The PCP could then round out the practice by accepting more capitation from other insurers or preserving the rest of the practice for fee-for-service patients.

In the case of Ridgeland, capitation denotes the same concept but has a much larger consequence. RHMC only recently began accepting capitation contracts and is just beginning to understand the financial impact on its operations. Only two years ago, the organization accepted its first capitation contract, a Medicare HMO arrangement with a local health plan that is a certified Medicare HMO insurer. The insurer was required to contract with health care providers for provision of care and so approached RHMC, which was eager to break into the Medicare HMO business and saw capitated reimbursement as a new and attractive revenue stream that also made it possible to learn the nuances of capitation on a small scale. After ascending the learning curve, RHMC presumed that it wanted to move into capitation in a big way. It expected that it could provide defined services at a cost below that of its premium revenue (if it could carve out the pharmacy benefit).

The Medicare HMO laws have one particular feature that makes them quite different from traditional Medicare. Under Medicare HMO rules, Medicare pays its insurers a PMPM depending on the specific county in which the Medicare enrollee lives. In the United States, these PMPMs vary from just over $400 to just under $800—a significant variation—and are based on 95 percent of the average adjusted per capita costs (AAPCC) within each county. The AAPCCs represent the average spending of all the traditional Medicare beneficiaries in these counties.

The PMPMs represent the total for all health care services that must be supplied by the insurer to assume the initial risk. The amount has to be parceled out to providers of hospital care, primary and specialty physician care, skilled nursing, and home health care. Because of the variability in rate, it is clear that the Medicare residents of some counties are spending a great deal more money on health care than those elsewhere. In general, the counties where traditional Medicare health care spending is highest are populated with a disproportionately high share of Medicare-age residents (notably Dade and Broward counties in South Florida).

Although RHMC is not in one of the higher-level AAPCC counties, it still thinks itself capable of turning a profit on Medicare HMO (or Medicare risk) business. RHMC committed itself to building its Medicare HMO business. In RHMC's county, the Medicare insurers have chosen to reimburse their hospital providers through capitation methodology rather than a methodology of per diem or discount from charges.

RHMC has therefore projected that 4.5 percent of its payor mix would be Medicare HMO within the time frame of the five-year strategic plan. Because of this, the financial impact has to be estimated and projected for both the premium revenues as well as variable expenses. RHMC believes it can garner fifteen hundred Medicare members within a three-year time frame, thus earning an additional $300,000 per month ($200 PMPM times fifteen hundred members), or $3.6 million a year. (The $200 PMPM is the allocated hospital portion of the AAPCC in RHMC's home county.) At the same time, the physicians, both primary care and specialists, get to split as much as $150 PMPM (or a total of $2.7 million). RHMC administration considers this a considerable sum and well worth the trouble to achieve.

Implications for Operating Expenses

Projecting operating expenses over a five-year time horizon carries the same high risk of uncertainty as was encountered in projecting gross revenues. In the case of expenses, at least two main assumption sets must be determined: volume and inflation. Like revenues, all variable expenses are a function of projected volume. Therefore, it is appropriate to use the projected volume changes that have been previously accepted as one multiplier for variable expense change.

There is also a need to project change in inflation for all operating expenses, whether variable or fixed. Some may consider this nothing more than a guessing game. Prior-year inflation rates, arrayed by major expense category, can be found in a number of places. It is somewhat harder to find any company or service, whether proprietary or in the public domain, that projects the inflation rate by category over a coming five-year time frame. However, RHMC has found a service that does these projections over five years and across various major expense categories, and it has shaped a reasonably good crystal ball (see the *Rate Controls* newsletter, available from Rate Controls Publications, 800-975-8100). These external projections are then used as the source for predicting inflation in the strategic financial plan.

An underlying and unyielding assumption that needs to be determined before finalizing the five-year plan is the margin target that the organization requires annually. This is necessary for the organization to determine whether its assumptions will produce the results that it desires. Every organization has its own margin target, depending on a variety of factors including but not limited to the following:

- Organization culture
- Board requirements
- Demographics of the organization's service
- Payor mix
- Service mix
- Tax status (exempt or for-profit)

RHMC has determined that the appropriate annual operating margin required for the five-year plan is 4 percent, a figure that is relatively in the range of average profit as a percentage of revenue for all Fortune 500 organizations after taxes and before dividends, which was 6.5 percent in 1999 and 6.2 percent in 2000 ("Fortune 500," 2001). It therefore closely aligns with the kind of financial return generated by corporations in other industries and is supportable at the board level and within the community. Assumptions on operating expense for RHMC are thus expressed in the strategic financial plan this way:

- We expect salaries and wages to increase at a rate of 3.5 percent per year over the following five years
- Controllable nonsalary inflation increases are assumed to be 3 percent per year
- Pharmaceutical supply inflation is expected to increase by 10 percent per year
- Additional reductions of $500,000 per year in nonsalary expense must be assumed to achieve targeted goals
- As a result of net revenue reduction, to meet a targeted level of a 4 percent operating margin, the staffing level needs to be reduced by 15 percent, from one thousand FTEs to nine hundred at the end of the fifth year

In addition to the assumptions listed in the strategic financial report to the finance committee and the board of directors, the organization's administration also takes the opportunity to supply an analysis and conclusion. In the case of RHMC, the summary and conclusion for the upcoming five-year period show the following:

- The ability to generate the targeted bottom line results is compromised by the expected impact of managed care growth and capitated reimbursement plans. In addition, achieving the projected outpatient growth is a critical factor.
- The anticipated onset of capitated reimbursement and declining noncapitated reimbursement requires dramatic reduction in operating expense to maintain targeted margin and cash requirements. The magnitude of these cost reductions is consistent with those presented in the previous plan.
- Compared to the prior plan, the level of planned capital expenditure has been reduced by more than $5 million.
- The baseline strategic financial plan is essentially an operating plan assuming current market share. Market share is an integral part of the strategic plan. If successful, increased market share dramatically improves the results of this financial plan.
- Concern about possible community reaction to real or perceived reduction in customer service or patient care quality as staff reduction occurs may override the realization of cost reduction and margin targets.

Ratio Analysis

The assumptions used by administration lead to several financial and operational conclusions. Specifically, to meet the 4 percent operating margin target, the strategic financial plan indicates a number of directions that the organization may take. If it is unable to improve the future financial condition through volume and revenue assumptions, then it must take appropriate action on the expense side. In addition, the five-year future financial statements that are developed through this process create a series of ratios that are essential to the analysis and action plans being prepared. Finally, the analysis can be used to determine that future ratios will exceed the level required by bond covenants.

Ratios force the user to take two seemingly unrelated bits of data and create a result that has deeper meaning. The result often allows the information user to trend and benchmark the result, shaping a direction for action. For example, a simple ratio that validates this notion is the net margin ratio. The net margin ratio is net margin divided by total revenues, both of which are taken from the statement of operations. The result, expressed as a ratio, has more meaning than the two underlying numbers.

Consider these points:

- In 1999, RHMC had a net margin of $4.7 million on total revenue of $100.8 million. In 2000, its net margin was $6.4 million on total revenue of $103.1 million. By themselves, these numbers may not have much meaning.
- If all you knew about an organization was that it earned $4.7 million or $6.4 million, would you think the organization did well financially? Well, what is the base of revenue these earnings represent? Those earnings on $100 million in total revenues would be better than the same earnings on $1 billion of revenue.
- Consequently, developing a ratio that reflects the underlying value of the equation is important. In this case, running the numbers through the equation results in net margin ratios for 1999 and 2000 respectively of 4.7 percent and 6.2 percent.
- This is better, but it still does not give us final information for decision making. For this we need to see the results over time (trends) and against competitors and peers (benchmarking). However, determining the ratio itself does complete the first step.

In health care, several external services use ratio analysis to make decisions for their clients or themselves. The most likely use of ratios for an external user is to determine how well the organization did in relation to others. This is always done by bond rating agencies (Moody's, Fitch, Standard & Poor's), usually annually and occasionally quarterly. The ratings are continuously updated to evaluate the ongoing financial health of the organization with bonds that have been issued and are still outstanding.

There are literally dozens of ratios available for computation. Perhaps the best source of ratio analysis available in this industry is the annual *Almanac of Hospital Financial and Operating Indicators,* published by the Center for Health Information Performance, or CHIPS (Ingenix, 2001). This book, usually running to more than five hundred pages, presents current financial ratios against a variety of peer groupings. There is also commentary, analysis, and explanation of the various ratios.

Bonding-Related Ratios

For the health care financing community, as already mentioned in Chapter Two, the three most important ratios involved in bond repayment are long-term debt to capitalization, debt-service coverage, and cash flow to total debt. These were fully described and their calculations shown in Chapter Two.

EXHIBIT 3.1. OTHER FINANCIAL RATIO FORMULAS.

$$\text{Operating margin} = \frac{(\text{total operating revenue} - \text{total operating expenses})}{\text{total operating revenue}}$$

$$\text{Net (excess) margin (\%)} = \frac{(\text{total operating revenue} - \text{total operating expenses}) + \text{nonoperating revenue}}{(\text{total operating revenue} + \text{nonoperating revenue})}$$

$$\text{Current ratio (X)} = \frac{\text{total current assets}}{\text{total current liabilities}}$$

$$\text{Cushion ratio (X)} = \frac{(\text{cash and cash equivalents} + \text{board-designated funds for capital})}{\text{estimated future peak debt service}}$$

$$\text{Cash on hand (days)} = \frac{(\text{cash and cash equivalents} + \text{board-designated funds for capital}) \times 365}{(\text{total operating expenses} - \text{depreciation and amortization expenses})}$$

$$\text{Average age of plant (years)} = \frac{\text{accumulated depreciation}}{\text{depreciation expense}}$$

$$\text{Capital expense (\%)} = \frac{(\text{interest expense} + \text{depreciation and amortization expenses})}{\text{total operating expenses}}$$

$$\text{Accounts receivable (days)} = \frac{\text{net patient accounts receivable} \times 365}{\text{net patient revenue}}$$

$$\text{Average payment period (days)} = \frac{\text{total current liabilities} \times 365}{(\text{total operating expenses} - \text{depreciation and amortization expenses})}$$

Other Ratios

Still, there are other ratios that are always evaluated in the mix of bond rating because of their influence in the overall financial health of the organization (Exhibit 3.1 shows the actual equations):

- Operating margin
- Net margin
- Current ratio
- Cushion ratio
- Days cash on hand
- Average age of plant
- Capital expenditures as a percentage of total expenses
- Days in accounts receivable
- Average payment period

There are benchmarks for all of these ratios. They are usually reported as the median value of a list of organizations somewhat similar to yours. The median is usually defined as the organization in the sample that is exactly in the middle of the pack when the values are arrayed highest to lowest. Several rating organizations collect and disseminate benchmarks; see Table 3.3 for some of the values they report.

Operating Margin and Net Margin. Operating margin and net margin ratios involve either the operating results or net results as a function of net revenue. These are widely used indicators of profitability. Unfortunately, they are not always comparable. The controversy involving the placement of interest income above the line has already been discussed in Chapter Two. Still, the operating margin ratio can be considered useful when trended against itself. This allows the organization to determine if its financial direction is positive or negative. Meanwhile, the net margin ratio can be trended against itself or else compared to local, regional, and national benchmarks to determine whether the organization's financial outcomes are favorable or not.

Current Ratio. Current ratio describes an organization's ability to use current assets to pay off current liabilities. As long as the ratio is above 1.0, the liabilities should be extinguishable without problem. Still, a current ratio closer to 2.0 is considered good. To achieve a higher current ratio (which is preferable), the organization needs to increase current assets or decrease current liabilities.

Cushion Ratio. Cushion ratio is used to determine the amount of cash and cash equivalents available to pay off future peak debt service (which is defined as the largest annual interest expense and principal payments on the existing debt). A high ratio—one that continually exceeds benchmarks—is always preferable.

TABLE 3.3. RHMC KEY HOSPITAL FINANCIAL STATISTICS AND RATIO MEDIANS AS OF NOVEMBER 2000.

	RHMC 2000 Actual	RHMC 2005 Strategic Financial Plan	Moody's All Ratings
Measure sample size			320
Operating margin	5.0%	1.2%	0.5%
Net (excess) margin	6.2%	4.1%	3.0%
Current ratio (X)	1.27	1.9	1.89
Cushion ratio (X)	12.19	16.40	10.38
Cash on hand (days)	525.87	643.45	146.57
Average age of plant (years)	6.55	9.2	8.55
Capital expenses	18.8%	19.3%	n/a
Accounts receivable (days)	63.3	55.0	67.6
Average payment period (days)	81.9	62.0	64.8
Long-term debt to capitalization	64.6%	54.78%	37.9%
Debt service coverage (X)	2.28	2.9	3.30
Average length of stay (days)	4.07	5.10	4.85

Days Cash on Hand. Another ratio that is used in determining total cash available to liquidate or pay off annual operating expenses is days cash on hand. The available cash includes long-term investments that can be converted to cash in less than one year (generally without decreasing the value of the investment). Bond investment managers and holders of the organization's tax-exempt bonds are interested in this ability to meet short-term obligations. If the benchmark is approximately 150 days of cash on hand, then it is important for the organization to meet, if not exceed, this. A high ratio compared to benchmarks is always preferable.

Average Age of Plant. Average age of plant is an important and underrated ratio that represents the relative age of the organization's plant and capital equipment. In this case, a low result compared to benchmarks is preferable because it designates the equivalent of a new or at least more modern physical plant. Even if the organization does not build a completely new plant, this ratio accounts for all capital renovations and equipment replacement that have taken place.

Capital Expenses as a Percentage of Total Expenses. Capital expense as a percentage of total expense is linked to the average age of plant because any capital expenditures affect both ratios.

Standard & Poor's All Ratings	Fitch IBCA	HCIA	Data Advantage	Ingenix/ CHIPS	Solucient/ HBSI
552	140	1,298	4,024	1,372	448
0.7%	1.0%	1.6%	−2.1%	n/a	4.91%
3.1%	3.3%	3.4%	5.8%	3.1	7.2%
1.87	n/a	1.99	1.89	1.97	2.37
9.40	10.10	n/a	n/a	9.55	n/a
135.00	144.00	n/a	35.89	102.50	n/a
8.90	8.80	9.89	4.39	9.42	n/a
8.4%	n/a	7.0%	6.8%	7.3%	8.8%
87.9	69.8	66.5	87.3	67.9	61.7
65.5	n/a	60.1	76.9	59.2	51.7
37.0%	39.3%	31.0%	31.3%	26.8	0.5%
2.80	n/a	4.17	n/a	3.40	5.12
4.80	n/a	4.03	4.89	4.27	4.89

There are differing views on the value of this ratio. One school of thought suggests that because higher expenses for capital lead to higher depreciation expenses and thus lower operating and net margins, any expended capital should pay for itself through a return-on-investment calculation. The thinking is that any capital that does not pay for its annual depreciation may well need to be paid for by decreasing FTEs. Trading FTEs for capital purchase may be a good idea only if it is done with foreknowledge. However, it is not uncommon in this industry for capital purchases to be made without enough financial analysis.

Still, the Advisory Board has made a case that organizations with higher-than-average capital expenses as a percentage of physical assets, as well as higher capital expenditures per bed, create an enduring advantage if the capital purchases are made to expand or establish new services (Advisory Board, 1996). Thus the Advisory Board highlights Columbia/HCA and suggests that heavy reinvestment of profit in plant and equipment is likely to magnify an advantage over time.

Days in Accounts Receivable. Days in accounts receivable is used by bond rating agencies and internal operational management to assess the value of potential cash tied up in accounts receivable. There are also numerous opportunities to benchmark this ratio, which allows administration to determine if accounts receivable management is effective. The concepts behind accounts receivable management and the implications of this ratio are explored in Chapter Five.

Average Payment Period. The average payment period is somewhat tied to those ratios that assess cash level and the organization's ability to pay its debts. In this case, the debt being liquidated specifically refers to current liabilities. The largest current liability is usually trade vendor payables. A bond rating agency would review this ratio to determine whether the organization is in line with industry standards for payment periods. This is not a detailed review of the payable balance but rather a result derived from financial statement information. If either the investment manager or the organization is interested in getting behind the numbers, an external rating agency such as Dun and Bradstreet will give details.

Operating Ratios

There is more to ratio analysis than just bond rating. Ratio analysis can be extremely useful in understanding the organization's operations. Some useful operating ratios:

- Full-time equivalents (FTEs) per adjusted patient days (APDs)
- Salaries, wages, and fringe benefits as a percentage of net revenues
- Expenses per APD
- Expenses per adjusted discharge (EPAD)
- Revenue per FTE
- Length of stay

Exhibit 3.2 shows the ratio calculations.

FTEs per APD. The most common ratio used in the health care industry to measure overall productivity is FTEs per APD. Full-time equivalent represents the wages being paid to an employee who is designated as full time, which in most organizations means the employee is paid (but does not necessarily work) for 2,080 hours annually (fifty-two weeks, forty hours per week). APD is a calculation that attempts to convert outpatient revenue into an equivalent inpatient day.

Some controversy surrounding this widely used equation has sprung up in recent years. FTEs per APD has become an established benchmark throughout the industry. Yet it is fraught with inconsistency. The numerator (FTEs) is highly susceptible to manipulation, while the denominator is a poor equalization factor for converting outpatient services into an inpatient equivalent.

EXHIBIT 3.2. OPERATIONAL RATIO FORMULAS.

Adjusted patient days	=	$\dfrac{\text{total revenue} \times \text{inpatient days}}{\text{inpatient revenue}}$
Adjusted discharges	=	$\dfrac{\text{total revenue} \times \text{inpatient discharges}}{\text{inpatient revenue}}$
FTEs per adjusted patient day	=	See Table 3.4
Salaries, wages, and fringe benefits as a percentage of net revenues	=	$\dfrac{(\text{salary expenses} + \text{total fringe benefit expenses})}{\text{total revenues}}$
Expenses per adjusted patient day	=	$\dfrac{\text{total expenses}}{\text{adjusted patient days}}$
Expenses per adjusted discharge	=	$\dfrac{\text{total expenses}}{\text{adjusted discharges}}$
Revenue per FTE	=	$\dfrac{\text{total revenues}}{\text{total FTEs}}$
Average length of stay (days)	=	$\dfrac{\text{patient days}}{\text{total discharges}}$

In the case of the numerator, the total number of paid (or worked) hours is divided by the number of hours in the period under study (for instance, if a week is 40 hours, a biweekly period would be 80 hours, and a year would be 2,080 hours). The problem is that most organizations collect and report only the hours paid to employees, but not the hours paid for contract labor or purchased services. So if an organization wants to manipulate the FTEs per APD calculation to make overall productivity look better, it can outsource many of its services to nonemployees.

Inpatient and outpatient revenues consist of different service components and levels of severity. They are not comparable. Most hospital charge masters (which generate the list price for every service and supply) are not completely based on any established costing methodology. Instead they have evolved over time without ongoing review for consistency. Because of this, outpatient services may have become overweighted or underweighted, making the denominator a poor factor for such an important benchmark.

In the case of the denominator, the equation used to convert outpatient revenue into inpatient day equivalents is significantly flawed. This equation was created many years ago, when 85 to 90 percent of hospital revenues were derived from inpatient services and the remainder was outpatient. At the time, this equation did a moderate job of conversion. But by the late 1990s, when outpatient revenues equaled or exceeded 50 percent of total revenues in hospitals and integrated delivery systems, the service equivalent no longer worked.

Salaries, Wages, and Fringe Benefits as a Percentage of Net Patient Service Revenue.
Salaries to net service revenue is a better ratio to measure overall productivity than FTEs per APD. It was popularized by Columbia/HCA, which saw the problems inherent in the FTEs per APD equation. With 350 hospitals, they needed a ratio that was reliable and consistent. This one removes the question of whether all outsourced hours have been accounted for and whether or not the APD equation does a good enough job in converting outpatient services.

The ratio includes all salary dollars paid out plus all dollars paid to contract labor and service companies for staffing expenses. Further, it includes all dollars paid out in fringe benefits because they are fully attached to salaries. The resulting ratio measures the level of labor costs in relation to the revenues being generated by the organization. A downward trend is preferred. Better financial performance usually results when labor costs can be minimized.

RHMC decided to take a compromise position in the controversy. Although it is aware that the FTEs per APD ratio has consistency problems, the organization still wants to capture the data and at least measure the trends against its own performance over time. Continuing to use the ratio against its own prior performance eliminates one of the two problems plaguing the ratio: the contract labor component. It does not, however, eliminate the problem that the conversion factor is flawed. At the same time, RHMC has adopted the salaries, wages, and fringe benefit ratio as an adjunct.

When RHMC started to use the ratio, it went back three years to see whether it was trending favorably or unfavorably. In fact, although FTEs per APD was trending favorably downward, salaries, wages, and fringe benefits as a percentage of net revenue were trending unfavorably upward. This is another indication of the problem inherent with the FTEs per APD ratio. Table 3.4 summarizes the input and output of the two equations.

RHMC's FTEs per APD in 2000 were recorded as 4.10. According to various reputable benchmarks published around the country, this would be considered very good, from the standpoint of productivity measures and cost containment. But as an example of how this ratio is often falsely portrayed, it is important to

TABLE 3.4. RHMC ANALYSIS OF FTES PER APD VERSUS SALARIES, WAGES, AND FRINGE BENEFITS AS A PERCENTAGE OF NET REVENUES FOR THE YEARS ENDED 1998–2000.

	1998	1999	2000
FTEs per adjusted patient day			
FTEs	880	1,000	980
Patient days	46,000	45,500	44,200
Inpatient revenue	$73,000	$74,000	$78,000
Outpatient revenues	$65,000	$69,000	$76,000
Total revenues	$138,000	$143,000	$154,000
Calculation of adjustment to patient days			
$\dfrac{\text{Total revenue}}{\text{Inpatient revenue}} \times \text{inpatient days}$	1.89	1.93	1.97
Total adjusted patient days per year	86,959	87,926	87,267
Number of days in the year	366	365	365
Number of adjusted patients per day	237.6	240.9	239.1
Ratio, FTEs per adjusted patient day	3.70	4.15	4.10
Salaries, wages, and fringe benefits as a percentage of net revenues			
Salaries	$32,000	$34,000	$36,000
Contract labor	$1,300	$1,500	$1,000
Fringe benefits	$4,900	$6,800	$5,800
Total staffing costs	$38,200	$42,300	$42,800
Net revenues	$92,800	$92,800	$93,400
Ratio, salaries, wages, and fringe benefits as a percentage of net revenues	41.2%	45.6%	45.8%

know that RHMC outsources its laboratory services. It has been estimated that these services are equivalent to 105 FTEs for the organization. If they were accounted for in the equation, the FTEs per APD for the year 2000 would increase from 4.10 to 4.54, still a respectable ratio but not as good as before. The salaries, wages, and fringe benefits as a percentage of net patient service revenue ratio are similarly affected because the expense is treated as a purchased service, not as contract labor. This highlights how any ratio can be distorted.

Expenses per Adjusted Patient Day and Expenses per Adjusted Discharge. The EPAPD and EPAD expense ratios are closely related. The numerator is the same while the denominator is either inpatient patient days or discharges adjusted for outpatient services provided. Because this is primarily an operational ratio and not one used by bond rating agencies, there are fewer external services having benchmarks. However, the EPAD ratio is available annually through the Mercer/ HCIA Top 100 analysis, usually published in December in *Modern Healthcare*. Expanded information and analysis is also available directly through HCIA. Other services such as McFaul and Lyons produce proprietary expense per APD ratios established through analysis of more than one thousand clients.

These ratios are particularly important to administration because they demonstrate actual cost performance. In addition, because they can be benchmarked and trended, they are extremely useful as an overall indicator of how well or poorly the organization is performing over time and against like organizations.

Revenue per FTE. Revenue per FTE is an interesting ratio because it is one of the few that cut across other industries. Most other industries routinely capture and report revenue per employee as an operational productivity value. In this service industry, a health care organization generally earns less revenue per employee, but this should not deter evaluation of this ratio. By capturing the ratio, the organization can strive to continuously improve its revenues.

Length of Stay. Length of stay is one of the most ubiquitous ratios in health care. Almost every segment of the industry uses it. Hospitals, psychiatric facilities, skilled nursing facilities, and children's hospitals all capture this measure and use it to continuously compare themselves against prior measurements as well as outside benchmarks.

It should be recognized however, that this ratio is only one component of operational understanding. Organizations have been attempting (successfully) to reduce length of stay since Medicare changed its method for reimbursing hospitals in 1983. They went from paying costs per diem to paying for the type of diagnosis for which the patient was being treated. Because it was not in the organization's best financial interest to keep patients for a long period of time, care plans were established to allow the patient to be discharged sooner than before DRG reimbursement was adopted.

Still, there is a big issue that needs to be analyzed in reviewing the length of stay ratio or in benchmarking length of stay against other organizations or your own organization. The length of a patient's stay is often a function of the severity of the illness. The industry has spent many years developing numerical equivalents for patient severity or acuity. The most common statistic used as a proxy for severity is called the Case Mix Index (CMI). CMI is the accumulation of the case weights for all the Medicare inpatients who have been discharged from the hospital over a defined time period. The average CMI is 1.00, but it varies from 0.40

for the most common case of labor and delivery to over 16.00 for a tracheostomy. When looking at length of stay statistics, it is also important to incorporate a severity indicator.

The Capital Plan and Its Relationship to the Strategic Plan

The annual strategic financial plan compels the organization to continuously update its capital plan to determine capital requirements and its relationship to available cash and investments. These steps are performed concurrently with operating projections. The process used to execute the capital plan is often organized in seven basic steps:

1. Defining the institution's capital position
2. Identifying ongoing capital requirements
3. Quantifying the debt capacity and identifying the level of risk capital
4. Defining the primary funding and financing problems and setting key goals
5. Developing and evaluating financing alternatives
6. Establishing a master capital plan
7. Preparing an implementation plan*

RHMC believes in these steps and follows them closely. It performs an annual update of the capital plan in conjunction with the strategic financial plan update.

The centerpiece of the capital plan is identification of ongoing capital requirements (item 2). To do so, the medical center has to make a series of capital assumptions linked to the strategic plan and the strategic financial plan, which are moving along just ahead of the capital plan. These assumptions relate to decisions on whether to purchase, lease, or build necessary capital. In any case, the dollar value associated with acquisition is the critical feature after the organization decides what to acquire.

Table 3.5 illustrates the RHMC's ongoing capital requirements. As can be seen, it is a five-year plan that summarizes various types of planned capital acquisition. In addition to the budgeted routine capital items, special, nonroutine capital items are featured. These special line items consist of information technology and facility upgrades, typically the two largest contributors to capital purchase. In addition, there are separate budget categories for land acquisition as well as physician recruitment and physician medical office space.

---

*An excellent discussion of capital planning and its implication for the health care organization is presented in Kaufman and Hall, *The Capital Management of Healthcare Organizations* (1990).

TABLE 3.5. RHMC FIVE-YEAR CAPITAL BUDGET (IN THOUSANDS OF DOLLARS).

	Budget 2001	2002	2003	2004	2005	Five-Year Total
Routine capital budgets	$ 5,000	$ 6,000	$ 7,000	$ 7,000	$ 7,000	$32,000
Information technology	3,000	5,000	3,000	3,000	3,000	17,000
Facility improvements and upgrades	2,500	2,500	2,500	2,500	2,500	12,500
Property acquisitions	500	500	500	500	500	2,500
Physician recruitment	1,000	1,000	1,000	1,000	1,000	5,000
Physician medical office space	500	500	500	500	500	2,500
Total	$12,500	$15,500	$14,500	$14,500	$14,500	$71,500

Routine Capital Items

The line item for routine capital budgets generally consists of much of the equipment that is needed in areas such as laboratory, radiology, and cardiology as well as the nursing floors. As stated in Chapter Two, this is applicable only for purchases where the price exceeds whatever is stipulated in the organization's capitalization policy and has an estimated useful life greater than one year.

Information Technology

The capital line for IT has gotten much more respect over the past few years. Prior to the mid-1990s, the health care industry spent less than 2.5 percent of its capital for information technology. This compares unfavorably to the 5 to 7 percent spent by the manufacturing, insurance, and banking industries. Being behind these other industries meant that the right amount of information was not collected, reported, or analyzed in either the financial or the clinical side of the health care business. This created an opportunity for those in the health care industry to gain a competitive advantage over one another through technology. Toward the end of the 1990s, most health care providers got the message (aided by the year 2000 problem).

At RHMC, the administration started to understand its lack of effective information technology support in 1996, when it began to allocate a greater portion of scarce capital resources to IT. As such, it now makes a point of separately breaking out this line and spending for IT in the most appropriate manner. Some of the allocated money is projected to be spent on upgraded IT infrastructure such as new fiber optic cabling and distribution closets—costing $1.2 million. In addition, post-Y2K implementation, RHMC plans to upgrade all HIPAA-noncompliant software. This is budgeted at $2 million. Finally, purchase of a new organization-wide clinical and financial system is expected over the next three years, at a price of $9 million. The issue of information technology in health care is discussed in great detail in Chapter Ten.

Facility Improvement and Upgrade

As in other industries, health care needs to remain reasonably current with physical plant. Thus RHMC projects the amount of money it believes will be need over the next five years to keep its plant modern. In addition, this line is used to allocate capital funds for new major projects that involve acquisition of new or expanded facilities, whether through construction, purchase, or capital lease. RHMC has allocated funds for projects such as major renovation of two of its medical/surgical units, projected to cost $2 million each; a new renal dialysis unit with sixteen patient stations, projected to cost $1.6 million; and a newly expanded emergency department that is projected to cost $2.5 million.

Land Acquisition

Land acquisition is an important and often overlooked line, particularly dependent on the location of the health care facility. In the case of RHMC, it is land-locked, surrounded on all four sides by residential housing. To expand, it must allocate funds to buy up all of the single-family housing that comes on the market within the target area designated by the administration and approved by the board. This policy also allows solicitation of the homeowners in the target area to sell to the organization based on the appraised market value. RHMC's target area consists of two streets directly adjacent to the campus. Once it acquires all the houses along the block, the organization will be able to incorporate the area into the existing health care zone, tear down the houses, and expand service offerings. It is important to note that this is a long-term strategy that has the opportunity to succeed for the next administrator.

Physician Recruitment

Another line item that has sprung up since the early to mid-1990s, when hospitals began in earnest to employ physicians, is recruitment. This helped change the face of the industry in a fundamental way. Hospitals began to recruit and employ physicians in response to the rapid buildup of managed care health plans throughout the country. The defining feature of the managed care plan was its insistence that covered beneficiaries (members) always see a primary care physician (PCP) before any advanced care would be covered (paid for) by the plan. Hospital care, whether inpatient or outpatient, was considered specialized care. Hospitals wanted to remain in some control of their volume and knew that physicians they employed would refer their hospital business to them.

So hospitals began to employ physicians, some in a bigger way than others. There are two primary ways to acquire a physician practice: buy an existing practice or establish a new one by employing young physicians just out of residency programs.

Each method has its own issues. However, the hospital spends capital money in either case. Purchasing an existing practice requires the transfer of funds from the hospital to the physicians in the group to pay for their existing assets. Establishing a new practice requires the hospital to fund significant start-up costs, sometimes for as long as three to five years until the practice is self-sustaining.

In any case, the capital needs for physician recruitment became significant for health care entities in the late 1990s and show no signs of slowing down any time soon. RHMC was caught up in the physician employment frenzy, as were its immediate competitors. They all found themselves having to allocate considerable sums in their long-term financial plan. However, it needs to be pointed out that the balloon burst on hospital-based physician practice acquisition sprees in many areas of the country in 1998 and 1999. This coincided with the devastation of investor-based physician practice management companies. Nevertheless, RHMC and its competitors still feel the need to continue their acquisition policy in the community. We examine physician practice management issues in detail in Chapter Eight.

Physician Medical Office Space

If your organization is going to employ physicians, you will obviously need to find them a place to practice. RHMC has allocated funds to either build or capital-lease new facilities for physicians to practice. Even if you don't employ physicians, your organization may want to build medical office space to attract physicians to practice there.

Capital Affordability

An important aspect of this five-year capital budget is the cumulative total, which is used to determine if the organization can indeed afford all of it. There are several ways to determine how much money the organization can afford to spend on capital equipment. RHMC uses:

- Spending equivalent to annual depreciation expense
- Spending equivalent to a percentage of annual depreciation expense
- Spending equivalent to adequate cash flow

The first form of spending in the list is a tried-and-true method used by organizations in many industries. Because depreciation is a noncash expense on the statement of operations, most administrators believe it is acceptable to spend depreciation money on capital acquisition—and many do. It is the equivalent of turning capital funding into operational funding every year.

As for the second form of spending, even though many health care organizations allocate and spend 100 percent of their annual depreciation expense on capital acquisition, this may not be the most efficient or effective use of these funds. We saw earlier in the chapter that the RHMC administration is currently proposing a $5 million reduction in its five-year capital expenditure plan because of the negative impact these purchases would have on the bottom line.

In fact, there are organizations that routinely spend only 70 to 80 percent of their depreciation expense on capital purchase to maintain a lower future depreciation expense. This is done knowingly because these organizations do not want to trade FTEs for depreciation, as we already reviewed earlier in the chapter.

Spending pegged to cash flow is a variation on spending equivalent to annual depreciation. It reflects, as does the depreciation calculation, annual depreciation but further takes into account any principal (and possibly interest) payments that the organization is already committed to making. Thus the calculation is designed to compensate for the extra cash outlays previously approved by hospital administration.

◆ ◆ ◆

To conclude, understanding these three methods at least allows a health care organization to make an informed decision regarding which method to use and the various implications.

In summary, the capital plan is the culmination of the strategic plan process, setting the stage for the approved capital acquisitions that the organization will be permitted to make in the coming years. RHMC's diligence in preparing and updating the strategic plan, the strategic financial plan, and the capital plan has allowed it to maintain healthy margins. It has also aided projecting both the best and the worst into the future. In doing so, this diligence has turned plans into action with forethought. This is the mark of good management.

With all the work that had been performed by the RHMC staff, and the quality of the analysis presented by its administration, the board of directors approved the updated five-year strategic financial and capital plan at its special March meeting. Specific application of the capital plan will be implemented during the annual capital budgeting process, which commences in June. See Chapter Six for initiation of the annual capital budget.

CHAPTER FOUR

APRIL

Sam Barnes pants as he lunges at a well-placed kill shot delivered with pinpoint precision by his opponent, Joel Hogan.

"Ugh! Missed again," Sam grunts.

"Sam, what's the matter with you?" asks his friend and racquetball partner of the past several years.

"I don't know. Well, OK, maybe I do know. Even though you know I love to play racquetball and it keeps me in decent shape, I've been unable to find enough energy to maintain my conditioning over the past several weeks."

"Well, I've noticed that you seem to have lost a step or two over the past couple of months," Joel says with an air of pleasure in his voice. "So what the heck is going on with you?"

"I've been thinking a lot about what I do at work. And it sure seems like things are closing in on this industry. A few years ago, the biggest thing that came down the pike was the Balanced Budget Act. It cost the industry plenty of money, and yet it seems as if the general public had no concept of the major changes that took place because of it. It was true that the feds needed to save a lot of money to keep the Medicare trust fund solvent, but doing it on the backs of hospital and home health providers led to a host of service cuts. That made services less accessible to the very people who need them—the sick, the old, the poor."

"OK," Joel replies, "but the feds are going to do this with or without your approval. And didn't I hear that they gave back some of the money in 1999 and 2000 anyway? Why are you letting this sap your energy?"

"Yeah, you're right. The industry did get some of the cuts in the Balanced Budget Refinement Act, in 1999, and then in the Budget Improvement and Protection Act in 2000. But it wasn't enough. I'm convinced that the policy makers don't have a complete picture of the provider's role. And sometimes I can't really help how I feel. You know I'm pretty passionate about my work. It's more than a job with me. I care about the quality of the services we offer at Ridgeland. Just as important, I care about the perception of quality throughout the industry. If one provider gets a bad name, it usually paints a black mark on the rest of us. And it's been a real struggle to maintain the quality. We were cut close to $200 billion since 1998, throughout the industry."

Joel is perplexed. "So what do you plan to do about it? Are you planning to take any action or just wallow in pity and despair?"

"That's just the problem. At the moment, I haven't quite figured it out, but I know I'll keep working on it till I do. Right now, though, I plan to refresh myself by beating your sorry body at this game."

April Fools Day at Ridgeland Heights Medical Center should be a time for some practical jokes and a little bit of frivolity, but at RHMC this is not so. The medical center is continuing to reduce expectations, as a result of some significant decreases to revenue. The lowered expectations are having a negative impact on employee morale. Although the administration is trying to counter the prevailing mood by creating a positive environment, it is not working. The administration makes a point of staying in close touch with staff to explain the revenue changes, but the fact remains that the changes have added new pressure to the organization.

Most of RHMC's constituency is well aware of the belt tightening that has taken place. The medical staff have noticed. They perceive there are fewer nurses on the floor to take care of patients. The nurses have noticed, recognizing that employees who resign are not being replaced as fast as before. They know this because they are being asked to work quite a bit more overtime. They believe it to be the effect of tightening staff. The remainder of the clinical staff have noticed too; they are aware that the nurses are more tired and more critical than before as they work ever longer hours.

The administration has noticed. The prized patient satisfaction scores, which everyone in the organization was once so proud of, are in decline. Over the previous two years, the organization has managed to maintain scores in the range of the 90th percentile across a set of four hundred peer hospitals. RHMC had in fact managed to move into the high nineties during several of those months, in all three rated areas (inpatient, outpatient ancillary services, and emergency department). Yet over the past few months, satisfaction was starting to show some obvious deterioration.

Unfortunately, though the effects are obvious, the constituents are misdiagnosing the causes. Coincidentally, in the middle of revenue-reduction efforts by many of the third-party payors, the industry is in its third major nursing shortage in twenty years. As RHMC's administration assembled much of the staff over the past three months to explain the revenue-reduction problem, it made a great effort to communicate its commitment to patient care and patient satisfaction. In fact, the current year's budget included an increase to the nursing staff, not a decrease. However, the message has been lost in the continuing depression caused by ongoing overwork.

At RHMC, the reduction in revenue was a function of its payor mix. RHMC identifies its payor mix to analyze and understand the source of its revenues. Payor mix is based on gross revenues. For the current year, it stands as follows:

Medicare	38 percent
Medicaid	6 percent
HMO managed care	16 percent
PPO managed care	14 percent
Worker's compensation	4 percent
Commercial insurers	8 percent
Other	14 percent

In this case, in all of its payor mix RHMC is fairly representative of the national average except for Medicaid. Because of its location in a relatively affluent community, there are not as many Medicaid-eligible residents. Table 4.1 shows the RHMC payor mix and how it compares to the national average. Because RHMC has almost 40 percent of its total revenue stream coming from Medicare, it is extremely important for the administration to understand the roots of the reimbursement reductions. Even more important, they must make decisions on how to operationalize changes that need to be made because of the current and continuing revenue reductions.

The roots of revenue reduction were set many years ago during creation of the federal Medicare and Medicaid programs, as well as the more recent rise of managed care.

Medicare and Medicaid Net Revenue Concepts

Medicare and Medicaid reimbursement dollars are crucial to the financial health of America's health care system. The following discussions reflect the policies, processes, and procedures surrounding these programs.

The History of Medicare and Medicaid

Medicare and Medicaid, known legally as Title XVIII and Title XIX of the Social Security Act, were enacted in 1965. Medicare* was created to provide health insurance to most American citizens age sixty-five and over and to certain disabled people under sixty-five. Medicaid was created as a state-operated program to provide publicly financed health care coverage for the poor. These programs, which were signed into law by President Johnson on July 31, 1965, became effective on July 1, 1966.

*An interesting and short history of the Medicare program with extensive bibliography and citation listings was reviewed for this section (Pearman and Starr, 1988).

TABLE 4.1. PAYOR MIX, RHMC TOTAL COMPARED
TO NATIONAL AVERAGES FOR HOSPITALS.

	RHMC (percentage)	1998 National Average (percentage)
Medicare	38	32.4
Medicaid	6	15.9
Other government	2	12.5
Private health insurance and other private funds	42	35.8
Out-of-pocket	12	3.4

Source: National Center for Health Statistics, *Health, United States, 2000,* tab. 119.

Over the last three decades, the Medicare program has received considerably more publicity and press than Medicaid. This may well be the result of two particular factors. First, Americans over sixty-five, through experience, have learned to use the system to their advantage, meaning they have more political clout than Medicaid patients. In addition, Medicare costs more than Medicaid and is thus more likely to contain the impact of expenditure savings and entitlements. Finally, Medicare is a single federal government program, applied equally across all beneficiaries throughout the country, while Medicaid is a federal and state program that is really fifty distinct programs.

Medicare actually has two components. Part A (called the hospital insurance program) primarily covers inpatient hospital and surgery services, posthospital skilled nursing care, home health services, and hospice care. In 1972, the Part A fund also began covering patients with end-stage renal disease (ESRD) and certain organ transplants. Medicare Part B (called the supplemental medical insurance program) primarily covers physician services, outpatient medical and surgical services, and independent laboratory services.

Each coverage type is financed independently and differently. Part A services are paid through a trust fund financed by a special form of Social Security tax on earnings. The money is accumulated and collected through employer and employee contributions. The Medicare tax is equal to 1.45 percent of salaries and wages payable by both the employer and the employee, for a total of 2.9 percent. (Self-employed individuals are required to pay both parts of the tax.) In addition, although non-Medicare Social Security taxes have an annual maximum above which the taxes end, there is no annual maximum for the Medicare contributions.

Part B services are financed through patient premiums and general federal tax revenues. When Medicare was started, 50 percent of the Part B services were financed through premiums. Over the years, as increases in patient premium failed to keep up with increasing cost of service, the percentage of the Part B services financed by premiums dropped to approximately 25 percent. Therefore the federal treasury now finances 75 percent of Medicare Part B services.

Getting passage of the Medicare bill was President Johnson's number one priority in 1964 and 1965. Several previous presidents had tried and failed to get some form of legislation passed that offered health insurance to various segments of the American population. President Truman proposed a national health insurance program during his term; it was defeated by Congress. Presidents Eisenhower and Kennedy advocated some form of national health insurance. In fact, Kennedy campaigned on a promise that he would propose a national health insurance program that would protect the elderly regardless of their finances.

Given the long-standing advocacy of national health insurance by various presidents, and the failure to pass it, obviously there were heavy political forces arrayed against programs of this kind. The two greatest opponents to federalized health insurance were the American Medical Association, representing the nation's physicians, and the American Health Insurance Association (now known as the Health Insurance Association of America), representing the nation's private insurance companies. Physicians were concerned that federalization of health insurance would lead to a decline in quality of care, while private insurance companies were concerned that federalization would drive them out of business.

Still, Johnson's landslide victory in the 1964 election and his single-mindedness in adopting his Great Society programs allowed him to push Congress hard for passage. Ultimately the Part A program was adopted to pay primarily for the hospital inpatient services; Part B was adopted as a way of separating physician payments from the hospital side. Finally, to appease a number of constituencies that wanted means-based health insurance, Medicaid was adopted as a state-operated, income-based supplemental plan.

Impact of Medicare and Medicaid on Provider Net Revenues

One interesting aspect of both Medicare and Medicaid is that they had an explosive financial effect on the industry. Medicare and Medicaid were expansive and expensive. Prior to these programs, small hospitals and individual solo physician practices dominated a cottage industry. There was a lot of charity care given by and to health care providers because many patients were very poor and could not afford the care they needed. Passage of the Medicare and Medicaid programs turned health care into a true industry.

All of a sudden (on July 1, 1966), money was plentiful. It was as if a gigantic spigot opened. Dollars gushed, so much so that within six weeks of Medicare's birth Johnson ordered an inquiry into the rising cost of medical care. Figure 4.1 shows the rise of Medicare outlays and beneficiaries from 1967 through 1998, while Figure 4.2 shows the rise of Medicaid outlays and enrollees from 1972 through 1998.

FIGURE 4.1. MEDICARE EXPENDITURES AND ENROLLEES, 1967–1998.

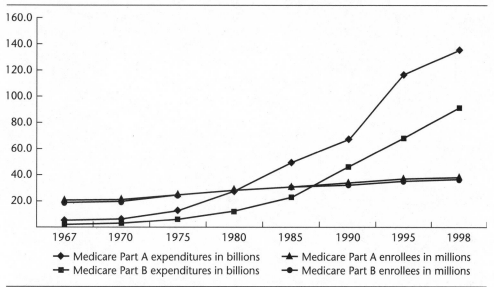

◆ Medicare Part A expenditures in billions ▲ Medicare Part A enrollees in millions
■ Medicare Part B expenditures in billions ● Medicare Part B enrollees in millions

Source: National Center for Health Statistics. *Health, United States, 1996–1997,* tab. 138; *Health, United States, 2000,* tab. 133.

The only constant is a significantly upward slope on the cost lines. Medicare went from paying out just under $5 billion in 1967 to expenditures of $213.4 billion in 1998, a forty-twofold increase over this thirty-one-year time-span (National Center for Health Statistics, 1997). Meanwhile, Medicaid expenditures increased from $6 billion in 1972 to $142.3 billion in 1998 (National Center for Health Statistics, 2000). This is a significant element in why health care is now a $1.2 trillion industry.

In addition, it should be noted that Medicare calls for patients to pay a deductible to the provider of service for the health care rendered. Insurance deductibles are generally developed to discourage usage because these fees are supposed to be paid directly by the consumers of service out of their own pocket. The Medicare hospital deductible is meant to represent the cost of a first-day stay in a hospital. Therefore, to further understand the caliber of hospital cost increases between 1966 and 2001, it is interesting to note that whereas the original inpatient hospital deductible was $40 in 2001 it is $792—a twentyfold increase over thirty-five years (*Federal Register,* Oct. 19, 2000).

Medicare and Medicaid fueled the great expansion of health care inflation in the country. As previously stated in Chapter One, when it was a sleepy industry prior to 1966, health care absorbed just 5.7 percent of the gross domestic product (GDP) in the country. In the intervening thirty-five years, the percentage of GDP

FIGURE 4.2. MEDICAID ENROLLEES AND EXPENDITURES, 1972–1998.

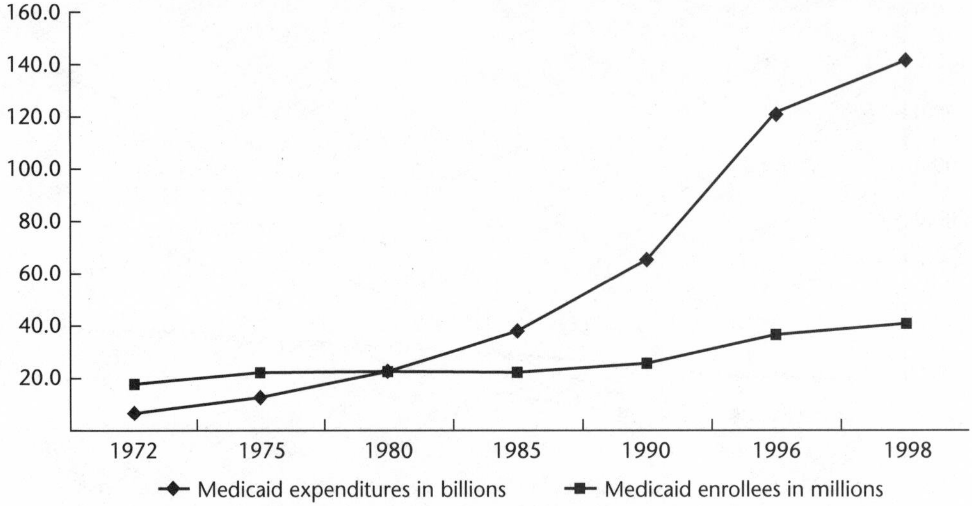

◆ Medicaid expenditures in billions   ■ Medicaid enrollees in millions

Source: National Center for Health Statistics. *Health, United States, 2000,* tab. 136.

has grown to 13.0 percent (http://www.hcfa.gov/stats/nhe-oact/hilites.htm, Mar. 12, 2001), a 228 percent increase. There have been three beneficiaries of this increase:

- Providers, who have been able to expand access to patient care (and make money doing so)
- Patients, most of whom have never had greater access to high-touch, high-tech health care
- The community, which has saved many of its most valuable resources; and its residents, who, because of the increased access to medical care, no longer die prematurely

Implication for Ridgeland Heights Medical Center

RHMC's growth over the past thirty-five years imitates that of Medicare. Once a sleepy community hospital, like many of its competitors RHMC expanded exponentially when Medicare opened up the floodgate of money. Previously, a hospital could not count on full payment for many of its services. Now, Medicare was guaranteeing payment for basic services as well as a whole new set of care. Skilled

FIGURE 4.3. DEATH RATES PER 100,000 RESIDENT POPULATION, AGES 65–74.

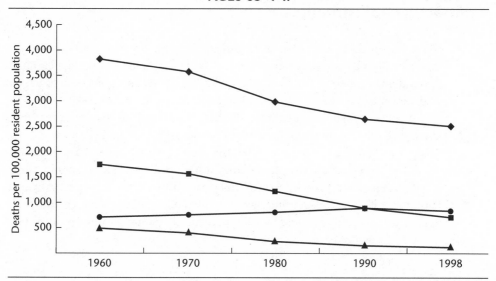

Source: National Center for Health Statistics. *Health, United States, 2000,* tabs. 36–39.

nursing home care for one hundred days and unlimited home health care services would now be reimbursed from a payor with seemingly unlimited resources (Medicare). Medicaid would now guarantee the rest of the skilled nursing home care, after depletion of the patient's financial resources. In either case, the provider of care knew it would be paid.

In the case of physician services, the new revenue streams were enormous. Before Medicare, physicians often wrote off bills for the elderly because these patients could not afford to pay. Even worse, there were many patients who did not want to accept charity and would therefore not present themselves for needed care. They would get sicker and often die. In fact, the advent of Medicare in 1966 had a dramatic and positive effect on the death rate in America. According to government records, the death rate for all causes dropped by 34.7 percent between 1960 and 1998 for all persons aged sixty-five to seventy-four. Figure 4.3 shows declines in the death rates overall as well as for heart disease, cerebrovascular causes (strokes), and malignant neoplasms (cancers).

Interestingly, as the population increased over this time period, and the death rates for some of intransigent diseases declined, the death rate for cancer increased.

Calculation of Medicare and Medicaid Contractual Adjustments

With the advent of Medicare and Medicaid in 1966, hospitals and other health care providers began to do something they had never done before on their financial statement: they recorded contractual adjustments on the income statement and allowances for these contractual adjustments on the balance sheet.

A contractual adjustment is the discount the provider agreed to accept from the insurance company (the third-party payor) for providing health care to that company's beneficiary. Prior to 1966, the most prevalent third-party payor was the Blue Cross plans across the country. Blue Cross offered "indemnity insurance" coverage for its beneficiaries, which meant that Blue Cross generally paid the entire bill that was submitted without discount. Medicare changed the rules. If providers wanted to serve Medicare patients, they were required to accept the payments being offered.

Medicare Net Revenue Concepts

Medicare started off as a cost-based payment system. It agreed to pay the total "cost" of services given to beneficiaries. But there were no caps on these costs originally, so there was an incentive for health care providers to take on new costs and grow their businesses. And they did. Meanwhile, Medicare developed a plethora of reimbursement methodologies for paying for the disparate services that it covered.

Table 4.2 summarizes the many ways that Medicare reimburses, prior to and subsequent to the 1997 Balanced Budget Act (BBA). The biggest change, until 1997–98 and the BBA, was in inpatient reimbursement.

As previously stated, Medicare originally reimbursed all services on cost. But as costs exploded, Medicare quickly moved to put a cap on them—unsuccessfully until 1983, when it adopted a new prospective payment system (PPS) reimbursement methodology for inpatient services. It was called diagnostic-related group (DRG) reimbursement.

DRG reimbursement had a dramatic effect on how the industry operated. It changed the provider's incentive. Prior to DRGs, Medicare reimbursed all of the provider's costs at the percentage of Medicare patient utilization. DRGs reimbursed the provider a fixed price per case, regardless of the cost of providing the care. Therefore providers had to adapt to a new reality, become more cost-conscious, and really begin to understand their cost structure for the first time.

TABLE 4.2. MEDICARE'S PAYMENT METHODOLOGY PRIOR TO AND SUBSEQUENT TO THE 1997 BALANCED BUDGET ACT.

Medicare Covered Service	Payment Method (Prior to 1997 Balanced Budget Act)	Payment Method (Subsequent to 1997 Balanced Budget Act)
Inpatient hospitalization	Diagnostic-related groups (DRGs)	Prospective (1983), diagnostic-related groups (DRGs)
Capital-related costs	Limited cost-based through 2001, quasi-prospective reimbursement	Prospective (2000), 100% federal case rate
Outpatient surgery, radiology, and diagnostic services	Blend of hospital-specific costs and national rates	Prospective (2000), ambulatory payment classifications (APCs)
Physician services	Resource-based relative value scale	Prospective (1992), resource-based relative value scale (RBRVS)
Skilled nursing care	Cost-based with "reasonable cost limits"	Prospective (1998), resource utilization groups (RUGs)
Home health services	Cost-based with per-visit limits	Prospective (2000), home health PPS
Organ transplants	Cost-based	Retrospective, cost-based
Hospice care	Four types of reimbursement depending on service	Mixed, four types of reimbursement depending on service
End-stage renal disease	Per-treatment fee	Prospective (1972), per-treatment fee
Prospective payment systems (PPS) exempt hospitals and units, such as:	Cost-based, but limited to special "target" rates	Retrospective, cost-based, but limited to special "target" rates

- Psychiatric
- Acute rehabilitation (Prospective 1/1/2002)
- Children's hospitals
- Hospitals outside the United States
- Distinct part hospitals

DRGs: How They Work. DRG reimbursement takes approximately 12,500 individual diagnoses available to physicians in the United States (available through the *International Classification of Diseases,* ninth edition, clinically modified for the United States—also known as the ICD-9-CM codes) and looks at whether surgery was associated with the case. It also takes into account the patient's age, sex, and whether or not there were additional complications or comorbidities. Then, through use of a computer program, called a grouper, all of these data are crunched to determine which one of five hundred or so DRGs the patient belongs to.

Interestingly, the DRG was not originally developed to be used as a reimbursement tool for the Medicare program. It was developed by researchers at Yale University and Yale–New Haven Hospital in the mid-1970s to facilitate clinical analysis. All of the ICD-9-CM codes that fall into each individual DRG are supposed to use approximately the same amount of resources. They are supposed to act similarly. But in actuality, many DRGs are not homogeneous and therefore the average price assigned to a DRG by the Medicare program creates problems for the provider.

Still, as we have now seen, the feds were looking for a way to contain total Medicare reimbursement for inpatient services and move away from cost-based reimbursement. Ultimately, they selected the DRG methodology and established pricing equivalents for each of them. As we can see from Figure 4.1, this does not appear to have been successful in containing costs.

Under the PPS, case weights are assigned to each DRG. These case weights are then multiplied by the individual hospital's base rate, to determine each DRG price for each hospital. It does not matter what the hospital charged for all of the services rendered during the patient's stay; if the patient was a Medicare beneficiary, the hospital is paid only the DRG rate. The difference between the gross charges (hospital prices) and the DRG payment (Medicare reimbursement) is recorded as a contractual adjustment on the income statement and as a Medicare contractual allowance (discount) to accounts receivable on the balance sheet.

For example, assume that RHMC had a base rate of $4,000. Mary Smith, the patient, generated gross charges of $10,000 for her stay in the hospital. The DRG for her stay had a case weight of 1.5. Therefore, RHMC expects to be paid $6,000 (1.5 × $4,000) for her stay. Medicare will pay 100 percent of this DRG amount to RHMC minus Smith's annual deductible of $792.

The accounting debits and credits for this case are represented as follows.

| Dr. | Accounts receivable (balance sheet) | $10,000 |
| Cr. | Various gross charges (income statement) | $10,000 |

To post the various gross charges as the fee for services rendered to the patient

| Dr. | Contractual adjustment (income statement) | $4,000 |
| Cr. | Contractual allowance (balance sheet) | $4,000 |

To record write-down of Mary Smith's account to reflect the expected reimbursement, *at the time of billing* (continued on next page)

Dr.	Cash—received from Medicare	$5,208
Dr.	Cash—received from Mary Smith (patient)	$792
Cr.	Accounts receivable—Mary Smith	$6,000

Record cash received from Medicare and the patient to zero out the patient's account.

APCs and How They Work. After viewing and reviewing the positive financial outcomes of the DRG system for inpatient acute hospitalization, Congress mandated that outpatient hospitalization also be brought under a prospective payment system. The federal government, through the 1997 BBA, determined that an Outpatient Prospective Payment System (OPPS) would go into effect on October 1, 1998. Although neither that date nor a series of subsequent "live" dates were met, the OPPS did become effective August 1, 2000.

HCFA determined that the prospective payment methodology that would be used to reimburse hospitals was the Ambulatory Payment Classification (APC) system. It was a dramatic departure from the prior cost-based system of reimbursement, and it caused a big change in how hospitals had to register, charge, code, and bill for Medicare outpatient services.

The APC categorizes outpatient procedure codes into clinically and financially homogeneous groups. To do this, the system uses outpatient procedure, visit, and supply codes taken from the HCFA's Common Procedure Systems (HCPCS) and the Physician's Common Procedure Terminology (CPT-4) coding schemes. Each APC is assigned a fixed payment amount for the facility fee or technical component of a patient's visit. The provider of service receives the amount of this APC as payment in full, after it is adjusted for the hospital's wage index.

There are some exceptions to the outpatient services that are assigned APCs. These exceptions generally involve outpatient services that were already being reimbursed on either a fee schedule or some other prospectively determined rate satisfactory to the government. APC-excluded services include the following:

- Ambulance services
- Physical and occupational therapy
- Speech language pathology services
- Renal dialysis services paid under a composite rate
- Laboratory services paid under the clinical diagnostic laboratory fee schedule
- Nonimplantable durable medical equipment and prosthetics
- Services and procedures that require inpatient care

To create a uniform and homogeneous set of APCs, the system needed to create a large number of APCs. When the system was turned on in August 2000,

TABLE 4.3. SUMMARY OF APC TYPES, AUG. 1, 2000.

Payment Service Indicator	Type of Service	Total Number of APCs	Service Examples
G	Current drug or biological agents paid under the transitional pass-through	352	New drugs or biologic agents whose costs are significant in relation to APC payment amounts
H	Device paid under the transitional pass-through	15	New medical devices whose costs are significant in relation to APC payment amounts
J	New drug or device paid under the transitional pass-through		Drugs or devices determined to be eligible for APC payments after August 1, 2000
P	Services that are paid only in partial hospitalization program	2	Psychiatric outpatient day treatment programs
S	Outpatient significant procedures not subject to multiple procedure discounting if procedure is performed on the same day	89	CT scans, MRIs, other major diagnostic services
T	Outpatient significant procedures eligible for 50 percent multiple procedure discounting	149	Most traditional ambulatory surgery
V	Medical visits for which payment is allowed	8	Emergency department and clinic visits
X	Ancillary services	47	Radiology tests, EKGs, pulmonary tests
	Total	662	

there were 662 of them arrayed across eight major categories. Table 4.3 is a summary of the APCs that appear in each category.

Each APC is assigned a weight by the government. This weight is then multiplied by the national APC payment rate and hospital-specific wage index to determine the provider's reimbursement for the services rendered or supplies dispensed. For the year 2000, the unadjusted rate was $48.47. The rate increased to $50.24 on April 1, 2001, thanks to adjustments legislated by the Benefits Improvement and Protection Act (BIPA) of 2000. There are several other nuances to the APC rules, but this summary is a starting point from which to understand its complexities. Providers needed to take dramatic steps to minimize possible reimbursement losses under APCs, particularly through poor operational procedures and processes. A terrific and readable guide to APC operational improvement processes is *Understanding and Managing Under APCs* by Julie Micheletti (2001).

From the contractual adjustment prospective, APCs work like DRGs. The amount of reimbursement expected by the provider must be subtracted from the gross price generated on the charge description master to write down the posted charges to realizable value. As we have already seen in this chapter, DRGs and APCs are just one of many payment methods that may be used to reimburse health care providers. Medicare has several other methodologies for various types of providers (see Table 4.2).

Medicaid, which is a state-run program, allows each state to determine the payment method to providers and uses many methods according to patient type (inpatient, outpatient, physician, home health, skilled nursing care, and so on). Managed care payors also use a variety of payment methods when determining the provider's net revenues. Still, the concept of contractual adjustment remains the same. Once you know and understand that there are various reimbursement methods, it is simple to prepare contractual allowances monthly for the financial statements. We examine the various types of managed care reimbursement later in this chapter.

Medicaid Net Revenue Concepts

Over the years, Medicare has received considerably more press than Medicaid. This is primarily because Medicare is a national program administered with mostly consistent rules across the United States, affecting a politically astute constituency, the elderly, who have been known to vote politicians in or out of office. Medicaid, in contrast, is a national program but controlled and administered by the fifty states in widely differing ways. Although the federal government mandates the specific entitlements that each and every state must give to Medicaid recipients, the states are allowed to determine the socioeconomic level of their residents who will be eligible. Because Medicaid is a program designed for the poor, beneficiaries are generally disenfranchised to a greater extent than politically connected Medicare beneficiaries.

Medicaid differs considerably from Medicare in its required benefits and level of payment to the provider. Because it is state-administered and state-financed, the states are continuously struggling to balance the level of provider payment with their own budget constraints. In fact, in the past states struggled with federally inspired "unfunded mandates," which require specific entitlements to be included in the Medicaid program but do not include any new money coming from Washington.

FIGURE 4.4. MEDICAID RECIPIENTS, PERCENTAGE BY CATEGORY, 1972–1998.

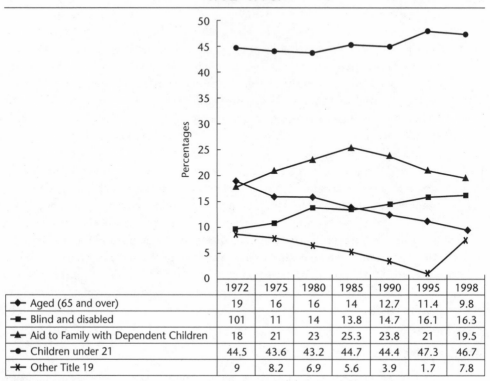

	1972	1975	1980	1985	1990	1995	1998
◆ Aged (65 and over)	19	16	16	14	12.7	11.4	9.8
■ Blind and disabled	101	11	14	13.8	14.7	16.1	16.3
▲ Aid to Family with Dependent Children	18	21	23	25.3	23.8	21	19.5
● Children under 21	44.5	43.6	43.2	44.7	44.4	47.3	46.7
✳ Other Title 19	9	8.2	6.9	5.6	3.9	1.7	7.8

Source: National Center for Health Statistics, *Health, United States, 2000,* tab. 136.

There is one particularly surprising revelation in the Medicaid program that is not generally reported. Figure 4.4 shows the twenty-seven-year trend of Medicaid recipients according to eligibility type as a percentage of the total (1972–1998). In addition, Figure 4.5 isolates the 1998 year and compares and contrasts recipients as a percentage of total versus recipient payments. As can be seen, in 1998 patients sixty-five years of age or older made up only 9.8 percent of total Medicaid beneficiaries. Yet they accounted for 28.5 percent of total Medicaid expenditures.

The primary reason for this is that though Medicare pays for only the first one hundred days in a skilled nursing facility, Medicaid pays for any unlimited stay that is deemed medically necessary. It is often the case that someone of Medicare age, when finally requiring chronic care in an SNF, exhausts the assets accumulated throughout a lifetime after Medicare pays for the first hundred days. The individual then becomes Medicaid-eligible. Because the chronic illnesses treated in

FIGURE 4.5. 1998 MEDICAID RECIPIENTS AND PAYMENTS
AS A PERCENTAGE OF TOTAL, BY BASIS OF ELIGIBILITY.

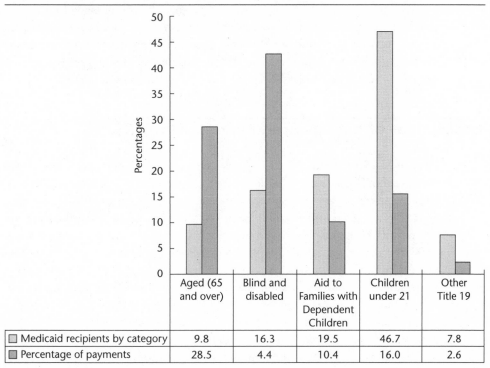

	Aged (65 and over)	Blind and disabled	Aid to Families with Dependent Children	Children under 21	Other Title 19
☐ Medicaid recipients by category	9.8	16.3	19.5	46.7	7.8
☐ Percentage of payments	28.5	4.4	10.4	16.0	2.6

Source: National Center for Health Statistics, *Health, United States, 2000,* tab. 136.

an SNF are often costly and may very well last until death, Medicaid has become the largest individual line item in the budget of almost every state, averaging more than 15 percent of the total. By contrast, children under the age of twenty-one, who make up 46.7 percent of Medicaid-eligible recipients, account for only 16.0 percent of Medicaid expenditures (National Center for Health Statistics, 2000).

In any event, Medicaid programs around the country have been notorious in underpaying for the services rendered to their beneficiaries. Providers have had to scramble to make up the net revenue shortfall engendered by providing services to Medicaid patients. The hospitals and physicians particularly affected are generally located in inner-city and rural areas, where economically challenged citizens live. These hospitals may have a Medicaid payor mix approaching 40 to 60 percent. Added to their Medicare payor mix, which could average 30 to 40 percent, they often suffer in maintaining operating margins that would allow for capital replacement or expansion, paying properly to maintain their workforce.

In some cases, they may even have to close their doors, thus complicating access to health care in their community.

RHMC, on the other hand, is in the enviable position of being located in a socioeconomically advantaged area. Its Medicaid payor mix is only 6 percent, and it has been able to offset Medicaid shortfalls relatively easily; thus the expected net revenues from Medicaid and the ensuing contractual adjustments do not have a major detrimental effect on the organization's bottom line.

Implications of the Balanced Budget Act of 1997

Despite Medicare's attempt to reign in payment to providers, particularly with the advent of DRGs in 1983, it was deemed unsuccessful. The continuing upward spiral of provider payments was having a detrimental impact on the Part A trust fund. Remember that the fund is financed through a Social Security (Medicare tax) payment from employers and employees. It turns out that between 1966 and 1996, the Part A trust fund accumulated an excess of almost $120 billion. This was net inflow from workers minus net outflow to providers. Still, Medicare prognosticators actuarially estimated that the trust fund would be depleted within five years.

The problem was not particularly on the inflow side. It was estimated that the Medicare trust fund would continue to take in as much in ensuing years as before. It was clear, however, that the outflows were about to dramatically increase because of perception of alleged provider fraud and abuse, increasing health care options available to Medicare beneficiaries, and improving benefits for staying healthy (Balanced Budget Act of 1997, http://www.hcfa.gov/init/bba/bbaintro.htm).

In addition, there was great concern over growth in the population over sixty-five, characterized by the march of the baby boomers approaching the age of Medicare eligibility. Consequently, members of Congress came together to pass the most dramatic piece of health legislation since the inception of Medicare in 1966. Called the Balanced Budget Act (BBA) of 1997, it changed the way Medicare reimbursed for all the services provided to its beneficiaries. This included outpatient services, home health care, skilled nursing care, hospice, graduate medical education, rural providers, and physicians. The BBA also changed some of the reimbursement concepts within the Medicaid program.

The legislation was designed to save the Part A trust fund $116.4 billion over the five-year period of October 1, 1997, to September 30, 2002. Savings were expected to be generated in certain areas:

Hospitals	$ 44.1 billion
Skilled nursing facilities	$ 16.2 billion
Home health agencies	$ 9.5 billion
Beneficiary premium increases	$ 13.7 billion
Medicare+Choice	$ 18.5 billion
Physician services	$ 5.3 billion
All other	$ 9.1 billion
Total BBA savings	$116.4 billion

The initial savings generated in the very first year (calendar year 1998) had a significant impact. There were three big changes:

1. *Zero increase in the annual update factor.* In 1983, at the advent of the DRG system, Medicare promised to update each provider's base rate by an inflation factor predicated on a market basket of health care goods and services. However, over the years Medicare generally allowed an increase in the market basket of hospital goods and services *minus* about 1 percent. At the birth of the BBA, to produce the needed savings Congress further determined that there would be no increase in the annual update factor for the 1998 fiscal year. Future updates in fiscal years 1999, 2000, and 2001 were to be at the market basket minus 1.8 percent, 1.1 percent, and 1.1 percent, respectively.

2. *Correction of a formula-driven overpayment.* This item, included in the BBA, is a correction of a calculation error. Expected to save more than $2 billion alone, it was instituted immediately, on October 1, 1997, and reduced provider payment proportionately.

3. *Change in home health services reimbursement.* The BBA represented a significant change to the cost-based reimbursement system that existed for home health services for so many years. Although Congress ultimately wanted home health services for Medicare beneficiaries to be reimbursed on a prospective system by fiscal year 2000, it created an interim payment system (IPS) as of fiscal year 1998 to begin capturing savings immediately.

Keep in mind that government figures show that of the 2.4 million home health patients in 1996, 73.0 percent are sixty-five years of age or older (National Center for Health Statistics, 2000). Providers are therefore receiving a majority of their home health service reimbursement from the payor that cut their payments 15 to 20 percent. In addition, the IPS puts new restrictions on the number of visits

FIGURE 4.6. PERCENTAGE CHANGE IN HEALTH CARE INDUSTRY REVENUES BETWEEN 1997 AND 1998.

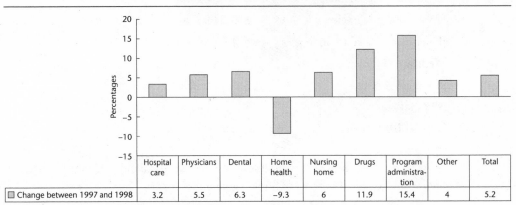

	Hospital care	Physicians	Dental	Home health	Nursing home	Drugs	Program administration	Other	Total
Change between 1997 and 1998	3.2	5.5	6.3	−9.3	6	11.9	15.4	4	5.2

Source: National Center for Health Statistics, *Health, United States, 2000,* tab. 118.

Medicare reimburses and a new cost limit per beneficiary. The combined effect of these reductions significantly hurt both the free-standing and the hospital-based programs through closure of more than 750 home health programs in the first nine months of the IPS.

The devastation of the home health service sector of the industry was evident. As can be seen in Figure 4.6, between 1997 and 1998 alone the home health agency segment of the industry lost more than 9 percent of its revenue, while the hospital industry experienced a paltry 3.2 percent increase. Congress took notice; between early 1999 and late 2000 it passed two major bills, which were signed by the president, designed to reinstate some of the more onerous cutbacks engendered in the 1997 BBA.

Balanced Budget Refinement Act of 1999 (BBRA)

The first of the reinstatement acts was known as the Balanced Budget Refinement Act of 1999. It was designed to restore approximately $11.9 billion over five years to hospitals, health systems, and other providers that had been cut in the BBA. In addition, the Medicare+Choice payors had $4 billion restored. Still, some of the restoration was just a freeze in additional cuts that were scheduled to take effect during fiscal years 2000–2002. A small measure of relief was granted for skilled nursing facility and therapy services, home health services, and some hospital inpatient services, such as a delay in cuts for indirect medical education scheduled for 2000. Here is an analysis of the act in this context:

Hospital outpatient	$6.1 billion
Skilled nursing facilities	$2.7 billion
Home health care	$1.3 billion
Rural hospitals	$800 million
Teaching hospitals	$600 million
PPS exempt hospitals	$300 million
Disproportionate-share hospitals	$100 million
BBRA total	$11.9 billion

Still, the biggest relief that was granted in the BBRA was the significant amount of additional funding assigned by Medicare to what was then the upcoming APC program. In its initial representations to the hospital industry, Medicare budgeted an average *5.7 percent loss* for outpatient reimbursements affected by the Outpatient Prospective Payment System. With the dollar amount assigned under the BBRA, the government now stated that rather than a loss, each hospital would earn an average of 4.6 percent on the APC program. The mechanism for this increase was a transitional payment system that reimbursed hospitals in addition to their OPPS payments during the first three years of the PPS, if their payments were less than their pre-PPS payments in 1996 (determined according to formula). These payments did begin a process of relief that helped many hospitals and other health service providers start a financial rebuilding process.

Benefits Improvement and Protection Act of 2000 (BIPA)

After the passage of the Balanced Budget Refinement Act, the industry immediately began a further lobbying campaign to restore additional cuts that had been made in the original Balanced Budget Act. Restoration of $11.9 billion was not considered to be sufficient. Thus, beginning in early 2000, a variety of provider-based advocacy groups carried on further lobbying in the halls of Congress. They pointed out to lawmakers that the industry had still absorbed more cuts than were originally intended and further relief was needed. The end result was passage, late in 2000, of the Benefits Improvement and Protection Act of 2000 (BIPA.)

This act had a continuing positive impact on improving revenues for health care providers. It was worth an estimated $11.55 billion to providers over five years as well $11 billion to Medicare+Choice payors. There were several areas of relief for the providers:

- Restoration of the full market basket index for hospital inpatients for fiscal year 2001 (October 1, 2000–September 30, 2001). The return of the 1.1 percent reduction in FY 2001 (from 2.3 percent under BBA to 3.4 under BIPA), along with a reduction of the market basket of *only* 0.55 percent in FY 2002 and 2003, returned $3.7 billion to hospital providers.
- Restoration of the full market basket for hospital outpatients for fiscal year 2001 of 1.0 percent (from 2.4 percent to 3.4 percent), which was worth $1.1 billion over five years.
- Increase of the indirect medical education adjustment back to 6.5 percent. This is worth $1.0 billion over five years.

There are several other adjustments in the BIPA law, the entire impact of which can be seen in this list:

Financial Analysis of the BIPA of 2000

Hospital inpatient	$3.70 billion
Hospital outpatient	$1.10 billion
Medicaid disproportionate-share hospitals	$1.45 billion
Medicare disproportionate-share hospitals	$1.25 billion
Teaching hospitals	$1.00 billion
Medicare bad-debt increase	$700 million
Home health care	$680 million
Rural hospitals	$630 million
Long-term care hospitals	$300 million
Skilled nursing facilities	$350 million
Rehabilitation hospitals	$200 million
Hospice	$130 million
Psychiatric and mental health hospitals	$300 million
Increased renal dialysis composite rate	$50 million
BBRA total	$11.55 billion

In general, however, the impact of both BBRA and BIPA was to restore confidence to many providers and provider types in 2001.

Impact of the Balanced Budget Act on Medicaid

The BBA also had some effect on Medicaid reimbursement. Although not as extensive as the Medicare impact, there are a few changes worth noting. The most interesting was the decision by Congress to repeal the Boren Amendment to Medicaid administrative rules, which required state Medicaid programs to reimburse providers at a "reasonable and adequate" rate. During the early and middle years of the 1990s, SNFs and hospitals had used the Boren Amendment to successfully sue states for higher Medicaid fees.

The SNFs had the most at stake because Medicaid paid for almost 50 percent of all SNF care in 1995, while it paid for only 15 percent of hospital costs in the same year. As was previously mentioned in this chapter, Medicaid has traditionally underpaid for services rendered to its beneficiaries, and in the 1990s the Boren Amendment was the only tool that providers had to rectify the situation.

Some other changes that the BBA made to Medicaid include clauses to pay providers at the lower Medicaid rate when patients have dual eligibility for Medicare and Medicaid and expansion of Medicaid eligibility and benefits. Finally, there was an increase of $4 billion to extend health coverage to five million low-income, uninsured children. Under this program, formally known as the State Children's Health Insurance Program and dubbed by some "KiddieCare," the states were granted significant discretion in how to spend this money. In fact, since inception of the program in late 1997, there have been improvements in Medicaid coverage for children under twenty-one. The Kaiser Commission on Medicaid and the Uninsured released a report in February 2001 to explain the reasons for a 1.8 million drop in the number of uninsured nonelderly Americans in 1999. It found that increasing public health insurance coverage acted in concert with expanding employer-sponsored insurance coverage to bring about the reduction. In addition, stabilizing Medicaid enrollment and implementation of the State Children's Health Insurance Program played a large role (http://www.kff.org/content/2001/2229/).

Overall Impact of the Balanced Budget Act on RHMC

Most providers throughout the industry initially felt the pressure of lowered operating margins caused by lower BBA-generated Medicare reimbursement. A *Modern Healthcare* article reported that 1998 was shaping up as the first time in the thirty-two-year history of Medicare that the outflow to providers would be less than that of the previous year (Weissenstein, 1998). As expected, the Medicare payment reduction was affecting all providers, but particularly those with a high

Medicare payor mix of patients. In addition, it was having a compounded negative effect on those organizations that provided inpatient and outpatient services,
home health services, skilled nursing care, and physician services.

Ridgeland Heights was just such a provider. It had been able to beat its 4 percent budgeted operating margin for a number of years with some ease, given its
location and favorable payor and service mix. Yet the 1998 budget year was the
beginning of a three-year downward spiral in operating margin, induced in part
by the BBA. For the 1998 budget year, the administration recommended to the
board that the operating margin be cut to 3 percent (a reduction from the prior
year of only a single percentage point but a reduction of 25 percent from the previous year's 4 percent budgeted target—1 percent divided by 4 percent equals 25
percent) to account for expected BBA revenue reductions. The organization's financial analyst estimated that the reduction from Medicare cuts alone would be
more than $1 million in the first year. This was just over 1 percent of operating
margin. In addition, the administration was not able to devise expense reductions
on the short notice given by the federal government for the 1998 budget year.

In the three years following inception of the BBA, RHMC experienced declining profitably that was mirrored throughout the industry. Many providers
were unable to effectively adapt new strategies to offset some of the revenue decreases associated with the act. To maintain or increase the bottom line during
the Medicare BBA era, providers needed to do the following:

- Develop new programs
- Initiate new services within existing programs
- Adjust their payor mix
- Adjust their case mix
- Cut their expenses

Yet most not-for-profit providers were unable to implement many of these
items. In fact, in early December 2000 the American Hospital Association reported that nearly half the nation's hospitals did not make enough money in 1999
to maintain operations and stay competitive. The AHA reported that the aggregate hospital profit margin sank to 4.7 percent, its lowest level since 1994. The report, *Hospital Statistics 2001,* stated that 48.6 percent of hospitals reported profit
margins of less than 3 percent, which compared with 42.2 percent reporting
profits below that threshold in 1998. Finally, 32.1 percent of hospitals lost money
in 1999, compared with 26.6 percent that were in the red in 1998.

The medical center attempted to initiate a series of steps to return profitability to the board-mandated 4 percent. It will be aided by additional reimburse-

ments to be received thanks to BBRA and BIPA. We review the budget steps in detail starting in Chapter Six, when RHMC kicks off its annual budgeting process.

Managed Care Net Revenue Concepts

Medicare and Medicaid shortfalls from the BBA were not the only thing affecting the bottom line of many health care entities. The continuing rise of managed care in America was having negative financial consequences for many providers. Managed care is generally defined as a range of utilization and reimbursement techniques designed to limit costs while ensuring quality of care. To reduce costs, a managed care plan must focus on price, volume, and intensity of service. These cost reduction techniques (noted in Chapter One) have played havoc with the operating margin of many a health care provider.

Health insurance of the managed care type has overwhelmed and overtaken the traditional indemnity plan that was the primary form of health insurance in this country over the past fifty years. Although managed care has been around almost as long, it was mostly confined to the Kaiser plans in the western United States. Throughout the rest of the country, insurance companies were paying providers close to or at 100 percent of their submitted charges. However, as stated in Chapter One, these charges by providers and payments by the insurance companies were having a detrimental effect on the real health care payors: employers. In the late 1980s, employers revolted against the continuing rise of health insurance premiums and switched to managed care plans. The results, as seen in Figure 4.7, were dramatic. Managed care plans came from almost nowhere in 1976 to give coverage for over eighty million Americans by 1999.

The managed care plan has a variety of methods for reimbursing the providers servicing the plan's enrollees:

Methods for Managed Care Company Reimbursement of Hospitals

- Per diem (defined dollar amount per day; most common method)
- Percentage of charges (second-most-common method)
- Charges (not common)
- Diagnosis-related groups (DRGs)
- Medicare plus *x* percent
- Carveout of various services
- Case rate
- Bundles for hospital and physician services
- Bed leasing

FIGURE 4.7. GROWTH OF MANAGED CARE IN AMERICA, 1976–1999.

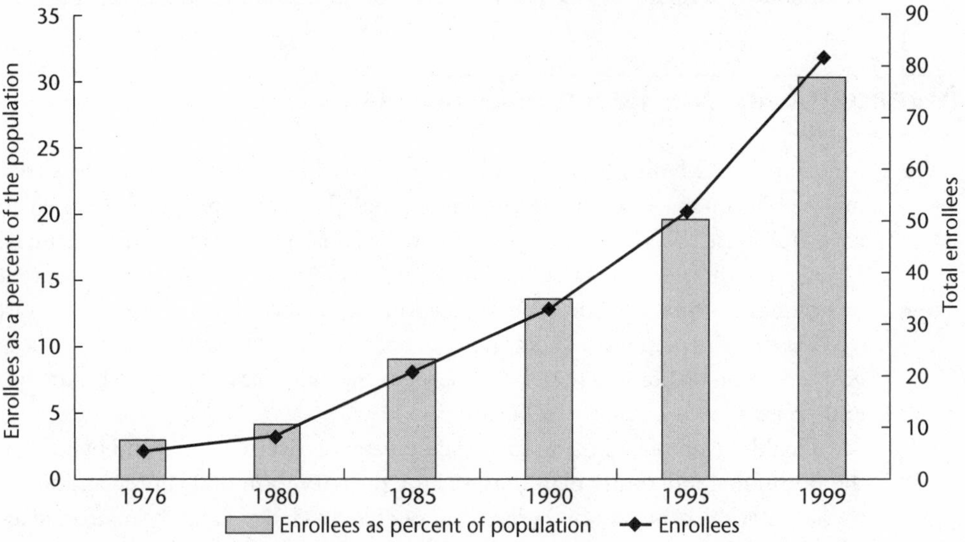

Source: National Center for Health Statistics, *Health, United States, 2000,* tab. 131.

- Capitation
- Periodic interim payment or cash advance (cash flow implications only)
- Penalties and withholding, to create incentives for shorter stay or lower level of care
- Ambulatory payment classifications (APCs) and ambulatory patient groups (APGs) for outpatient care

Methods for Managed Care Company Reimbursement of Physicians

- Capitation (most common method for primary care physicians), including withholds, penalties, and bonuses
- Fee schedule by CPT code (most common method for specialty physicians)
- Charges (not common)
- Percentage of charges
- Medicare plus *x* percent
- Carveout
- Retainer
- Salary

- Hourly rate
- Global fee
- Bundled case rate
- Outpatient and professional DRGs or ambulatory patient group
- Modifying reimbursement on the basis of performance (quality measures, patient satisfaction measures)

In every case, reimbursement for services is less than what the providers received previously.

Not only do managed care companies have all of these ways to reimburse providers, but the providers could contract with dozens of managed care companies during any given year. This means that the provider, whether a hospital, a physician, a home health agency, or an SNF, needs a mechanism or tool to keep track of the type of deal being signed. Otherwise, it cannot prepare monthly financial statements that include managed care contractual adjustments.

Providers have had to make significant adjustments in operating structure to accommodate the decreased reimbursements from MCOs. Because an MCO offers less expensive premiums to its subscribers, it must procure services from a provider at less expense. So it negotiates a contract with a provider offering payments. At the same time, the MCO offers a plan to subscribers (beneficiaries) that generally limits the benefits. A plan of this sort generally comes in three flavors:

1. *HMO plans.* This is a formally organized health care system that combines delivery and financing functions. The fixed monthly premiums paid to the HMO are generally lower than those for a traditional indemnity plan. In return for these lower premiums, the members of the plan must use the providers stipulated by the plan in the plan's network. It is a limited-choice plan for members, requiring that a primary care physician (PCP) be the gatekeeper for all other specialty services.

2. *PPO plans.* This is a health care financing and delivery program that creates a financial incentive to the consumer to use a select panel of preferred providers. The difference between an HMO and a PPO is not always significant. The HMO absolutely locks the member into using its panel of providers, but PPO members are more likely to be steered to use the PCP that they select at their initial visit through lower deductibles and copayments. The PPO also often has a clause allowing the member to use specialist providers outside the preferred panel. When this occurs, the member has to pay additional fees for the services.

3. *Point-of-service plans.* Also called an open-access product, here the members (enrollees) are permitted to choose a provider outside the main panel, without

referral from a PCP. In fact, most POS plans do not even require the member to sign up with a PCP. Coverage is offered under a financing mechanism similar to traditional indemnity and is available any time service is desired. Benefits for services received outside the HMO network are typically less comprehensive than HMO benefits, are significantly more expensive than the HMO managed care product, and include a deductible or copayment.

The original managed care model was the HMO type of plan. In the early 1990s, the PPO plan appeared as employers were looking for some additional choice in health insurance options for their employees. The POS plan was offered in the mid-1990s; it accelerated in the late 1990s as employees began complaining about the lack of choice offered in provider panel plans. The most interesting aspect of this movement to POS is that it looks, feels, and operates much like the traditional indemnity plan that employers rejected in the early 1990s because of the high price of the premium.

It is a simple equation: *the greater the choice, the higher the insurance premium. The more limited the choice, the lower the insurance premium.*

Still, the biggest difference between POS and indemnity is that under POS the provider no longer receives charges as a payment. Instead, some kind of negotiated discount has been agreed to by provider and payor.

Finally, at the dawn on the twenty-first century, many employers offer all three types of plan to their employees, leaving it to them to choose the type they want, and the amount of premium the employee is willing to pay.

Regardless of the type of plan offered, the provider has to determine the final payment for the services rendered and record the difference as a contractual adjustment. The total contractual adjustment applied to the monthly gross charges gives the provider a clear idea if it is doing a good or bad job of negotiating contracts with the various managed care organizations with whom it does business. For example, suppose that an analysis of managed care contractual adjustments looks like this:

For Years Ended 1999 and 2000, Respectively

Managed care contractual adjustments	$ 28,000,000	$ 33,000,000
Total gross revenues	$143,000,000	154,000,000
Managed care contractual adjustments as a percentage of total gross revenues	19.6 percent	21.4 percent

Providers can learn a lot about themselves by performing appropriate analysis of their managed care payor mix. For example, in this summary data set, the managed care contractual adjustment increased by 1.8 percentage points. On first impression, this seems like a small amount. Yet the percentage increase between years is actually 9.2 percent (1.8 divided by 19.6). This is, in fact, a substantial increase between years, and it negatively affects the bottom line by $2,816,000 ($33,000,000 minus $30,184,000, the latter amount being the managed care contractual adjustment that the organization would have discounted if it had been able to maintain a 19.6 percent contractual adjustment percentage).

Clearly, there are many steps that the organization can take to analyze this increase. The ultimate purpose of the analysis is to make an informed decision on the need for the organization to meet its changing revenue streams. Some questions that could be asked:

- Was the change in contractual percentage a result of a change in the mix of MCOs with which we contract?
- Was the change a result of poor inpatient utilization of services? For example, did the length of stay increase beyond the budget?
- Was there a change in the mix of inpatient and outpatient utilization of services beyond what was projected?
- Are we, as an organization, being paid appropriately by the MCOs? Have they properly performed their own contract analysis?

Providers may be contracting with two MCOs or two hundred. This usually depends on the level of managed care penetration in a particular geographic region. The greater the penetration, the more sophisticated the provider must be to be able to negotiate, bill, collect, and analyze the various contracts. Most providers have found that they need an automated system into which they can load the terms of contracts to get accurate and timely information on the net revenue expected to be generated per case, whether it be inpatient or outpatient.

These various automated systems, usually called contract payment analyzers or contract management systems, may be attached to the organization's main computerized billing system or freestanding and interfaced with the billing system. The output from these systems is the primary source for posting managed care contractual adjustments. The difference between gross charges and contractual adjustments becomes the posted net revenue for all the managed care accounts. These systems also allow the provider to determine if the managed care company has made accurate and timely payment of the net amount expected.

Preparation of the Medicare and Medicaid Cost Report

The Medicare and Medicaid cost report is the primary means for the federal government to monitor hospital costs. The following section highlights the major issues surrounding this report.

Who, Why, and How?

For a hospital fiscal year ending in December, April is the month when processing of the Medicare and Medicaid cost report heats up. HCFA rules require that the cost report be filed with the fiscal intermediary within 150 days of the end of the fiscal year. The purpose of the cost report is to allow Medicare to properly pay for outpatients, SNFs, and other specialty care services rendered by health care providers to Medicare beneficiaries.

Filing the cost report has been required since the beginning of the Medicare program in 1966. It was particularly necessary because back then Medicare reimbursed all of its services at cost. This remained true until 1983, when Medicare changed its reimbursement for inpatient services from a retrospective cost-based methodology to the fixed prospective payment of DRGs. The cost report continued being required in 1983 because reimbursement for all of the other hospital services was still at cost. The only way to determine the cost apportionment for these services was to continue preparing the cost report. The big difference was that a year-end payable or receivable for inpatient services no longer applied. Another major change occurred in 2000, when outpatient reimbursement was converted from cost-based to prospective reimbursement.

The Medicare cost report is designed in a reasonably logical way to allow the preparer (provider) and the payor (Medicare) to understand the development of each year's report. Table 4.4 shows the various major elements of the cost report. Each element assists in progress toward understanding an organization's Medicare cost.

The Medicare cost report has had a significant impact on the health care industry. Medicare mandated provider preparation of the cost report to determine its required settlements, but the cost report and its costing methodology became a de facto standard for cost accounting in the industry. Before 1966 and the advent of Medicare, most of the industry had no need for any type of cost accounting system, sophisticated or not. Most hospitals were small, and much of their revenue was generated from a small set of charges and a lot of donations. Medicare and Medicaid reimbursement ushered in the era of health care as a business nationally. Consequently, the Medicare cost report primarily required that hos-

TABLE 4.4. MEDICARE AND MEDICAID COST REPORT, MAJOR ELEMENTS, AND INDEX OF WORKSHEETS.

Worksheet	Purpose
A	Determine Medicare allowable costs
B	Step-down costs of nonrevenue (overhead) departments to revenue-producing departments
B-1	Statistics used to allocate overhead department costs
C	Determination of the ratio of costs to charges (RCC) used on worksheet D to develop Medicare's proportionate cost
D	Determination of Medicare's total portion of provider's cost (including pass-through items, TEFRA limits, outpatient ancillary costs)
E	Determination of Medicare's "final settlement" with the provider
F	Calculation of return on equity capital (for-profit providers only)
G	Presentation of the provider's audited financial statements
H	Determination of hospital-based home health agency "final settlement"
I	Determination of hospital-based renal dialysis costs
K	Determination of hospital-based hospice costs
L	Calculation of final capital payments
S	General information, including wage rates used to determine regional wage indices

pitals use a specific type of cost-finding technique called *step-down*. The very name is representative of how the technique looks. (It is interesting to note that cost reports using the step-down allocation methodology were developed by New York Blue Cross in its contracting with providers in the 1950s and later adopted by Medicare in 1966.)

The step-down method of cost finding organizes the health care facility's costs so that overhead expenses are properly allocated to revenue-producing cost centers. Those departments that most likely have costs (overhead) related to the other are allocated (or closed) earlier than others. The allocation is based on statistics that have been refined over the years to permit the best apportionment of overhead.

Table 4.5 displays the step-down methodology. As can be seen, the actual step-down (worksheet B in Medicare parlance) looks like a descending staircase

TABLE 4.5. RHMC STEP-DOWN COSTS FOR
THE TWELVE MONTHS ENDED DEC. 31, 2000.

Cost (and Allocation Methodology)	Salaries	Non-salaries	Total	Depreciation, Building (Square Feet)	Depreciation, Equipment (Dollar Value)
Depreciation, buildings		2,500,000	2,500,000	2,500,000	
Depreciation, equipment		2,000,000	2,000,000		2,000,000
Employee fringe benefits		3,243,000	3,243,000		20,000
Administration and general	1,500,000	2,500,000	4,000,000	200,000	20,000
Maintenance and repairs	200,000	400,000	600,000	125,000	50,000
Operation of plant	400,000	300,000	700,000	50,000	100,000
Laundry and linen	200,000	500,000	700,000	50,000	20,000
Environmental services	300,000	200,000	500,000	50,000	30,000
Medical records	200,000	150,000	350,000	25,000	15,000
Total, nonrevenue departments	2,800,000	11,793,000	14,593,000	500,000	255,000
Inpatient medical/ surgical nursing	3,500,000	500,000	4,000,000	500,000	50,000
Inpatient intensive care nursing	2,000,000	400,000	2,400,000	150,000	100,000
Skilled nursing facility	500,000	100,000	600,000	150,000	20,000
Operating and recovery rooms	900,000	800,000	1,700,000	200,000	200,000
Anesthesia	300,000	300,000	600,000	50,000	50,000
Laboratory	1,200,000	1,200,000	2,400,000	200,000	300,000
Radiology	600,000	800,000	1,400,000	200,000	350,000
Cardiology	300,000	200,000	500,000	150,000	150,000
Physical and rehabilitation medicine	500,000	150,000	650,000	50,000	75,000
Central supplies	200,000	1,000,000	1,200,000	150,000	150,000
Drugs	300,000	1,500,000	1,800,000	50,000	100,000
Emergency department	1,000,000	200,000	1,200,000	150,000	200,000
Total, revenue-producing departments	11,300,000	7,150,000	18,450,000	2,000,000	1,745,000
Total costs	14,100,000	18,943,000	33,043,000	2,500,000	2,000,000

Employee Benefits (Gross Salaries)	Reconciliation	Administration and General (Accumulated Cost)	Maintenance and Repairs (Square Feet)	Operation of Plant (Square Feet)	Laundry and Linen (Pounds of Laundry)	Environ-mental (Square Feet)	Medical Records (Gross Revenues)	Step-Down Costs (Totals)
3,263,000								
347,128	4,567,128	4,567,128						
46,284	821,284	131,722	953,006					
92,567	942,567	151,174	21,908	1,115,650				
46,284	816,284	130,920	21,908	26,251	995,363			
69,426	649,426	104,159	21,908	26,251	100,000	901,743		
46,284	436,284	69,974	10,954	13,125	0	11,133	541,469	
647,972	3,665,844	587,950	76,679	65,626	100,000	11,133	0	
809,965	5,359,965	859,663	219,082	262,506	250,000	222,653	167,712	7,341,579
462,837	3,112,837	499,255	65,725	78,752	105,363	66,796	95,835	4,024,562
115,709	885,709	142,055	65,725	78,752	50,000	66,796	23,959	1,312,995
208,277	2,308,277	370,215	87,633	105,002	100,000	89,061	43,126	3,103,314
69,426	769,426	123,405	21,908	26,251	80,000	22,265	14,375	1,057,630
277,702	3,177,702	509,659	87,633	105,002	40,000	89,061	57,501	4,066,558
138,851	2,088,851	335,022	87,633	105,002	30,000	89,061	28,751	2,764,320
69,426	869,426	139,444	65,725	78,752	30,000	66,796	14,375	1,264,516
115,709	890,709	142,857	21,908	26,251	20,000	22,265	23,959	1,147,949
46,284	1,546,284	248,002	65,725	78,752	20,000	66,796	9,584	2,035,141
69,426	2,019,426	323,887	21,908	26,251	20,000	22,265	14,375	2,448,112
231,418	1,781,418	285,714	65,725	78,752	150,000	66,796	47,918	2,476,323
2,615,028	24,810,028	3,979,178	876,327	1,050,024	895,363	890,610	541,469	33,043,000
3,263,000	28,475,872	4,567,128	953,006	1,115,650	995,363	901,743	541,469	33,043,000

as it moves from left to right. This example is a summary of a complete step-down. It does not include all the lines or all the columns but is instead presented to illustrate how the initial step-down methodology works.

The following list identifies sample nonrevenue departments whose costs must be allocated to a revenue-producing department on a statistical allocation basis:

Nonrevenue Department and Statistical Allocation Method

Building depreciation	Square feet
Employee benefits	Full-time equivalent staff
Human resources	Full-time equivalent staff
Information services	Total expenses
Plant operations	Square feet
Environmental services	Square feet
Cafeteria	Full-time equivalent staff
Administration	Total expenses
Financial services management	Total expenses
Materials management	Supply expenses
Laundry	Laundry pounds
Patient accounting	Inpatient and outpatient units of service
Medical records	Inpatient and outpatient units of service
Planning and marketing	Total revenues
Medical staff	Total revenues
Central transportation	Adult admissions
Food services	Adult patient days
Care management	Nursing labor
Community services	Total revenues
Overhead	Total expenses
Bad debts	Total revenues

Ratio of Costs to Charges

The purpose of the step-down is to allocate overhead costs in order to create total costs for the revenue-producing departments so that ultimately these total costs can be compared to the total charges for each revenue-producing department. This comparison is known as the cost-to-charge ratio (or the ratio of cost to charges, RCC). The charges for those services provided to Medicare patients are then multiplied by this ratio to determine the cost of rendering care to Medicare patients.

Here is a summarized version of this calculation:

Cardiology direct costs (per Worksheet A)	$5.0 million
Cardiology allocated costs (per Worksheet B)	$4.0 million
Total cardiology costs (final column, Worksheet B)	$9.0 million
Total cardiology charges (per Worksheet C)	$18.0 million
Overall cost-to-charge ratio	0.50
Outpatient cardiology charges for Medicare beneficiaries	$4.0 million
Outpatient Medicare cost for cardiology services	$2.0 million

Implications and Sensitivity of Medicare Cost Reporting

In this example, outpatient services were used instead of inpatient services because, as we now know, inpatient services have not been reimbursed under a cost-based system since 1983. By 2001, Medicare will have phased out almost all remnants of the cost-based system. As we have already seen, the 1997 BBA required Medicare to adopt prospective, non-cost-based reimbursement for hospital-based outpatient (ambulatory) services, home health services, skilled nursing facility, and rehabilitation services.

Yet it is certain that the Medicare cost report will survive. At the moment, this report is the most comprehensive financial statement required for every hospital provider in the United States. There is no other source that combines overall charge information with high-level cost and statistical information. Data of this sort are invaluable to competitors in tracking their neighbor's operation because it is fully available through the Freedom of Information Act to anyone requesting it. When these data are coupled with billing information from the Medicare Medpar file (an accumulation of all the financial and clinical data included on the bills submitted to the Medicare program for reimbursement), health policy experts and analysts are able to spot trends that would not be obvious without such data.

Each year, RHMC's financial analysts gear up to collect the required information. Cost and charge information is assembled from figures available on the hospital's books. Statistical information is collected and prepared using time-honored techniques; all information is double-checked for accuracy. Like a tax return filed with the government, the cost report is an official document that supports the claim that payment was made to the provider by Medicare. The RHMC financial analysts take this preparation seriously. They have had heavy-duty training, attending many continuing education seminars over the years. They study the literature and pay attention to all the new pronouncements issued by Medicare throughout the year. Most of these pronouncements are published in the *Federal Register,* now available daily on the Web at http://www.access.gpo.gov/su_docs/fedreg/.

Furthermore, the financial analysts and their bosses are well aware of recent government efforts to review cost report submissions for fraud. Since its inception in 1966, each hospital's Medicare fiscal intermediary has reviewed cost reports for reasonableness and completeness. Where errors were found during the audit that affected the final annual reimbursement, either positively or negatively, the intermediary made the changes; payments without interest were made, by either the health care organization or the government; and the cost report year was closed. Recently, however, the federal government has staged some high-profile raids on the corporate offices of major for-profit providers, alleging that two sets of books were being kept, the regular set and a "reserve" set.

As with income tax policy and practice, there are gray areas in the Medicare regulations. Many providers in the health care industry believe it is permissible to submit a cost report that includes items that have not yet been deemed black or white by the government. Yet it is uncertain whether a submitted request for additional reimbursement will ultimately withstand government scrutiny. Conversely, GAAP requires that organizations take a conservative approach in booking revenues. This is essentially where an irresistible force meets an immovable object. Most hospitals that take an aggressive or disputed position in filing the cost report also book a reserve against the amounts that they are uncertain of receiving. Section 115 of the *Provider Reimbursement Manual* (HCFA Publication 15-2, titled "Cost Reports Filed Under Protest") states that "you are permitted to dispute regulatory and policy interpretations through the appeals process established by the Social Security Act. Include the nonallowable item in the cost report in order to establish an appeal issue, and the disputed item must pertain to the cost reporting period for which the cost report is filed." Yet at the moment, the government has taken the position that these reserves represent the equivalent of a second set of books, on the basis of action it has taken against a couple of large integrated delivery systems.

Thus, providers that believe Medicare regulations allow them to report certain disputed expenses would be well advised to send a cover letter with their annual cost report submission explaining that a disputed position has been taken. The industry continues to monitor developments in these and other cases because of its applicability to most health care providers.

Presentation of the Audited Financial Statements to the Finance Committee

As members of RHMC's administration continue to monitor and respond to ongoing revenue-reduction issues, the bimonthly finance committee meeting is upon them. Although operations are currently being maintained through a mix of small expense reductions, the operating margin is nonetheless being negatively affected.

Meanwhile, the centerpiece of the April finance committee session is once again the presentation of the previous year's audited financial statement by the partner of the external accounting and auditing firm retained by RHMC. The audit partner has a particular agenda that she wants to present to the committee. A tried-and-true format with which the auditing firm is comfortable, it includes an overview of the health care industry as well as some of the current risks inherent in the business. The partner then reviews unusual circumstances, if any, surrounding the audit. Finally, she presents the financial results of the audit. From the point of view of management, the most important finding is the lack of any audit adjustment. This means that the financial statements that have been presented monthly by the finance administrator are valid and fairly presented. This allows the board finance committee to continue to place trust in current management.

Implications of Management Letter Comments Proposed by the Auditors

Each year, as part of the scope of their activity, the auditors prepare a review of the internal controls of the organization. This review is made into a report and submitted to the finance committee, commenting on any material weaknesses in financial controls that have been uncovered. This is an essential part of the audit and is given great weight by the board members. It is one of the few times that the board gets to see behind the curtain through independent eyes whether management is doing what it says.

Management of RHMC is quite aware of the weight given to this report by the finance committee. But the finance administrators have always welcomed publication of this report. They have been trained to understand the importance of internal controls right down to the detail level (where the auditors dwell). They know that the best way to avoid any type of misappropriation is to maintain proper internal controls. RHMC's finance administrators have a history of performing various types of operational and financial review proactively, to understand their systems, uncover any problems, and fix them. Operational reviews that have been performed in the recent past include the following:

- Information system risks and control assessment
- Treasury management risk assessment
- Cost report risk assessment
- Materials management risk assessment
- Accounts payable audit and assessment
- Patient registration and accounts receivable process assessment

This year, as in the past several years, the auditors did not discover any significant financial or operational issues to present. This reaffirmed for the finance committee that management was acting properly in preserving the assets of the organization. The auditors did, however, comment on the organization's fraud-and-abuse compliance efforts and the need to continue being diligent in its efforts. Other than that important comment, the auditors stated they were pleased with the controls.

Finally, as is done every year, the organization's entire management, which includes the president and chief executive officer, the chief operating officer, the chief financial officer, and the chief strategy officer, were dismissed from the meeting so that the audit partner could give the members of the finance committee—acting in their capacity as the audit committee—a private assessment of management. Because this particular management group had been together for more than ten years, it is presumed that the audit partner was giving the board members the same clean bill of health in private as that given in public.

CHAPTER FIVE

MAY

*Sam is working on a presentation to the finance committee when his phone rings.
Angela Renfro, the organization's patient accounts manager, is on the line.*

"Angela, what's up?"

"Sam, I've got this problem that I want to talk to you about."

"OK, tell me about it."

Angela is a little tentative. She seems unsure how to begin.

"Well, I don't know if you've noticed, but the accounts receivable balance has been
going up the last several weeks."

"Actually, Angela, I did notice," *Sam replies, somewhat amused.* "I was going to
call you tomorrow to see what's going on. On my first quick review, I thought I noticed
the percentage of accounts older than 120 days from discharge was growing, but I
haven't done a complete review yet."

"That's just my point," *she fairly screams.* "It's not the older accounts that are the
problem. In fact, if you look at the accounts stratified by age, you'll find, as I did, that
the receivable dollars in all the billed accounts are decreasing. The trouble is in the accounts where the patients have been discharged but no bills have been produced."

"What? Oh my gosh. You know, I haven't been looking at the discharged, not-final-
billed category recently because it was doing so well. I just forgot about it for a while. Do
you know why all of a sudden it's out of control?"

Angela is agitated; Sam imagines her squirming in her seat.

"Well, ever since the organization restructured management and moved responsibility for the medical records departments from you to the operations director, I've noticed they lost some of their focus on the financial aspects of the medical records function.
Then the manager told me that he lost some of his coding staff to out-of-state moves
and pregnancies. With limited staff, they thought they'd concentrate on some other
clinical medical records issues, not the coding and abstracting completion, which I need
before the bill can drop. This is even more critical since August 2000, when Medicare
APC took effect."

Aaaarrrgghhhh! Sam thinks. He says, "I hate to use this expression, but you know,
I told them so. When they restructured, I warned them this could—and probably
would—happen. Management is really just a function of focus. Unless the finance division is responsible for all aspects of the finance function, there's no accountability. OK,
so how many receivable dollars are tied up just waiting for the coding to take place?"

"It's already almost $5 million. This is just about ten extra days in the accounts re-
ceivable balance at our average revenue of $500,000 a day."

"OK, so I'd better have a talk with the medical records manager and her boss to make sure we get a whole lot of focus back on this issue, pronto. I sure do hate to have responsibility for something without the authority."

"Yep. I know what you mean."

May in the northern regions of the United States is a time of great promise. The frost of winter is finally gone. The April rains have subsided, and the flowers are beginning to bloom in earnest. A rebirth takes place among the frigid-fingered inhabitants of the northern climes. At RHMC, this reemergence from winter's cold is usually cause for celebration. Men start to bring out their spring suits, shedding the wool of winter. Women are happy to put away some of their warm-weather outfits and replace them with lighter-weight and more flexible fashions.

The accounting and finance staff continue to do the jobs for which they are responsible. It is one of the two times of the year when there is traditionally a slightly lighter load of work. The year-end functions are behind them and the budget has not yet really begun. This is a purging month for the staff as they perform their own spring cleaning, rifling through the files (electronic and paper) to delete and reorganize as appropriate. This, however, is not the case for staff and managers responsible for billing and collecting patient accounts.

Fundamentals of Accounts Receivable Management

The month of May typically holds no particular milestone in the world of accounts receivable management at RHMC, which is an hour-by-hour, day-to-day task that involves dozens of small but important transactions. Managers of the accounts receivable function are most often task-oriented and driven to achieve the various goals set down by the organization's administration. These goals are often an aggregation of important aspects of management. At RHMC, the goals are as follows:

- Improving patient service and satisfaction
- Improving employee satisfaction (morale)
- Improving the quality of the department's outcomes
- Reducing the dollars in overall net accounts receivable in relation to the net revenues being generated (called "days in accounts receivable")

Achieving these goals is hard, but not unlike achieving the goals of any other management position. One difference is that the accounts receivable manager is among the few management positions that hold the fate of the rest of the organization in their hands. Numerous health care organizations live from hand to mouth. Said another way, the only way the organization may be able to meet its payroll or pay its vendors is for the accounts receivable manager to collect cash on the outstanding bills. No collections, no payroll.

The accounts receivable manager (hereafter called the patient accounts manager, or PAM) understands this. It is true because accounts receivable production is constantly monitored by the administration, often daily. Although the administration is primarily concerned about daily cash receipts, the PAM has a significantly more complex set of productivity measures, which, once met, turn generation of patient bills into cash.

Here is a summarized listing of the major elements of accounts receivable management. Each item has significant implications for the nature and quality of ultimate cash collection.

Accounts Receivable Management Issues

- Policy, planning, and evaluation (*planning*)
    Establishing objectives and goals
    Internal and external auditing policies
    Performance standards and measurements
    Third-party relationships (for example, Medicare, Medicaid, managed care)
- Admission and registration policy and procedures (*inputs*)
    Inpatient and outpatient registration policies and procedures
    Precertification
    Preadmission or preregistration
    Insurance verification
    Registration
    Customer relations
- Patient financial services policies and procedures (*throughput*)
    Charge capture issues
    Documentation capture
    Coding and reimbursement issues (ICD-9-CM and CPT-4 coding)
    Revenue maximization activity (lost charge recovery efforts)
    Medical records, quality assurance, and utilization review
- Postdischarge account management (*output*)
    Bill preparation and mailing
    Billing audits and fraud abuse and controls

Third-party and self-pay follow-up techniques

Patient cost sharing, inpatient and outpatient

- Collection policy and procedures (*follow-up*)

Bad-debt expense and charity care policy

Financial counseling

Financing of self-pay patient accounts

Payment policy

Selection of collection agencies

Monitoring performance of collection agencies

- Legal aspects

Bankruptcy

Contracts

Federal rules and regulations

Litigation policy

Workers' compensation

Patient and hospital rights and obligations

- Managed care organizations (MCOs)

Arrangements and negotiations between providers and MCOs

Contractual obligations between the two parties

Capability of the provider to meet managed care requirements

Competition

Monitoring results

Future trends

Within all of these items, there are six areas that must be specifically highlighted because of their overriding importance:

1. Precertification, preadmission, and insurance verification
2. Documentation capture
3. Coding and reimbursement
4. Fraud-and-abuse issues
5. Managed care arrangements and negotiation
6. Monitoring results

Precertification, Preregistration, and Insurance Verification

Of all the important concepts in accounts receivable management, precertification, preregistration, and insurance verification are *the most important*. The quality and speed of the collection process at the time of billing and thereafter is *completely dependent* on the quality and skill exhibited during precertification and insurance verification at the time of preregistration. In a later discussion in this chapter regarding which division the patient registration department should report to, the importance of overemphasizing these areas is demonstrated if the organization wants to hold down days in receivables.

Precertification and insurance verification are important because it has become imperative to recognize and capture the patient's or employer's policy information, which is usually located on the patient's insurance card. The registration department is responsible for determining the preauthorization requirements for every patient who presents for services, whether as an inpatient or outpatient, and verifying benefits with the appropriate managed care company. Determining accurate demographic (name, address, telephone number, next of kin, and so on) and insurance information (guarantor's name, address, telephone number, exact policy number, and so on) is the most important function the patient registration department performs. The patient accounting department relies completely on the quality of this information to be able to perform timely billing and collection activity.

Documentation Capture

The ability of the medical records department to ensure optimal reimbursement within the revenue cycle for inpatient or outpatient accounts is wholly dependent on the quality of documentation. Documentation is the written record of care provided during a patient's stay. An old saying in the industry states, "If it isn't documented, it didn't happen." That sums it up perfectly. Documentation of services and the distinctions made by clinicians (physicians and nurses) contemporaneously during the stay are critical to the ability to maximize reimbursement.

This is also a legal distinction. More and more, health care organization coding of services is being challenged. There is a much stronger presumption of innocence if the organization is able to document the level of clinical services required by the patient and provided by the organization.

One of the best ways to ensure capture of quality documentation is to make available ultratraining for all the people involved in this effort. The most important people involved in documentation are the floor nurses, the utilization review nurses (sometimes called care managers), and the physicians. The toughest group to train is the physicians, because they usually do not work for the organization, they may believe they have no stake in improving documentation, and they were never taught in medical school that documentation equals better reimbursement and generally do not want to learn it now.

But it is absolutely necessary to make sure that this training is carried out appropriately and effectively. The difference between, for example, a DRG without a comorbidity or complication (CC) and a similar case with a CC could be several thousand dollars. Physicians who understand these distinctions are actually creating a better medicolegal record of the case. Thus any documentation training needs to emphasize that improved documentation is always worthwhile for all the participants involved.

RHMC is fully aware of these distinctions and understands that improved documentation equals improved reimbursement. It is also aware that the best way to improve documentation is to invest heavily in training. Therefore, several years ago, after the inception of the DRG program for inpatient reimbursement by Medicare (1983), an outside consulting firm was hired that specializes in documentation training. The hospital then made the training mandatory for utilization review nurses and medical record coders. It also included in the training a number of physicians who have substantial practices at the hospital. In addition, the hospital made sure to offer this same training to any new employees who started in these areas subsequent to the original training.

Finally, RHMC contracted with this same consulting firm to perform quarterly sample reviews, to determine that all documentation was properly included and that coding for reimbursement purposes was accurate. The consulting firm used the same coding books and rules employed by Medicare to do so. Because it had taken these steps, RHMC was comfortable that it was complying with the difficult billing requirements required by the Medicare program, even though reimbursement for its inpatient cases had improved. It was a case study in how to do better by doing better.

Because of the significant success of the inpatient program, the hospital brought back a consulting firm in 1999 to review steps of this same type for the APC program, which was scheduled to begin in August 2000. Once again, documentation training was performed for the crucial employees and physicians who would most affect the quality of the billing. This was done to ensure that all the legal requirements were being met and that the hospital was receiving proper reimbursement for the services that were being rendered.

Coding and Reimbursement

One of the primary functions of the finance division is to maximize reimbursement. The best way to do this is to maximize the quality of clinical documentation. This gives coders the best opportunity to apply for the highest level of reimbursement, where appropriate. In addition, every health care organization needs to give coders the best available tools, such as up-to-date coding books and automated software.

It is definitely appropriate for any health care organization to maximize reimbursement. Notwithstanding the federal government's current focus on what it characterizes as health care billing fraud, it is legal, moral, and proper to apply for the best available reimbursement so long as the documentation is reflective of the care provided, it supports the coding, and the coding supports the billing.

There are many technical aspects to the coding function. The most important detail is the ability to convert clinical documentation into clinical coding. Coding comes in many forms. The most prevalent coding formats are the following:

• ICD-9-CM. *International Classification of Diseases,* ninth edition, clinically modified (for the United States). In Chapter Four, we saw that ICD-9 codes are the most important element in creating the diagnostic-related group (DRG), and the DRG is how Medicare reimburses a hospital for an inpatient stay.

• HCFA's Common Procedure Coding System. ICD-9-CM creates reimbursement for Medicare inpatients. The Health Care Financing Administration (the regulatory body that the Medicare program falls under) uses HCPCS, a uniform method for health care providers and medical suppliers to code for their professional services, procedures, and supplies and thus create reimbursement for Medicare outpatients.

• RBRVS. The Resource-Based Relative Value Scale is the method Medicare has defined to reimburse for physician office services. It is based on HCPCS codes.

• CPT-4. The *Physician's Current Procedural Terminology,* fourth edition, is a systematic listing of procedures and services performed by physicians. It is the most widely accepted coding methodology in America.

Whether the coder works for a hospital, a physician's office, or any other health care entity that receives part of net revenues from use of coding, it is always important to remember the primary significance of coding to reimbursement maximization. When the patient accounting staff prepare to send out a bill to any third-party payor that reimburses for services using these codes, the staff are always aware of the revenue implications of coding.

Timeliness of Coding

There is one other specific and critical aspect within the coding cycle of patient accounting and billing. The patient's bill cannot be sent out to the third-party payor until the coding is completed and validated. Here are the specific steps involved in this procedure:

1. The physician documents the patient's final diagnosis.
2. Various service units (radiology, laboratory, cardiology) complete all the written (documented) test results and they are received by the medical record coders.

TABLE 5.1. DHHS OFFICE OF INSPECTOR GENERAL, FISCAL YEAR 2001 WORK PLAN, SELECTED AREAS OF REVIEW IN BILLING AND CLAIMS PROCESSING.

Area of Concern	Issue
Hospitals	
Hospital discharges and subsequent readmission	Examining Medicare claims for beneficiaries who were discharged and subsequently readmitted to the same acute care PPS hospital. Also reviewing claims processing procedures to determine effectiveness of existing system edits used to identify and review related admissions.
Payments for related hospital and skilled nursing stays	Determining the extent of Medicare payments for short- and long-stay hospital and skilled nursing facility care that was provided sequentially to the same beneficiary.
Home health	
Payment based on location of service	Evaluating the implementation of a relatively recent change in paying for home health care. Effective October 1997, home health services are to be paid based on the location where the service is provided (in the patient's home), rather than where the service is billed (typically the urban location of the parent home health agency).
Skilled nursing home care	
Ineligible stays in skilled nursing facilities	Quantifying improper payments for SNF stays that did not meet Medicare's coverage conditions. (A three-day hospital stay must precede the SNF stay.)
Consolidated billing requirements	Determining the extent of overpayments during calendar year 1999 for Part B services subject to consolidated billing provisions of SNF PPS. Under BBA 97, consolidated billing requires that SNFs bill Medicare for virtually all services rendered to residents during Part A stays. Prior OIG work found that for more than one-third of claims reviewed, Medicare contractors made separate Part B payments to outside suppliers for services subject to consolidated billing.
Physicians	
Physicians at teaching hospitals (PATH)	Verifying compliance with Medicare rules governing payment for physician services provided in the teaching hospital setting and ensuring that claims accurately reflect the level of service provided to patients.
Critical care codes	Examining the use of two critical care codes that may be billed to Medicare only if the patient is critically ill and requires constant attention by the physician. Payment for critical care is based on the time spent with the patient.

3. All clinical information relevant to the most proper coding of each patient's stay is abstracted from the medical chart.
4. The coding itself is performed by the coder, who now has all the relevant information.

Regarding step three, information often becomes available just after the patient's discharge. A lab test can add significantly to the severity of the case by necessitating an additional ICD-9 code. This extra code could make a big difference in the final DRG that may improve the organization's reimbursement.

Managing this medical records function (coding) has great bearing on the ability of the billing department to send out a timely bill. Another truism of the health care industry is that the PAM is responsible for the entire accounts receivable balance, whether or not the individual has control over all the functions described in the earlier list. In many cases, the PAM does not always have control over all those functions. Therefore, he or she has to use excellent management skills to become best friends with the manager of medical records and the coding supervisor in order to accomplish the primary goal of timely billing. The reality is that untimely coding can cause unbilled accounts to skyrocket and add millions of dollars and many days to the accounts receivable. (There is further discussion of the issue of timeliness and control, particularly related to patient registration issues, later in this chapter.)

Fraud-and-Abuse Issues Related to Billing

Issues of fraud and abuse in billing for services are multifaceted and complex. The Medicare and Medicaid programs want to be sure that they are paying only for the services required for and used by their beneficiaries. Yet they have estimated that several billion dollars are being squandered in payment to providers. The Office of Inspector General, which is an arm of the Department of Health and Human Services, has created a work plan of what it believes are the biggest areas of fraud and abuse in claims processing. The areas they have targeted for substantial review in 2001 are summarized in Table 5.1.

It is pretty obvious that the government is serious about fraud and abuse in billing. The table is not comprehensive, yet some of the areas listed are given more weight than others. It is not known which of these areas is considered most highly weighted, but some supposition can be gleaned from the OIG's work in the recent past and the probability of a greater monetary return for the government (Gardner, 1998). Since the appearance of Gardner's article, the OIG has continued to bring charges against many health care providers and contractors. In fact, in its semiannual report published in January 2001, the OIG reported savings of $15.62 billion for FY00 (ending September 30, 2000). This total comprises

- $14.4 billion in implemented recommendations and other actions to better use funds
- $142 million in audit disallowances
- $1.23 billion in investigative receivables

In addition, the OIG excluded 3,350 providers for fraud and abuse, convicted 414 providers for "crimes against departmental programs," and undertook 357 civil actions.

Finally, in the four full years (FY97 through FY00) since the Healthcare Fraud and Abuse Control Program was implemented under the 1996 Health Insurance Portability and Accountability Act (HIPAA), the OIG has reported overall savings of more than $47.3 billion:

- $665 million in audit disallowances
- $43.3 billion in savings from implemented legislative or regulatory recommendations and action to better use funds
- $3.4 billion in investigative receivables

More than twelve thousand individuals or entities were excluded from the Medicare program. The report is available at http://oig.hhs.gov/semann/index.htm.

It is principally because of extraordinary results of this kind that the government's focus on fraud and abuse, with strong emphasis on Medicare billing issues, will not abate. Thus, the PAM and the organization's billing staff need to be aware of all the billing rules all the time to stay legal in this important operation.

Several areas probably represent the risk of greatest exposure. The first is upcoding of patient bills. This usually involves an inpatient or emergency department case and is a function of claiming higher reimbursement than is deserved because the clinical documentation does not support the claim. This is unlike the situation mentioned earlier involving RHMC, where improved documentation led to higher reimbursements.

Upcoding achieved prominence when a *Wall Street Journal* article in early 1997 highlighted how it works and why it can cost Medicare so much money. In a nutshell, the article explained that the DRG system, and the codes needed to drive it, is so cumbersome that the DRGs, codes, and guidelines fill two volumes totaling more than twenty-six hundred pages, thus making it extremely difficult to claim proper reimbursement. In fact, health care providers often downcode as well as upcode because of the difficulty that these issues entail (Lagnado, 1997).

The federal government is currently reviewing the issues of upcoding for pneumonia cases involving DRGs 89 and 90 and the significant difference in their case weights. The article pointed out that DRG 90 (simple pneumonia, which has no secondary complication) might have a reimbursement rate of $2,791, while DRG 89 (pneumonia with complications) may have a reimbursement rate of $4,462, a difference of $1,671, or 60 percent. This amount can be "earned" by adding a complication, where appropriate, to the patient's chart; it is often only an issue for the provider, whether physician or utilization review nurse, to pay a little more attention to some of the secondary clinical issues and test results. Health care organizations have been hiring consultants to teach documentation and coding maximization to improve their reimbursements. As the chief financial officer of a major academic medical center said in the article, "It is like hiring a tax expert to make sure you took all your deductions."

A second area is nursing home implementation of consolidated billing. This is ripe for fraud and abuse because of the potential for double billing. A major change in the billing rules rendered by the 1997 Balanced Budget Act mandated that for nursing home stays not paid by Medicare Part A, nursing facilities are responsible for submitting bills to Medicare contractors for most Part B services. Except in a few specialized areas, only the SNF is able to directly bill Medicare. The possibility of other providers continuing to bill the program, while these services are now bundled into the consolidated bill, is the concern of the OIG. It plans to monitor this area closely.

Third is accuracy and carrier monitoring of physician visit coding. As with the coding issues described for inpatient hospitalization, Medicare also reimburses physicians through use of codes. In this case, the codes are called evaluation and management (E&M). Also as with DRGs, physicians or their staff might code the visit at a higher level than is permitted based on the documentation. The OIG believes it has done enough sampling to indicate that this is a high-profile area to pursue.

It is imperative that health care financial managers who have responsibility for billing or reporting gross and net revenues and receivables should go annually to at least one continuing education class or seminar held around the country on the fraud-and-abuse billing topic; several sessions would be better. Along with staying abreast of the current literature, this is the best way to maintain knowledge and expertise in this highly volatile area. Expanded discussion of the non-billing fraud-and-abuse areas can be found in Chapter Seven.

Managed Care Arrangements and Negotiations

At this moment in the health care industry, managed care volume may amount to 20 to 50 percent of an organization's net revenues. This may well be the case in any large segment of the industry: hospitals, physician practices, SNFs, and home health agencies. Many of these organizations are large enough to have personnel responsible for negotiating managed care contracts and patient registration and billing. In such an organization, it is imperative that the departments responsible for these patient financial services be given a seat at the negotiating table. Their job at the table should be to ascertain that the negotiator agrees only to terms and conditions that can be appropriately administered by the departments. If this is not done, there is a very good chance that the organization will be stuck with lost revenue, increased accounts receivables, and increased bad debt.

These problems are the result of the organization's failure to properly pre-certify, preauthorize, or bill in a timely manner, which may be the result of lack of coordination between the managed care negotiator and patient financial services personnel.

Monitoring Results

Several accounts receivable management processes highlighted in this chapter suggest ways to improve department outcomes. They may seem terrific in theory, but the results may be quite different in practice. The primary method that is used to determine whether improvements have in fact been made is to first determine the baseline of the process you are measuring and then monitor the process outcomes periodically (daily, weekly, monthly). These outcomes allow the PAM and administration to understand in which direction the outcomes are heading: up or down.

Earlier in the chapter, RHMC's goals for its patient accounting department were presented:

- Improving patient service and satisfaction
- Improving employee satisfaction (morale)
- Improving the quality of the department's outcomes
- Reducing the dollars in overall net accounts receivable in relation to the net revenues being generated

Each goal can be numerically measured and monitored. One of the PAM's job requirements is to help set these goals and then achieve them. The best way to set goals in these areas is to use benchmarks, which can be used in various ways. In setting initial goals, for example, measuring the current year's results against prior results would be a good use of benchmarking. This is particularly appropriate if the organization is unable to find external benchmarks. The advantage of this process is that it allows the organization to gauge the direction of results—in other words, at least determine if things are getting better or worse against prior perfor-

TABLE 5.2. RHMC BALANCED SCORECARD MEASURES, PATIENT ACCOUNTING DEPARTMENT.

Measure	Goal
Improving patient satisfaction and service	
–Reduce patient complaints received	< 6 patient complaints per unit per year
–Improve scores on patient satisfaction survey	> 93rd percentile in all categories
–Improve closure on every patient query received by the department	> 98%
–Improve employee productivity in collection unit	40 quality calls per day per employee
Improving employee satisfaction	
–Improve employee satisfaction scores	> 80% score on employee opinion survey
–Reduce disputes brought to human resource department	Zero disputes brought to HR
Improving quality	
–Reduce billing errors	< 2% error rate
–Reduce time taken to post cash	Post all cash on day of receipt
–Improve timely posting of contractual adjustments	98% of contractual adjustments are posted within 24 hours after billing
Reducing days in accounts receivable	
–Reduce net days in accounts receivable	< 55 days

mance. The disadvantage of this process is that it does not allow an organization to determine if performance is poor, good, or excellent against the results of peers.

RHMC has set specific numerical goals in all four of the categories it has chosen to measure. Table 5.2 presents the various goals for RHMC's patient accounting department:

• *Improving patient service and satisfaction.* RHMC subscribes to a customer survey service company. More than four hundred health care organizations from around the country are part of the benchmark group. Three of the questions asked on the survey, which goes to all inpatients and outpatients who have been discharged, relate to patient accounting functions. The goals are set high to achieve a ranking in the top 10 percent of the group. The results are monitored monthly, feedback is presented to the staff, and improvements are constantly sought to improve the rankings.

• *Improving employee satisfaction (morale).* RHMC also subscribes to an employee opinion service benchmarking group. In this case, employee morale is measured through an ongoing survey process. The PAM is able to measure the satisfaction of the staff in two ways. First, it can be measured against scores from prior periods to determine the direction in which morale is trending. Second, satisfaction can be assessed against published national norms. RHMC's goal is to achieve an 80 percent satisfaction rating from its own employees.

• *Improving the quality of the department's outcomes.* These goals are extremely important to the organization's patient accounting department manager. This is one of the primary ways for the manager to set goals that improve the department's processes, thereby improving outcomes. Management has identified error rates as a critical quality outcome driver. Reduction in error rate always improves outcomes and productivity by obviating rework. Therefore major emphasis is always placed on identifying and then correcting areas where errors are caused. For example, a significant focus is production of clean claims (bills) to third-party payors. Clean claims are turned around and paid in much more expeditiously, so the patient accounting department spends time monitoring both electronic and manual claims production for errors. In general, the department strives to keep its error rate under 2 percent.

• *Reducing the dollars in overall accounts receivable in relation to net revenues being generated.* This is a commonly cited measurement and benchmark in the health care industry. There are many sources for the measure, popularly known as days in accounts receivable. The problem with this benchmark is that there are so many ways to calculate it. Accounts receivable is often cited as both gross receivable and net receivable; either may be used as the numerator. In addition, it is also possible to calculate the denominator using daily gross or net revenues. Finally, some organizations report only a portion of their receivable pay classes as gross and other pay classes as net. It makes for a confusing measurement and benchmark.

RHMC has solved this problem by using the only days in accounts receivable measure that is considered reliable as a benchmark: net accounts receivable divided by daily net revenues. These net amounts are available on the balance sheet and income statement. In addition, and more important, net figures are reported on the annual audited financial statements, where gross revenues have been reduced by contractual adjustments to net expected value and gross receivables have been reduced by allowance for doubtful accounts (ADA) and allowance for contractual adjustments (ACA) to the most likely value. Because these are audited figures, this is the most reliable set of measures available to create a benchmark for days in accounts receivable. RHMC's goal is to achieve fifty-five days in accounts receivable, which, according to several of the benchmark services, would place the organization favorably vis-à-vis the industry median.

Patient Registration: Which Division Should It Report to?

There is one issue not ordinarily discussed in print, but it has a major impact on managing accounts receivable. The question is to which division in the organization the patient registration department should report. The answer often goes a long way in establishing the level of days in accounts receivable. Around the time that Medicare came into being (1966), many patient registration departments reported to the operating division, not the finance division. There was good reason for this. As a cottage industry, the primary means of cash receipt was from the patients themselves or a handful of third-party payors. It was extremely easy to identify the payor and this did not require much training. In addition, there were no great financial implications to improperly identifying the correct payor because there were no preauthorization requirements or billing deadlines that would cause coverage denial for services rendered.

As already noted in Chapter Four, the commencement of Medicare turned health care-providing services from a cottage industry into a major one. Concurrently, identification of the actual payor became more critical because many payors, including the indemnity insurers, sold varying coverage to employers under the same policy name.

Many administrators throughout the industry recognized that with these changes came a shift in the responsibility of the patient registration department. Although still extremely concerned about customer satisfaction, it was clear that capture of insurance and demographic information became the critical aspect in effective accounts receivable management.

Over the next ten to fifteen years, many health care organizations—particularly hospitals, which usually separated the registration function from the billing function—moved the reporting responsibility of patient registration from the operating division to the finance division. It is a truism of the industry that the best way to turn accounts receivable into cash is to perform preregistration and registration functions correctly, accurately, and quickly. Put another way, the front end of the receivable cycle is considerably more important than the back end.

Precertification, preregistration, insurance verification, and registration represent the front end, while bill production, bill submission, third-party follow-up, and collection activities represent the back end. Good back-end processing is possible only if the front-end systems and procedures are faultless. Current contracts between providers and payors demand that the provider capture lots of specific data at the time of the patient's registration. Without correct capture, there is a good chance that the payor will delay or deny the claim (that is, not pay it because the provider did not meet the technical specifications of the contract).

The PAM is fully responsible for collecting accounts receivable and the level of bad debt being generated. If the patient registration function does not report directly either to the PAM or to a finance director, there is every possibility that accounts receivable will not be at the level required by the administration or board.

Yet, anecdotally, there appears to be a disturbing trend in recent years. Hospital administrators are moving the reporting responsibility of the registration department back under the operations division. The explanation most often cited is that admissions and registration functions are performed at the front door of the hospital for many patients, and as such the patient's experience as a customer begins there. Therefore, the reasoning goes, only the operations division can provide the kind of positive patient experience so highly sought.

There are two big fallacies in this argument. First, the operating division can collect demographic and insurance information that is equal to or better than what the finance division can do. Second, the finance division cannot provide customer service and satisfaction equal to or better than what the operating division can.

Neither of these notions is true. Most health care finance professionals will tell you that collecting accurate insurance information is extremely difficult. The reason for the difficulty is related first to the incredible complexity of rules and regulations inherent in Medicare inpatient and outpatient billing, and second to the number of managed care companies that currently populate the landscape. Every managed care company has a set of coverage provisions for its beneficiaries that often differ from its competitors. Thus, a different set of preverification steps and standards have to be followed. Making things even worse, within the same managed care company (as was shown in Chapter Four) there can be several kinds of plan. Because of this, when a registrar is presented with a patient's insurance card, there is no guarantee that payment is ensured. Different plans mean different benefits. Even the same employers may have three or four plans.

The first priority of the registration manager must be accurate and timely collection and processing of the patient's demographic and insurance information. The best way to accomplish this priority goal is through relentless staff training on insurance. This training should comprise all the nuances of the information contained on the insurance card. Additionally, it should emphasize the implications of various preauthorization, precertification, and second-opinion requirements contained in the diverse insurance plans within the organization's service area.

Although customer service must always be emphasized, there is an inherent conflict between properly collecting a patient's demographic and insurance information and the patient's desire to get immediate treatment. Health care organizations would like to register patients in the same manner as a hotel. But it is important to recognize that an insurance card is not a credit card. The finance division constantly tries to balance customer service requirements with the need to collect timely and accurate information. Unfortunately, the operating division simply does not grasp the seriousness of the financial implications inherent in maintaining vigilance in this area, as it generally places the patient's desire for speedy registration ahead of the requirements imposed by the insurance industry. After all, the operations division is not responsible for the accounts receivable at the board level. Thus, the level of accounts receivable is influenced by the decision of which division is responsible for this information collection effort.

Calculation of Allowance for Doubtful Accounts and Bad-Debt Expense

Doubtful accounts and bad-debt expense are key aspects of accounts receivable management. One aspect that has significant implications for the income statement is calculation of the allowance for doubtful accounts. On the balance sheet, the ADA is a contra account to the accounts receivable asset line. It reduces the gross receivable by the amount calculated to be uncollectible. Sometimes referred to as the reserve for bad debt, the ADA calculation encompasses some interesting twists; as stated in Chapter Two, it is one of the six extremely sensitive items likely to receive an audit adjustment if done poorly.

Bad-debt expense is the other side of the double-entry bookkeeping in the ADA calculation. (Bad-debt expense is another of the six most sensitive financial statement items.) Most health care organizations use a four-sided approach to ADA and bad debt reporting. The four financial statement accounts that are always involved in this calculation are accounts receivable, allowance for doubtful accounts, bad-debt expenses, and bad-debt write-offs.

The ADA is the key to the entire set of equations. Every health care organization needs to perform a detailed analysis each month to determine the proper ADA balance. The ADA calculation attempts to measure the projected amount of recorded accounts receivable that cannot be collected at that month's end. For financial statement purposes, it is the GAAP method used to write down the gross receivable to its estimated realizable value.

Table 5.3 represents an ADA calculation used by Ridgeland Heights. The most important features of the calculation are use of an aging schedule and stratification by major pay classes. These concepts value accounts by the length of time they have been outstanding and the quality of the payor class with which each patient was registered. In the latter example, it is a truism of the industry that some payors will surely convert the receivables of their beneficiaries to cash once the claim has been determined to be proper. This is the case even if the account ages beyond a reasonable period. RHMC has also stratified its receivables between inpatient and outpatient accounts because of the various payment methodologies that may be employed.

TABLE 5.3. RHMC DETAILED ANALYSIS OF ALLOWANCE FOR DOUBTFUL ACCOUNTS (ADA) FOR THE MONTH ENDED DEC. 31, 2000.

Inpatient Accounts	Unbilled	Less Allowance for Contractual Adjustment	Adjusted Unbilled	0–30 Days	31–60 Days
Medicare receivable	1,782,084	(1,015,788)	766,296	852,582	264,409
Allowance percentage			5.00%	5.00%	5.00%
Medicare allowance			38,315	42,629	13,220
Medicaid receivable	107,285	(432,972)	(325,687)	36,451	122,285
Allowance percentage			5.00%	6.00%	10.00%
Medicaid allowance			(16,284)	2,187	12,228
Managed care receivable	878,541	(556,180)	322,361	1,440,125	1,117,852
Allowance percentage			4.00%	6.00%	10.00%
Managed care allowance			12,894	86,408	111,785
All other receivable	256,895		256,895	118,947	64,698
Allowance percentage			30.00%	30.00%	40.00%
All other allowance			77,069	35,684	25,879
Total inpatient receivable	3,024,805	(2,004,940)	1,019,865	2,448,105	1,569,243
Inpatient reserve			111,993	166,908	163,113
Total inpatient reserve percentages			10.98%	6.82%	10.39%
Outpatient Accounts					
Medicare receivable	1,239,377	(2,335,665)	(1,096,288)	703,717	933,793
Allowance percentage			5.00%	5.00%	6.00%
Medicare allowance			(54,814)	35,186	56,028
Medicaid receivable	95,464	(264,174)	(168,710)	33,418	46,354
Allowance percentage			5.00%	5.00%	6.00%
Medicaid allowance			(8,436)	1,671	2,781
Managed care receivable	1,501,256	(900,256)	601,000	1,225,365	1,395,822
Allowance percentage			4.00%	6.00%	10.00%
Managed care allowance			24,040	73,522	139,582
All other receivable	925,652		925,652	475,812	544,813
Allowance percentage			30.00%	30.00%	40.00%
All other allowance			277,696	142,744	217,925
Total outpatient receivable	3,761,749	(3,500,095)	261,654	2,438,312	2,920,782
Outpatient reserve			238,486	253,122	416,316
Total outpatient reserve percentages			91.15%	10.38%	14.25%
Total receivables	6,786,554	(5,505,035)	1,281,519	4,886,417	4,490,025
Total reserves			350,479	420,030	579,429
Total reserve percentages			27.35%	8.60%	12.90%

61–90 Days	91–120 Days	121–150 Days	151–180 Days	Over 180 Days	Total Billed	Total
161,301	73,747	59,881	21,606	257,328	1,690,854	2,457,150
10.00%	20.00%	25.00%	35.00%	50.00%		15.80%
16,130	14,749	14,970	7,562	128,664		276,240
118,464	39,360	37,500	40,208	116,979	511,246	185,559
15.00%	20.00%	30.00%	50.00%	60.00%		17.50%
17,770	7,872	11,250	20,104	70,187	125,314	
558,417	429,685	230,325	161,410	989,547	4,927,361	5,249,722
15.00%	17.00%	25.00%	25.00%	30.00%		11.20%
83,763	73,046	57,581	40,353	296,864		762,694
103,719	53,770	18,899	16,491	137,418	513,942	770,837
50.00%	60.00%	70.00%	85.00%	98.00%		63.30%
51,860	32,262	13,229	14,018	134,670		384,669
941,901	596,562	346,604	239,715	1,501,272	7,643,403	8,663,268
169,522	127,930	97,030	82,036	630,385		1,548,918
18.00%	21.44%	27.99%	34.22%	41.99%		17.88%
408,121	249,968	185,515	89,856	436,316	3,007,286	1,910,998
13.10%	20.00%	25.00%	50.00%	70.00%		15.80%
53,464	49,994	46,379	44,928	305,421		536,584
52,374	17,530	21,100	3,385	54,593	228,754	60,044
9.00%	12.00%	18.00%	23.90%	44.80%		17.50%
4,714	2,104	3,798	809	24,458		31,899
751,254	648,952	482,541	315,965	2,152,748	6,972,647	7,573,647
14.00%	18.00%	30.00%	35.00%	41.00%		11.20%
105,176	116,811	144,762	110,588	882,627		1,597,108
364,785	287,596	215,874	135,896	842,095	2,866,871	3,792,523
50.00%	60.00%	70.00%	85.00%	98.00%		63.30%
182,393	172,558	151,112	115,512	825,253		2,085,191
1,576,534	1,204,046	905,030	545,102	3,485,752	13,075,558	13,337,212
345,746	341,466	346,051	271,836	2,037,759		4,250,782
21.93%	28.36%	38.24%	49.87%	58.46%		31.87%
2,518,435	1,800,608	1,251,634	784,817	4,987,024	20,718,961	22,000,480
515,267	469,396	443,081	353,872	2,668,144		5,799,699
20.46%	26.07%	35.40%	45.09%	53.50%		26.36%

TABLE 5.4. RHMC ANALYSIS OF ADA, BAD-DEBT EXPENSES, BAD-DEBT WRITE-OFFS FOR THE TWELVE MONTHS ENDED DEC. 31, 2000.

	Opening Balance, ADA	Ending Balance, ADA*	Total Change in ADA
January	5,600,000	5,650,300	50,300
February	5,650,300	5,680,244	29,944
March	5,680,244	5,734,135	53,891
April	5,734,135	5,849,672	115,537
May	5,849,672	5,726,047	(123,625)
June	5,726,047	5,870,367	144,320
July	5,870,367	5,806,077	(64,290)
August	5,806,077	5,916,173	110,096
September	5,916,173	5,884,859	(31,314)
October	5,884,859	5,700,357	(184,502)
November	5,700,357	5,752,043	51,686
December	5,752,043	5,800,000	47,957
Totals	5,600,000	5,800,000	200,000

*As calculated by the detailed Allowance for Doubtful Accounts worksheet.

Importantly, the results of this monthly analysis are the amount of dollars that will be recorded as the ADA on the balance sheet. Because of this, it is imperative that the patient accounting manager and the finance administrators review the changes in the ADA monthly to determine causes for any significant change to the ADA. This review may well highlight good or bad changes within various payor categories that need to be corrected immediately.

Meanwhile, Table 5.4 represents the analysis of a complete ADA, bad-debt expense, bad-debt write-off, and recovery of bad debt. This schedule is prepared following completion of the detailed ADA calculations. There are some significant implications in this schedule. It is important to note that the bad-debt expense reported on the income statement is a function of the other three columns: the calculated ADA, as well as the actual bad-debt write-offs and actual recovery of bad-debt write-offs.

To prepare this schedule, the organization must have already recorded the actual write-off of patient accounts, according to the bad-debt write-off policy. In addition, it must also record any cash collected by the agencies engaged by the organization to perform intensive collection work on accounts of patients who did not pay their bills. Using this methodology, the result of the equation yields the actual bad-debt expense (also called provision for bad debts) that is recorded on the income statement.

Add Write-Offs	Less Recoveries	Subtotal, Net Write-Offs	Provision for Bad Debts (Bad-Debt Expense)
381,284	71,483	309,801	360,101
366,704	59,648	307,056	337,000
397,964	82,288	315,676	369,567
325,659	81,815	243,844	359,381
347,965	66,027	281,938	158,313
398,836	62,172	336,664	480,984
395,683	48,892	346,790	282,500
396,589	76,539	320,050	430,146
365,754	70,494	295,260	263,946
520,376	57,874	462,502	278,000
521,569	86,546	435,023	486,709
446,987	101,098	345,889	393,846
4,865,370	864,877	4,000,494	4,200,494

RHMC management and finance administration review these schedules in detail every month because of the schedule's importance to both the balance sheet and income statement. In addition, it is the best set of summary schedules available for administration to determine the adequacy of the reserve for bad debt, as well as the performance of the collection agencies being used to back up the organization's regular set of in-house collectors. Because these schedules involve two of the six most sensitive types of account, this is a critical monthly review that is heavily weighted in importance.

Calculation of Allowance for Contractual Adjustments

The other major allowance that reduces the gross receivable is the ACA. Like the ADA, the ACA is an estimate. In this case, it results from determining the amount of money in the gross receivable that will not convert to cash because of stipulations in contracts with the organization's various payors, particularly Medicare, Medicaid, and managed care. GAAP requires that "the provision for contractual adjustments and discounts be recognized on an accrual basis and deducted from gross service revenues to determine net service revenues" (AICPA, 1996).

Again, as stated in the health care audit guide (AICAP, 1996):

Amounts realizable from third-party payers for healthcare services are usually less than the provider's full established rates for those services. The realizable amounts may be determined by the following:

- Contractual agreement with other plans (such as Blue Cross plans, Medicare, Medicaid, or HMOs)
- Legislation or regulations (such as workers' compensation or no-fault insurance)
- Provider policy or practices (such as courtesy discounts to medical staff members and employees or other administrative adjustments).

Table 5.5 is the analysis that RHMC uses to determine its monthly ACA. There are several points that need to be made regarding this schedule.

First, the Medicare portion of the unbilled account is higher than the other categories because of specific rules and regulations involved in billing Medicare inpatient accounts. The largest portion of the unbilled category, in this case, is known as "discharged, not yet billed." The unbilled category is made up of different types of account: patients who are in-house (for example, in their hospital bed) at midnight of the balance sheet date, and those who have been discharged but whose bill has not yet been produced by the organization.

TABLE 5.5. RHMC ANALYSIS FOR ALLOWANCE FOR CONTRACTUAL ADJUSTMENTS FOR THE MONTH ENDED DEC. 31, 2000.

Inpatients	Medicare	Medicaid	Managed Care
Unbilled accounts (in-house and discharged, not yet billed)	$1,782,084	$107,285	$ 878,541
Billed accounts	n/a*	511,246	710,544
Subtotal	1,782,084	618,531	1,589,085
Contractual adjustment discount rate	57%	70%	35%
Allowance for contractual adjustment	$1,015,788	$432,972	$556,180
Outpatients			
Unbilled accounts (discharged, not yet billed only)	$1,239,377	$ 95,464	$1,501,256
Billed accounts	3,007,286	234,754	1,961,267
Subtotal	4,246,663	330,218	3,462,523
Contractual adjustment discount rate	55%	80%	26%
Allowance for contractual adjustment	$2,335,665	$264,174	$ 900,256

*No allowance is necessary for Medicare inpatient billed accounts because 100% of these accounts are automatically contractualized at the time of billing by the computer system's DRG grouper.

Second, only a portion of the inpatient managed care billed accounts are being written down to the ACA because many of these accounts have already been written down to their estimated contractual net expected receivable at the time of billing (see table 5.3). RHMC uses a special software program that generates the actual net revenue figure. The software emulates actual provisions of each managed care contract and then reviews each inpatient discharge for those provisions and automatically calculates the reimbursement. Therefore, no additional accrual for ACA is needed because the account has already been written down.

Third, the contractual adjustment discount rate is supposed to represent actual average of all accounts that have been processed over the past month. These amounts change from month to month, but on a small scale. A large change may occur if a high-volume managed care contract is signed at a discount rate that is significantly higher than the average. The other big reason a change may occur is a large change in Medicare reimbursement rules. This would usually happen on October 1 of any year, which is the beginning of the federal fiscal year.

Fourth, there is no in-house category for outpatients because, by their nature, they are meant to receive services on the day they are registered and should not be categorized as occupying a bed.

Fifth and finally, it is clear that there is no ACA for the accounts called "all other receivables" on the ADA schedule. These are primarily self-pay accounts and as such there is no formal discount contract between the organization and its patients. Thus there is no allowance, provision, or need for self-pay contractual adjustment.

The results of the monthly ACA are used to reduce the total balances on the ADA schedule before an allowance for bad debt is calculated. If this were not done, then the organization would be double-counting some of its discounts against gross receivable.

Once again, RHMC staff and management spend significant time on this analysis each month because of its effect on both the balance sheet and the income statement. Variance analyses are also performed across time periods and against various pay classes to establish whether there have been any measurable changes, and if so, where.

In summary, management of accounts receivable is a crucial part of the overall management of any healthcare organization. The responsibility for timely and efficient collection of cash and under significantly strict regulatory requirements is not for the faint of heart. RHMC has had the good fortune to retain the same PAM for the last several years. She has maintained her technical ability to manage through constant reading of industry literature and attendance at continuing education seminars throughout the year. The rapid pace of change in the industry has demanded continued vigilance, particularly in this area. RHMC has been reasonably successful thus far.

CHAPTER SIX

JUNE

Rick Samuelson, the president and chief executive officer of Ridgeland Heights Medical Center, is in a quandary. His thirty-five years of experience in health care organizations in general, fifteen of them at RHMC, are not helping him at the moment. The organization is about to begin its annual budget process, and he knows he faces a dilemma.

"Sam," he barks at his finance officer, "what's our chance of doing good financially next year? I'm pretty concerned about some of the trends that we've been experiencing over the past few years. After the Medicare Balanced Budget Act blew up our net revenues and affected the hospital, skilled nursing facility, and home health services, we still haven't recovered to the extent we should."

"Well, you're right. It's absolutely true that our bottom line eroded because of all those issues. In fact, as you know, the Medicare BBA issues are only a part of it. We have been having more and more problems negotiating what we feel are appropriate rates with managed care companies. We know they've been having their own problems with the claims they're paying for medical services. So along with the premium increases they've passed through to subscribers over the past couple of years, they're also trying to make it up by asking us for additional payment reductions."

"OK, but what are we going to do about the current financial issues and the future budget planning we have to do now?"

Sam is happy to respond to the question.

"There are only a few ways that we can have a positive impact on the bottom line. They're all tried-and-true methods, but none of them is easy. The best way to improve our operating margin, now and in the future, is to enhance our inpatient admissions and outpatient volume. That'll generate additional gross and net revenues. As long as our variable expenses are less than net revenues, our margins will improve."

"But, Sam, we haven't been able to make the kind of progress in the area that we want."

Sam has heard it before.

"Rick, I know that. First of all, we need to be more innovative in this regard. More volume means we need to gain market share from other providers, especially since the population of our service area isn't growing. Second, we haven't tried hard enough to implement cost reductions in a logical way, using some very specific cost analysis tools that highlight possible areas of improvement. Finally, we haven't attempted to perform process improvements in a meaningful and effective way. This could free up many of our revenue-producing departments to accept additional volume, leading to additional income."

"OK, you're right. We've had this conversation more than once. But in the past, you wanted to do this before our bottom line eroded, so it was hard to convince our stakeholders to take these issues seriously."

"Yeah, well, if we'd done some of these things previously, because the strategic financial plan predicted it, we'd be in better shape for the near future. In any case, those three areas are what we need to do to survive and thrive now and in the future."

June, in northern Illinois, is lovely. Spring has sprung with full force, and warm breezes are easily felt on the bare arms and legs of joggers and the pedestrians strolling leisurely through the parks around the region. Summer is just three weeks away, and vacation plans are in full swing. It is sometimes hard to get people to concentrate on their jobs as they discuss their getaway destinations.

That, however, is not the case at Ridgeland Heights Medical Center. Because its fiscal year ends on December 31, June is the month that the budget process starts in earnest for the upcoming year. The finance division staff, who are responsible for the entire budget process, have geared up for initializing this important function. The amount of work ahead is daunting when taken as a whole. As a result, the process is broken down into smaller pieces that are more easily digestible. Starting in June, the budget process will keep the finance and accounting staff occupied until just before New Year's Day.

Budget Preparation: The Beginning

June is the month that RHMC begins its annual rite of passage, the operating and capital budgets. In its logical sequence, the annual budget follows the strategic financial plan (discussed and described in Chapter Three), which follows preparation of the strategic plan. The logic of the sequence allows the organization to

- Express its vision and long-term goals in the strategic plan
- Express the best numerical forecasting in the five-year strategic financial plan
- Develop that into a projection or budget, one year into the future

There are several steps to preparing and presenting the annual budget. Exhibit 6.1 is a representation of the steps usually needed in preparing an operating budget. These twenty-four steps require four and six months, depending on philosophy. They involve managers in every facet of operations. In addition, a critical set of stakeholders who must be accessed, solicited, and appeased are the

---

EXHIBIT 6.1. THE PROCESS OF PREPARING AN OPERATING PLAN AND BUDGET.

Item No.	Task	Reasoning/Thinking for Task
Strategic Planning Segments		
1	Environmental statement	Analysis of the organization's current operating environment.
2	General objectives and policies	Provides the budgeting effort a uniform direction for optimal use of available resources. Objectives assume a macro view focusing on broad goals. Policies have a narrower focus, aiming at clarifying the details of budget preparation and establishing basic internal operating parameters.
3	Assumptions	Statements that project future events and the resulting future environment.
4	Operating policy decisions	Setting program priorities and establishing funding guidelines.
5	Operating objectives	Translates operating priorities into specific measurable goals that are obtainable within the budget period.
Administrative Segments		
6	Budget preparation manual	Describes the mechanics of preparing the operating plan and budget.
7	Projection package	Package of information that is transmitted for purposes of communicating either the raw data necessary for decision or actual decisions between levels of management.
8	Projection package approval	Volume estimates are reviewed from preceding perspective and the impact of such factors as: Changes in the demographic character of the organization's service area; Technological changes; Historical trends; Managed care penetration and stage of development are estimated.
9	Administrative package	Basic package for communicating budget preparation instructions and information to departmental line management.
10	Administrative package approval	Sign-off of administrative package to ensure that revisions are included and the package is complete.
Communications Segments		
11	General budget meeting	Introductory meeting designed to formally initiate the annual planning and budget preparation process for departmental management.
12	Technical budget meeting	Focuses on the specific mechanics of the budget procedures and budget preparation; this usually involves a series of meetings with the revenue-producing service areas.
Operational Planning Segments		
13	Administrative meetings, level of revenue-producing department	Objective is to translate the environmental statement, assumptions, operating policies, and objective decisions into projects and activities at the level of revenue-producing departments.

Item No.	Task	Reasoning/Thinking for Task
14	Decision package preparation	Departmental management develops decision packages that identify the new activities being requested with their costs and alternatives based upon the decisions made in 13 above.
15	Rank order of decision packages	Involves a series of consecutive meetings wherein succeeding levels of management integrate and rank-order the various decision packages prepared in 14 above.
16	Revenue budget preparation	Data from the projection package is used to calculate the initial revenue budget, using the current charge structure.

Budgeting Segments

Item No.	Task	Reasoning/Thinking for Task
17	Detailed specifications	Department management specifies in detail the resources needed to carry out approved projects; these resource needs are converted into actual dollars.
18	Tentative budget completion	This step organizes and aggregates the data developed in 17 above. This is basically a clerical and computational step. These expense totals now need to be compared to the projected revenues. Expense or capital budgets may now need to be revised.
19	Final administrative review	Senior administration makes a series of decisions that bring the two sets of budgets into balance.
20	Budget completion	Clerical steps needed to generate the final revenue, expense, and capital budgets. A cash flow budget should also be generated from this step.
21	Board approval	Presentation to the finance committee and the board of directors for approval to carry out this operating and capital plan in the following year.
22	Communication of budget approval to department management	This step involves feedback to the department managers of their final approved budget for the following year. They are expected to meet the goals set for: Volumes Gross revenues Net revenues Expenses Departmental operating margins
23	Implementation	Turning the budget into reality.
24	Feedback	Periodic feedback (usually monthly) to the department managers in the budget year that follows. This feedback involves: Statistical reports Financial reports Performance reports Variance reports

physicians linked to the organization, either in an employment capacity or in an affiliate relationship.

Budget Calendar

The planning tool that RHMC uses to design and maintain this annual project is a budget calendar. Separate calendars are prepared for both the operating budget and the capital budget. The calendars make time-frame expectations clear to all those individuals participating in the project. Table 6.1 is the operating budget calendar used by RHMC. It is divided into four columns, each having an important function:

1. *Responsible parties.* This column shows who is involved in each individual step.
2. *Activity.* This column represents each of the budgeting steps to be followed.
3. *Date.* This is the critical column. Each date listed must be met or else the whole budget process will be unsuccessful, and that is never allowed to happen. This column is monitored incessantly to avoid any slippage.
4. *Meeting time and location of meeting.* This column lets the responsible parties know when and where to show up.

There is a critical reason the dates on the budget calendars are never allowed to slip. The budget is a plan designed by management that must be approved by the board of directors, to allow management to operate the organization on a day-to-day basis. The board and its finance committee have their own calendars with future agendas that also are strictly adhered to. In the case of RHMC, the calendars have been designed so that all affected parties are aware well in advance of the crucial meeting dates and activities, to clear their calendar accordingly.

In Which Month Should the Budget Be Presented to the Board of Directors for Approval?

An important concept to note in preparing the budget calendar is the actual and total times required. Ultimately, the preparers and the reviewers must have the budget ready for the designated finance committee meeting that precedes the board meeting where final approval will be requested.

An interesting question that this often raises is, "Which month before the beginning of the new year is most appropriate for presentation to the board for approval?" The answer is that it depends on the particular culture and needs of each organization. Still, there are some guidelines and issues that can be raised to try to answer the question.

The most common time frame used by health care organizations is to present the budgets in the first, second, or third month before the new budget year begins. There are pros and cons to each time frame (see Table 6.2). The organizational culture, in this regard, can be conservative or liberal, from the perspective of the board, senior administrators, or the finance division preparers.

The board may be more or less comfortable having the budget approval under its belt early rather than late, so that they can get on with other important business. Or they might like to know that the budget package they are approving is based on the absolutely latest volume information available. The finance preparers, on the other hand, aware of the mountains of data that go into preparation, and the amount of work still required to produce reports for the department managers, will opt for the longest time available before the new year begins. Finally, senior administrators are usually neutral, opting for the time frame that causes the least disruption on the part of department managers, without denying the wishes of the board.

Budget Calendar Time Frame

Once it is clear which month the budget needs to be ready by for the finance committee and the board, it is then important to determine all the steps that need to be taken to prepare and complete the budget. The RHMC budget calendar summarizes all the major activities that need to be completed.

Now, to determine when the very first budget steps have to be started in any given budget year, it is imperative to know three things:

1. The date that the budget must be presented to the board
2. The amount of time needed between budget activities
3. The amount of time needed during each activity

A key concept in budget timetable preparation is knowing the date the budget is needed and then calculating backward from that date. In the case of RHMC, which has a fiscal year end of December 31, the key dates revolve backward from the month in which the board wants to approve it. At RHMC, there is a tradition of going to the board for approval during the October finance committee-and-board cycle. There is a practical reason for this. At RHMC, the board and its committees meet only every other month, beginning in February and continuing in April, June, August, October, and December. Therefore, the only possible choice for this organization is October or December; they have concluded that the December time frame does not afford them enough time to prepare the budget results after board approval.

TABLE 6.1. RHMC 2002 BUDGET CALENDAR, OPERATING BUDGET.

Responsible Party	Activity	2001 Dates	Meeting Time and Location
Executive and administrative staff, selected nursing and ancillary department managers, finance staff	Kick-off meeting for volume projections	June 1	Meeting Room 1, 2:00–3:30 p.m.
Executive and administrative staff, finance staff	Approve projected 2001 and budgeted 2002 admissions, length of stay, and patient days by service; approve projected 2001 and budgeted 2002 outpatient trends by ancillary service	June 26	Meeting Room 1, 2:30–4:00 p.m.
Finance staff	Issue 2002 operating budget calendar	July 1	
Finance staff	Compute gross revenues and contractual adjustments	July 11	
Executive and administrative staff, finance staff, accounting staff	Review salary and nonsalary assumptions: Merit increase percentage Full-time equivalent (FTE) target level Benefit costs Inflation by category	July 14	Meeting Room 1, 10:00 a.m.–12:00 p.m.
Finance administration, finance staff	Review gross revenues and contractual adjustments; validate payor mix	July 15	Finance Department conference room, 12:30–2:00 p.m.
Executive and administrative staff, finance staff	Review 2002 budgeted income statement developed by Finance Department based on prior high-level assumptions; determine price increase targets; revise salary and nonsalary assumptions	July 18	Meeting Room 1, 8:00–10:00 a.m.
Finance staff	Issue 2001 projected and 2002 budget worksheets to department managers	July 25	

The board of a health care organization may be constituted to meet every month, every two months (as with RHMC), or as infrequently as every three months. Again, it depends on the organization's needs and culture. For a board that meets monthly, the likely approval point is the November meeting, which has the most balanced set of pros and cons. It is also possible for a board that meets every

Responsible Party	Activity	2001 Dates	Meeting Time and Location
Finance staff	Budget training	Various	Accounting Department conference room
Department managers	Complete budget work-sheets and return to appropriate vice presidents and administrators	Aug. 15	
Appropriate vice presidents and administrators	Review and finalize depart-mental budget revisions	Aug. 18–28	
Appropriate vice presidents and administrators	Return budget worksheet to Finance Department	Aug. 29	
Executive and administrative staff, finance staff	Validate or adjust 2002 budget projections; pre-liminary approval of budget	Sept. 9	Meeting Room 1, 1:00–3:00 p.m.
Executive and administrative staff, finance staff	Final review and approval of 2002 budget; review human resource com-mittee packet	Sept. 17	Meeting Room 1, 9:00–11:00 a.m.
Finance staff, executive and administrative staff (as appropriate for document and packet review)	Prepare drafts for human resource committee: First draft (Sept. 12) Final comments (Sept. 14) Final draft (Sept. 19) Mailing date (Sept. 26) Committee meeting (Oct. 3)		
Finance staff, executive and administrative staff (as appropriate for document and packet review)	Prepare drafts for finance committee: First draft (Sept. 30) Final comments (Oct. 2) Final draft (Oct. 7) Mailing date (Oct. 14) Committee meeting (Oct. 21)		

other month to set its schedule so that the cycle constitutes January, March, May, July, September, and November. This would obviously allow the organization to use the more practical November meeting for presentation of the budget. Finally, it is possible for the board and finance committee to hold a special meeting once a year, in November, with an agenda devoted only to the budget, if they so choose.

TABLE 6.2. IN WHICH MONTH SHOULD THE BUDGET BE PRESENTED TO THE BOARD OF DIRECTORS FOR APPROVAL?

Presenting the Budget 70 to 90 Days Before the Next Budget Year Begins

Pros	Cons
1. There is more time to prepare and deliver the results of the approved budget to the department managers.	1. The data and information used to prepare the budget, particularly the volumes, are not as current as most of the managers and administrators would like in projecting subsequent-year financials.
2. There is more time that can be used if the finance committee or the board decides not to approve the budget for any reason.	

Presenting the Budget 40 to 60 Days Before the Next Budget Year Begins

Pros	Cons
1. There is a reasonable amount of time available for the finance division to prepare and deliver the results of the approved budget to the department managers.	1. There may not be enough time, before the new year begins, to produce a remedial budget plan and package if the board decides not to approve the budget.
2. The data and information used to prepare the budget, particularly the volumes, are appropriately current, yet not too stale.	

Presenting the Budget 10 to 30 Days Before the Next Budget Year Begins

Pros	Cons
1. The data and information used to prepare the budget, particularly the volumes, are the most current available.	1. There is no time to prepare and deliver the results of the approved budget to the department managers before the new year begins.
	2. There is no time remaining to produce a remedial budget for the board before the new year begins if the proposed budget is rejected.

Budget Calendar Steps

Now that the end date is known and all the designated budget activities have been counted backward to determine the start date, it is important to know there is a definite order of activity to be followed so as to produce the best possible budget results. Certain activities must be performed before others. To proceed, several budget steps must be accomplished in the kick-off month of June. The calendar lists these opening-month activities in June:

- June 1: kick-off meeting for volume projections (hold meeting)
- June 26: approve projected 1998 and budgeted 1999 admission, length of stay, and patient days by service
- Also June 26: approve projected 1998 and budgeted 1999 projected outpatient trends by ancillary services (hold meeting)

These activities are discussed later in this chapter.

Volume Issues

Many activities are listed on the budget calendar. The most important one is to determine projected and budgeted inpatient and outpatient volume. Absolutely no other projection is as crucial to the overall budget outcome as volume. All of the gross and net revenues, as well as all of the variable expenses, are a function of the increase or decrease budgeted for volume.

Several methods can be used to budget volumes in a health care institution:

1. Historical trends
2. Demographic changes
3. New services
4. Physician issues and inputs
5. Wishful thinking

Historical Perspective

The most common method used to changes in project and budget volume is to review the current volumes and those in the recent past (say, the previous two or three years) and extend that trend line into the future. This forecasting can be done through regression analysis. Although this is the most common method used by health care institutions, it is fraught with danger. As they say in mutual fund advertising, past results are no guarantee of future earnings. Nothing that happened in the past (even just last month) may have any bearing on the future. It is important to be aware of past volume, but the organization also needs to add many other characteristics to its analysis—demographic changes, new services, physician inputs—to be confident that the budgeted volumes have a reasonable chance of being attained.

Demographic Changes

Adding any known or suspected demographic changes to the trend in historical volume contributes significantly to refining the validity of the budget. It is imperative that the organization be aware of population change in its service areas. This is necessary to redetermine community needs and evaluate which, if any, programs must be expanded, contracted, established, or closed.

Demographic changes can have wide-ranging impact on volume and the success or failure of various program offerings. For example, let's say that a real estate developer has just bought up a one-thousand-acre tract of farmland in the organization's service area, with the express intent of building two thousand single-family housing units meant to be marketed to young, growing families. It is important for the organization to be aware of this development. It can then attempt to determine inpatient and outpatient volume increases that may accrue to pediatrics, obstetrics, and labor room services and budget accordingly.

Another example of a demographic change that could decrease volume is closure of a major manufacturing plant in town. The health care organization, which may have come to rely on the volume and revenue generated from plant employees, now has to downsize services to reflect possible reduction in the area population. Any and all known demographic changes should be reflected in short-term budgeting. It is essential that the organization employ someone to monitor these shifts and report them back to the administration and the finance staff promptly. This function is usually the responsibility of the planning and marketing departments.

New Services

Another set of major items needing consideration in the historical perspective are volumes for any new services or programs, such as diabetes, sickle cell anemia, or chest pain clinics, that the organization has planned to add in the upcoming budget year. For example, adding an MRI system is supposed to produce new volume for the radiology department. Because most new services are required to present a pro forma projection of profit and loss before approval of the service, the volume will be available to add to the budget. In reviewing the pro forma for the MRI in Chapter One, it was shown that volume projections are the critical driver of revenues and expenses. Critical evaluation was performed to determine the most likely volume projection. This is necessary for any new service proposed and accepted.

Physician Issues and Input

Another element highly critical to successful volume budgeting is awareness of current physician satisfaction and any issues that may be affecting usage of services. All patient volumes are a function of physician referral to the health care organization. Physicians are, by their nature, analytical and skeptical. Their long years of training and their responsibility for a patient's life or death make them very demanding. They want the health care organization to be highly efficient and give them the latest state-of-the-art equipment so they can provide the highest level of patient care.

Physician issues can often complicate completion of the operating budget. It is important for the administration to constantly monitor the state of employed or affiliated physician office practices for any demographic, managed care, or structural changes, which could have an impact on the ability of the physician to continue a former referral pattern to the organization. Additionally, many physicians split their practice between two or more health care providers. It is important for the organization to know which physicians are splitters. Because they often have to drive between their practices, which can take a lot of time and effort, some of these physicians eventually decide to give it up. It is a great advantage for an organization to be the recipient of the splitter's full-time attention. This could have a major positive effect on the budget year volume. Conversely, should a competitor organization get all the business, the budget volume would have to be adjusted downward.

Wishful Thinking

A concept that is sometimes used in volume budgeting is wishful thinking. This is often employed as the means to balance a budget that does not come out right the first time. If the budgeted bottom line does not meet board expectations using the techniques we have described, wishful thinking may be employed to boost the volumes and revenues accordingly. Unfortunately, because it is not based on any established method, it is unsupportable. However, this does not always stop health care administrators from using it. Finance managers and their staff should be ever vigilant in attempting to discourage this form of volume budgeting. If used, it will only delay the inevitable decisions to properly size the institution.

June 1: Volume Kick-Off Meeting

With all of this information as a backdrop, the finance division staff assigned to the budget calls a meeting with administrative staff and selected ancillary department managers to discuss upcoming volume issues. The first thing they look at is the trend of historical inpatient and outpatient volumes. The key inpatient volume drivers are admission and length-of-stay statistics, which result in the total number of patient days. The key outpatient driver is usually the number of tests or examinations performed.

During this meeting, the clinical managers and the finance staff review historical trends, discuss the current status, and speculate on the future prospects for volumes. The primary issues are these:

- Any change in physician practices involving physicians currently on active staff
- Any known additional physician practices that may be entering the service area
- Any additional services that may be added based on newly acquired technologies
- Any other change in services that adds or subtracts volume

All of these items are instructive but not definitive. They aid the department manager in projecting next year's volumes. Still, the administration may well desire a specific set of budgeted volumes to achieve a certain measure of profitability. If all of these items do not equal the desired changes, the managers have to determine additional steps to achieve them. Generally, this means greater marketing and promotion within or outside the service area, more focused managed care negotiation leading to additional patient load or improved level of service, and the results of customer satisfaction in attracting new patients to the institution. All of these issues are discussed and debated during the volume kick-off meeting on June 1. No specific conclusions are drawn, but the meeting creates a framework for subsequent action.

June 26: Approve Projected 2001 and Budgeted 2002 Inpatient and Outpatient Volumes

Subsequent to the kick-off meeting, the finance staff hold several one-on-one meetings with various clinical managers to solicit specific feedback regarding where managers believe volume in their departments is heading. All of this input is incorporated into the analysis presented to the administration during the June 26 budget meeting to approve subsequent period volumes. The finance administrator presents the analysis developed by the staff to the assembled members. The clinical managers' assumptions are summarized, distilled, and explained at this time.

These assumptions are debated and discussed. Some assumptions may appear to be too high or too low, depending on the assembled members' knowledge and experience. The administrators are always interested in understanding any new service lines or ideas from physicians that have been projected by their clinical managers. In general, though, the budget assumptions presented by the finance staff are approved. Any changes generated at the meeting are incorporated into the next iteration of the budget package.

Table 6.3 shows the organization's 2001 projected actual volumes as well as those they are budgeting for 2002 by inpatient unit. Similarly, Table 6.4 illustrates 2001 and 2002 budgeted outpatient visits. This is the result of discussion involving all of the items described.

Overall, the clinical managers, along with the administration, believe that their overall inpatient days will increase 9 percent next year, while outpatient visits will increase 8.3 percent. These volume changes are fully incorporated into gross and net revenue budgets as well as the variable expense budget calculations. The one warning that always emerges from this meeting is that these projections and volumes are subject to change depending on the budgeted operating margins that emerge from using these numbers.

Capital Budgeting (June)

In the meantime, while the operating budget time line is being established and on its way to implementation, the capital budget process has also commenced. Because the operating budget bottom line includes depreciation expense, it is essential that the capital budget be completed prior to completion of the operating budget. The capital budget determines the capital equipment to be acquired; buildings to be renovated, built, or leased; amounts to be spent; and the estimated useful life assigned to each of these assets. These elements allow the finance staff to determine the depreciation expense that must be included in the following year.

In Chapter Three, capital plan development concepts were reviewed in some detail as they relate to the strategic financial plan. The various types of capital assets available for acquisition were discussed in that chapter. During the strategic planning process, the amount of money available for the annual capital budget was determined. Because the funding amounts and sources are already known, the main purpose of the annual capital budget is to identify the specific capital items to be acquired. The problem in almost all health care organizations is which capital projects should be funded. It is a classic question, and there have been few good solutions over the years. The issue is to determine reasonably and efficiently how to allocate scarce resources—money available for capital.

TABLE 6.3. RHMC 2001 PROJECTED AND 2002 BUDGETED INPATIENT VOLUMES.

		Admissions		
	Number of Beds	2001 Projected	2002 Budget	Percentage Variance
Medical, surgical	120	2,700	2,800	3.7%
Intensive care	24	1,800	1,900	5.6%
Pediatrics	10	600	660	10.0%
Maternity	24	2,000	2,200	10.0%
Births	26	1,950	2,145	10.0%
Psychiatric	20	1,000	1,200	20.0%
Skilled nursing facility	30	800	840	5.0%
Totals	254	10,850	11,745	8.2%

The most common method, past and present, is characterized by decision making in the proverbial smoke-filled room. Administrators would get together once a year with a wish list of items requested by department management. The list includes requests from various physicians who spend their time in those particular departments. Despite the amount of money being requested here, financial analysis may not be performed or required. In general, the administrator with the most clout, the loudest voice, the most enthusiastic performance may get a pet project approved, while worthy projects are bypassed because of a less-than-optimal backroom performance by its administrative champion.

TABLE 6.4. RHMC 2001 PROJECTED AND 2002 BUDGETED OUTPATIENT VISITS.

	Visits		
	2001 Projected	2002 Budget	Percentage Variance
Emergency department	19,000	20,000	5.3
Outpatient surgery	4,500	5,000	11.1
Same-day surgery	3,700	4,000	8.1
Observation patients	1,950	2,000	2.6
Home health services	26,000	30,000	15.4
Other outpatients	112,000	120,000	7.1
Totals	167,150	181,000	8.3

Patient Days			Length of Stay		
2001 Projected	2002 Budget	Percentage Variance	2001 Projected	2002 Budget	Percentage Variance
13,000	14,000	7.7%	4.81	5.00	3.8%
6,500	7,220	11.1%	3.61	3.80	5.2%
1,500	1,716	14.4%	2.50	2.60	4.0%
4,000	4,400	10.0%	2.00	2.00	0.0%
3,900	4,290	10.0%	2.00	2.00	0.0%
6,500	8,160	25.5%	6.50	6.80	4.6%
8,800	8,400	−4.5%	11.00	10.00	−9.1%
44,200	48,186	9.0%	4.07	4.10	0.7%

This is not, nor has it ever been, a good situation. Yet it persists, first because the powerful have had no incentive to change it and second because no really good alternative that incorporates financial and nonfinancial criteria has been presented to the industry. At RHMC, the finance administrators were tired of the infighting and lack of consistency exhibited at this annual rite of frustration. On the lookout for a better way to develop and control the capital funding process, they were recently introduced to a new method of criteria-based capital budgeting.

In a nutshell, the solutions involve innovative organizational processes with supporting quantitative evaluation tools. Criteria-based capital budgeting aids the health care organization in its need to allocate capital to maintain state-of-the-art clinical and facilities equipment while concurrently developing ambulatory facilities, physician networks, and information technology. It also involves many decision makers from across the organization as part of an ongoing strategic planning process. Finally, it allows the organization to objectively evaluate capital proposals against established criteria and against proposals competing for the same scarce resources. The following is a summary of the criteria-based capital budgeting process.

1. Evaluate decision criteria.
2. Classify proposed expenditures.
3. Collect information.
4. Evaluate proposals.
5. Set strategic priority weights.
6. Calculate value scores.
7. Sort proposals on benefit-cost ratio.

TABLE 6.5. RHMC 2002 BUDGET CALENDAR, CAPITAL BUDGET.

Parties Involved	Activity	2001 Dates	Meeting Time and Location
Executive and administrative staff, finance staff	Validate strategic plan criteria	June 1	Meeting Room 2, 9:00–10:00 a.m.
Proposal reviewers, accounting staff, facilities management, information systems management, materials management	Training for all staff assigned to review capital proposals	June 10	Meeting Room 2, 2:00–4:00 p.m.
Proposal writers, all department management	Review the capital budgeting software; train all department management on the data elements required for a clean capital budget request	June 13, June 20	Meeting Room 2, 3:00–4:00 p.m.
Proposal writers, all department management	Allow department managers access to capital budget software upon completion of training	June 20	
Proposal writers, all department management	Submission of 2002 capital budget by department managers through electronic software located on managers' desktop	July 11	
Finance staff	Review all capital proposals for completeness of all required information fields	July 12–23	
Proposal reviewers	Capital proposals reviewed within the established time frames; the review is performed online at the reviewer's desktop	July 24– Aug. 6	Reviewer's office computer
Proposal evaluators	Detailed discussion of all proposals over $100,000 and training of all proposal evaluators	Aug. 11	Meeting Room 2, 1:30–5:00 p.m.

Table 6.5 shows RHMC's budget calendar with all of these concepts incorporated. In addition, the calendar is designed to run concurrently with the operating budget and finish in time to be presented simultaneously. The key characteristic of the budget is incorporation of the key strategic plan criteria. These criteria become the principal drivers of the capital decision process. Rather than decisions based on the gut, in the old smoke-filled rooms, the organization now has a criteria-based capital decision process.

Parties Involved	Activity	2001 Dates	Meeting Time and Location
Pool evaluators	Discussion of pool proposals: Information systems 9:00–10:30 a.m. Construction and renovation 10:30 a.m.– 12:00 p.m. Patient care 12:30– 2:00 p.m. Medical technology 2:00–3:30 p.m. Market development 3:30–5:00 p.m.	Aug. 12	Meeting Room 2
Proposal evaluators	Evaluate proposals online at the reviewer's desktop	Aug. 12–15	Evaluator's office computer
Pool evaluators	Pool consensus meetings: Information systems 9:00–10:30 a.m. Construction and renovation 10:30–12:00 p.m. Patient care 12:30– 2:00 p.m. Medical technology 2:00–3:30 p.m. Market development 3:30–5:00 p.m.	Aug. 22–25	Meeting Room 2, various times (see attachment)
Proposal evaluators	Proposal consensus meeting, all proposals over $100,000	Aug. 25	Meeting Room 2, 3:00–5:00 p.m.
Proposal and pool evaluators	Revise ratings, if necessary, on the reviewer's desktop	Aug. 26–28	Evaluator's office computer
Proposal evaluators	Meeting to discuss results of evaluations; final review of 2002 capital budget	Sept. 4	Meeting Room 2, 9:00–10:00 a.m.

In the case of RHMC, the administration has to first validate its strategic plan criteria. Although an organization with board-approved strategic plan criteria should be making operational decisions on this basis, such is not always the case. Health care organizations often give lip service to the strategic plan without making financial resources available to achieve stated goals. In the criteria-based capital decision process, the strategic plan criteria create the foundation for ultimate outcomes: which capital assets are funded.

The remaining steps in the June capital budget calendar involve training various staff, both technical and administrative, on their roles. If the individual is a proposal reviewer, for instance, she is trained to ensure that each capital proposal contains all of the data required before it can be moved on to the proposal evaluator. The proposal reviewer cares about the technical aspects of the capital request, such as whether it involves certain tasks:

- It requires additional consideration (electrical, facilities)
- It needs special computer hook-ups or special training for the technical staff (information technology)
- It necessitates special negotiations on price or contract terms (materials management)
- It creates special funding requirements (accounting)

The proposal evaluators care about each of the proposals, how it stands up on its own merits, how it compares to all the other projects on a criteria basis, and whether the organization is well served in total commitment to the strategic plan.

Both groups are trained in the month of June on use of the software that resides on their desktop personal computers. The software itself is on a computer server attached to the organization's local area network (LAN). Every individual involved in the process completes his role by accessing the LAN. Using this software at RHMC creates a highly efficient situation. Everyone has access to the same timely information. Because the process eliminates paper, all proposals are consistently presented to the evaluator, are easy for the accounting staff to administer, and facilitate ongoing updating of each project by the proposal writer and the evaluator.

As the month of June moves forward, these initial steps in the capital budget are performed. In later months, the meat of the capital budgeting process becomes more evident.

The training steps allow the finance staff to properly instruct department managers in how to use the system to input all the required elements for each capital request. Upon completion of this training in June, the managers are given access to the actual software on their PCs. They are then expected to submit all of their capital budgets back to the finance staff by July 11.

Accounting and Finance Department Responsibilities

Lost in the shuffle of all the fundamental issues that have been reported is some of the routine business performed by the accounting and finance department. In many health care organizations (as highlighted at the end of Chapter Five), the accounting department is responsible for preparing an accurate and timely financial statement. In addition, it is also responsible for preparing and paying all the employees through the payroll function and all the trade vendors through the accounts payable function. It is also accountable for all financial analyses (which usually include the cost accounting function), maintenance of the price list (from which gross revenue is determined), and the reimbursement function (preparation of the Medicare cost report) and the budget. Here is a summary of the major responsibilities of the accounting department:

General Accounting

- Capture of all of the organization's financial transactions during each accounting period (usually monthly), carried out through use of paper accounting transactions or through an electronic interface to subsidiary ledgers and journals
- Production of accurate, timely, organizationwide financial statements
- Collection of information, completion and submission of all IRS tax returns, whether for-profit or not-for-profit returns
- Preparation and facilitation of financial analysis for the external auditors
- Facilitation of all appropriate internal auditing functions

Accounts Payable

- Timely collection of all invoices from trade vendors
- Three-way matching of purchase orders, receiving dock receipts, and invoices to validate that all goods were authorized for purchase, were received, and are being billed by the vendor correctly
- Timely payment to trade vendors within terms of payment, or sooner if a discount for prompt payment is being granted

Payroll

- Collection of all payroll hours being requested and authorized for payment during each of the organization's payroll periods; this may be carried out through paper time cards or electronic time and attendance systems
- Validation and verification of all payroll hours, determining that all payroll policies and procedures were applied correctly by all of the department managers
- Timely payment of salaries and wages to employees
- Timely payment to pension plans

Budgeting

- Development and timely completion of the organization's operating, capital, and cash budgets
- Compilation and submission of all board-level budget packages

Strategic Financial Planning

- Development of the five-year strategic financial plan
- Development of the five-year capital needs analysis and plan

Reimbursement

- Completion of Medicare and Medicaid annual cost reports
- Coordination of all government audits and reports, including census reports
- Modeling of all new and revised managed care contracts, to improve negotiation
- Monthly analysis of contractual adjustments
- Maintenance of highly accurate net revenue calculations for financial analysis
- Maintenance of the charge master (price list), and annual analysis of potential and actual price increase

Financial Analysis and Decision Support

- Development and maintenance of the cost accounting system, including determination of variable and fixed costs and direct and indirect costs
- Maintenance and reporting from the decision support system; this allows operating managers to have the financial information needed to make proper decisions
- Development of all pro forma financial analysis
- Development of all other financial analysis
- Coordination in gathering all data required by various health care associations and rating agencies (American Hospital Association, state and local health care associations, Standard & Poor's, Moody's)

Other Responsibilities

- Processing of property and casualty insurance programs
- Monitoring of the pension plan and program; accounting coordination with the actuary assigned to the plan

It is hard to say which of the items on the list are most important, but it is no understatement to suggest that being late with the payroll checks, even by ten minutes, is the quickest way to lose the confidence of the entire organization. This would be true of the chief executive officer all the way down to the nonskilled staff. Missing a payroll deadline causes all kinds of trouble between the organization and its employees. Even when there is clear and direct communication about the cause of the problem, rumors begin to run rampant. It is vital not to miss a payroll. There are only a few reasons the payroll would ever be late, and two that are somewhat common. First, the computer may break down. This is not likely, but it is possible. Payroll systems are extremely mature and stable. They were one of the first applications designed for computers more than forty years ago. Still, anything can happen. Good management suggests building redundancy into computerized systems. This could mean paying for a duplicate system and keeping it available if and when the initial system goes down. Or it could mean creating manual downtime procedures, which are typically less expensive than an automated solution but cause more work in the event they are needed.

The second (unfortunately) common reason for ever being late on payroll is if an organization runs out of money. It has been known to happen in some organizations having either temporary or long-term financial difficulty. This is a much more problematic situation than just having the computer break down.

Not paying employees on time has numerous detrimental impacts on the organization as well as the employees. Most employees count on their paychecks to meet basic needs for themselves and their families, such as paying for rent, food, clothing, and transportation. If their paychecks are not available as expected, particularly if they already know that the organization is having financial difficulties, they begin to question the long-term viability of the organization. This inevitably leads to the staff looking for new jobs in other organizations, which begins a negative cycle of staff defection that weakens an already shaky situation.

Good management in this situation suggests that the payroll is always the first payment priority. This seems obvious, but as a practical matter it is not always easy. For example, though it is possible to delay payment to trade vendors that supply the organization with medical and surgical supplies, there are times when those vendors demand payment or threaten not to ship supplies that may be needed for surgical cases on the schedule for tomorrow.

The other situation that a financially stressed organization should never allow itself to become involved in is not paying the government for withheld payroll taxes. It must always be remembered in collecting these payroll taxes for various government agencies, the organization is acting as the government's agent. These funds cannot be used to pay for anything else, including medical supplies or the payroll itself. Payroll taxes are usually owed to the government within two to three days of payroll distribution. Penalties and interests are assessed immediately following that time period. Also, it is important to note that the administrators and any other staff who are responsible for making decisions when to pay the payroll taxes are personally liable for the taxes, penalties, and interest if the organization is unable to satisfy the debt. This is true even if the organization or the individuals successfully discharge other debts in a bankruptcy proceeding.

June Finance Committee Special Agenda Items

The June meeting of the finance committee provides another opportunity for management to present important information.

Human Resources Report

There are several reasons for presenting the report of the board-level human resource committee at the June finance committee meeting. Most important is to allow management to present analyses of the level of local and regional salaries and employee fringe benefits to the committee, which is charged with making recommendations and approving annual changes in these areas.

It is important to have goals related to this requirement. There are significant issues surrounding recruitment and retention policies. RHMC strives to maintain a certain level of compensation and benefits compared to the rest of the region. It is able to make this decision by accessing a variety of local and regional health care associations and labor bureaus from other industries. It is then able to determine whether or not it is maintaining the desired percentile compensation level.

The human resource committee and human resource administrator are aware that it is in the organization's best interest to maintain a competitive position in the marketplace. In fact, many human resource professionals would prefer that their organization take an aggressive position in the marketplace, especially if it can be afforded. This allows the organization to recruit the best potential candidates, which helps to reduce the turnover rate, lower expenditures for help wanted advertisements, and improve overall employee morale.

The report given to the human resource committee in June is preliminary. It allows the committee to understand the current levels in the marketplace and ask any relevant questions. Committee members come together again in September to be asked to approve the levels recommended by management in final development of the budget.

Pension Status and Actuary Report Review

Once a year, RHMC's management gives an update on the organization's pension plan to the finance committee. This is important because the board has a fiduciary responsibility to its employees to maintain the pension funds in a sound manner while ensuring that the funds earn a return appropriate to the pension portfolio's risk. The finance committee is interested in whether or not the market value of the pension assets continues to exceed the present value of all accrued benefits. So long as this is the case, the organization is not in an underfunded position with respect to its defined benefit pension plan.

EXHIBIT 6.2. RHMC PENSION STATUS, 2001 ACTUARIAL REPORT.

The report of our actuarial consultant was updated effective January 1, 2001, for the defined benefit plan. The following key items are highlighted compared to the prior year's results.

1. Market value of assets increased by $3 million from $23 million on 1/1/00 to $26 million on 1/1/01.
2. Present value of all accrued benefits increased by $1 million from $20 million to $21 million.

   The present value of all accrued benefits is composed of:

	1/1/00	1/1/01
Active vested employees	$ 7,000,000	$ 7,400,000
Active nonvested employees	1,000,000	1,100,000
Retired employees	8,000,000	8,300,000
Terminated vested employees	4,000,000	4,200,000
Totals	$20,000,000	$21,000,000

3. Assets over accrued benefits increased by $2 million from $7 million to $9 million.
4. Normal cost (defined as the amount that is required to fund the benefits expected to be earned in the current year) increased by $40,000 from $680,000 to $720,000.
5. Normal cost as a percentage of compensation decreased by 0.10 from 2.40 to 2.30.
6. The minimum required contributions for 1999, 2000, and 2001 are $400,000, $700,000, and $0.
7. Actual beneficiary payments in 2000 were $800,000. Expected beneficiary payments in 2001 are $840,000.
8. Pension expense for the accounting years ending December 31, 2000, and 2001 were $600,000 and $750,000 respectively.

Exhibit 6.2 highlights the items of major interest to the finance committee. Presented in this format every year, the report helps the finance committee understand various aspects of pension obligations, including minimum and maximum funding requirements established by the federal government's ERISA laws (established in the Employee Retirement Income Security Act of 1974). It also includes the actuarially determined net periodic pension costs to be recorded on the income statement, as stipulated by Statement of Financial Accounting Standards (SFAS) number 87 as well as the present value of accumulated plan benefits (stipulated under SFAS no. 35).

Because the ERISA and SFAS methodologies are different, technically complex, complicated, and required, the annual report to the finance committee is meant to be a simplified analysis. RHMC's finance officer verbally reports on some of the key assumptions used as input by the actuary to produce the results.

Some of the key assumptions are the discount rate used, the expected rate of return on the plan's investments, and the expected rate of compensation increases.

In this case, the finance committee is pleased that the annual pension report shows an increase in assets over accrued benefits. The members are additionally pleased to learn that according to the previous funding level and interest income earnings over the past year, they will not be required to pay any cash into the pension fund next year.

CHAPTER SEVEN

JULY

"Dad, you were right. This is a long story. Is it over yet?" asks the reasonably perplexed eight-year-old Susie.

Sam takes a deep breath. He wants to explain the story in the simplest of terms but is apparently having little success at the moment. All he can say is, *"Oh, come on, honey. This story is just getting interesting. There's so much more to it than I've already told you."*

She smiles—such a cute kid.

"I'm glad you've been telling this to me as a bedtime story. It sure has helped me get to sleep a lot easier. I think I understand some of what you've told me. I guess I never knew how your place made money. I didn't know that your company had to make money so you could get paid. That's pretty cool. But I still don't understand why your company doesn't get paid all the money you charge to people when you take care of them. I know that when we go to the supermarket, we have to pay the lady at the checkout counter for the food and stuff we have in our cart."

"You're so right, and that's pretty perceptive of you."

"Dad, what does perceptive *mean?"*

"Oh, never mind; don't worry about that. In any case, I do have to pay the lady at the checkout counter the amount of money that she rang up on her cash register. But what you're forgetting is that some of the things we bought were already discounted by the store or by the people who made the food and gave it to the store to sell. My company is doing the same thing. We're agreeing to discount our services to the people who are paying for them—the insurance companies. The big difference between the supermarket and us is that we don't have any shelves to put our discounted prices on. Another difference is that we may only give those discounts to certain people who have insurance from companies that want to make a deal with us, not to everybody. It's kind of like people in the supermarket who have coupons. They pay less than other people for the exact same food because they have coupons."

"I think I get some of it. But from the way you've been telling the story, it still seems unfair. It sounds like they just want to pay you a lot less than you want from them," says the still perplexed youngster.

"Yeah, it's true that some companies want to pay us less. But that's probably OK for our family. You see, part of the reason that my company pays me is to make sure that they know how much money we can discount and still have a certain amount left over at the end of the year."

"Well, I sure am glad that you like doing it, because I'm not sure it sounds like a lot of fun to me."

Warm breezes waft off Lake Michigan, blowing thin, wispy clouds against a high, light blue sky. Sunbathers and sunburners are lying out across a hot, white sandy beach. Summer is in full swing in the northern climes. Young and old alike enjoy the nice change in the weather. They know that it is fleeting. Winter is always just around the corner, waiting to bring its cold arctic blasts down on the town.

So there is always great enjoyment this time of the year. Schools are out, temperatures are in the eighties, and for many vacation has begun or will begin soon. The reality rarely meets or exceeds expectations, but the psychology of summer is having its dazzling effect. People around town are smiling easily; the pace of life has slowed as many stop to enjoy the weather. That is, for all but the finance staff at Ridgeland Heights Medical Center.

Budget Preparation: The Middle Months

July is the month when the budget becomes the top priority of the accounting and finance department. June was devoted to preliminary work, but July is when the heavy lifting begins. There are several critical meetings scheduled that shape the financial prognostications for the upcoming year. The July operating budget calendar is abundant with weighty issues:

- July 1: Issue 2000 operating budget calendar
- July 11: Compute gross revenues and contractual adjustments
- July 14: Review salary and nonsalary assumptions (hold meeting)
- July 15: Review gross revenues and contractual adjustments and validate payor mix (hold meeting)
- July 18: Review 2000 budgeted income statement, determine price increase targets, and revise salary and nonsalary assumptions (hold meeting)
- July 25: Issue 1999 projected and 2000 budgeted worksheets to department managers

All of these steps require a great deal of effort; the finance staff are prepared to perform their tasks with rigor and vigor.

Which Is a Better Budgeting Technique: Top-Down or Bottom-Up?

Meanwhile, as the organization continues its annual budget process, an age-old question is once again revived: Which budgeting technique is better for the organization, top-down or bottom-up? The answer usually depends on who is re-

TABLE 7.1. TOP-DOWN OR BOTTOM-UP BUDGETING TECHNIQUE: PROS AND CONS.

Top-Down		Bottom-Up	
Pros	**Cons**	**Pros**	**Cons**
Administration maintains control of the assumptions that determine the targeted operating margin.	Department managers are not invested in the budget outcomes because they did not have any input into the process.	Managers who set their own budget will be more invested in process and the future outcomes.	Managers have no incentive to set aggressive or "stretch" budget targets for their own department.
There is less chance of the managers needing to redo their budgets one, two, or three times to "balance the budget" as the assumptions change.	Administration is perceived as autocratic, not participative.	The budgeted volumes may be closer to reality, therefore causing less budget variance in the upcoming year.	Managers have no idea of the overall hospital budget targets and therefore no way of knowing the bottom line required from their department for the organization to succeed as a whole.

sponding and the stake he or she has in it. It is a highly charged issue, of particular concern to department managers who have to live with the consequences of either answer.

Top-down budgeting is defined as revenues and expense levels imposed by the administration and directed down to the manager who is expected to achieve them. Bottom-up budgeting is defined as revenue and expense levels determined by each department manager and aggregated to establish the organizationwide budget.

There are several implications to using either technique. Table 7.1 highlights the pros and cons of both.

The key issue is control: Who's got it, and how are they going to exercise it? As is common in any hierarchical organization, control is held at the top. But in this case, control is not really the most important issue. The really big issue is information management. Who's got it, and how is it going to be used? The overriding problem in budget management is achieving a targeted operating margin that is acceptable to the finance committee and the board. When department managers are given control of their own departmental budgets, they often have no good way to know what amount of departmental bottom line is needed by the administration to achieve the financial targets.

Now the next logical question is, Why doesn't the administration tell each department what type of bottom line is needed and then just let the managers go and achieve it? Of course, the answer is obvious. If the administration tells managers this information, they are effectively mandating the bottom line, which is once again top-down budgeting. It is a circular argument. Although managers want to be able to control their departmental budgeted volumes, revenues, and expenses, allowing them to do so potentially compromises the bottom line.

There is another possible problem when managers are given control of producing their budget assumptions, particularly volume. Managers are hard working, diligent, loyal, and smart. Like all human beings, they are also focused on their own welfare. Whether or not they are permitted to participate in an incentive compensation plan, they all have an annual review of their performance for the purpose of determining their annual pay raise. The managers are always evaluated against established goals. Obviously, they will attempt to establish goals that are easily achievable to maximize their accomplishments during the annual review. Therefore budgeted volumes, which drive budgeted revenues, are not aggressive. This generally makes it more difficult for the formulated budget to produce the targeted volumes required by the board.

So, what's the answer? To minimize manager frustration from being asked to constantly change their own assumptions throughout the budget process, the top-down technique is favored. Top-down budgeting also measurably shortens the process by six to eight weeks because it minimizes reworking caused by unusable volume and revenue assumptions. Managers are often willing to accept and cooperate in the top-down budget process if the pros and cons are explained to them and the ongoing budget process is constantly communicated. They still may not like it, but they learn to live with it.

July 1: Issue the Budget Calendar

Although there was some considerable amount of preliminary work performed in June facilitated by the finance staff with input from many of the clinical managers, the budget calendar is first issued on July 1. As explained in some detail in Chapter Six, the purpose of the budget calendar is to create expectations of the duration and timing of the project for all involved participants. This is done through establishing meeting times and places for the various get-togethers that are required for good communication of some complicated and demanding issues. The calendar sets the agenda for the next four months' work.

July 11: Compute Gross Revenues and Contractual Adjustments

Between June 28 and July 11, one of the key steps in preparing and executing a valid budget process is being performed in the back room of the finance department by some of its most valuable members, the financial analysts. The current and subsequent year's annual gross revenues and contractual adjustments are being calculated on the basis of the volumes approved at the June 26 budget meeting. At RHMC, the finance staff members with expertise in these areas are determining volume, gross revenue, and net reimbursement.

This determination is built on many assumptions. In addition to the inpatient and outpatient volume, other items must be projected to develop a valid and viable revenue budget. First, there is the detailed payor mix, highlighting many of the various clinical service areas and the inpatient and outpatient service side. Second, the payment levels for the entire payor mix are projected. Every conceivable and known change in payment level is essential for this process to succeed. The financial analyst may need to rely on other individuals in the organization for help. For example, it is now common to have a full-time employee negotiating managed care contracts. This person has to make a best guess on the discount levels projected for the upcoming year, as the basis on which the organization develops the net revenue budget. Third, gross revenues are broken down by inpatient and outpatient services. This is required to develop projected contractual adjustments. As always, the calculation for contractual adjustments is gross revenue minus net revenue (or expected payment).

To determine the actual contractual adjustments, it is necessary to know gross revenue, segregated into actionable categories.

The organization takes the various financial and statistical elements available and arranges them into usable criteria for analysis. The output of this extensive analysis is a summary sheet, used by the finance administrator at the budget meeting scheduled with the entire administration for July 18. Table 7.2 shows the summary gross revenue, contractual adjustment, and net revenue worksheet.

From the worksheet, we see these net revenues (gross revenue minus contractual allowance), across the same five column headings of actual, budget, and projected periods:

2000 actual	$95 million
2001 budget	$94 million
June 2001 actual	$50.07 million
2001 projected	$98.55 million
2002 budget	$98 million

TABLE 7.2. RHMC REVENUE AND CONTRACTUAL ANALYSIS, 2001 PROJECTED AND 2002 BUDGET (IN THOUSANDS OF DOLLARS).

	Gross Revenue					Percentage of Gross Revenues				
	2000 Actual	2001 Budget	June 2001 Actual	2001 Projected	2002 Budget	2000 Actual	2001 Budget	June 2001 Actual	2001 Projected	2002 Budget
Inpatient										
Medicare	36,000	38,000	19,000	38,500	40,000	48.6%	48.7%	48.0%	48.2%	47.6%
Medicaid	2,000	2,000	1,050	2,000	2,400	2.7%	2.6%	2.7%	2.5%	2.9%
Managed care	30,000	31,500	16,200	32,600	34,000	40.5%	40.4%	41.0%	40.9%	40.5%
All other	6,000	6,500	3,300	6,700	7,600	8.1%	8.3%	8.3%	8.4%	9.0%
Total	74,000	78,000	39,550	79,800	84,000	100.0%	100.0%	100.0%	100.0%	100.0%
Outpatient										
Medicare	23,000	26,000	13,000	26,200	30,000	33.3%	34.2%	32.9%	33.7%	34.9%
Medicaid	1,000	1,000	520	1,050	1,000	1.4%	1.3%	1.3%	1.4%	1.2%
Managed care	36,000	38,000	20,000	39,000	42,000	52.2%	50.0%	50.6%	50.2%	48.8%
All other	9,000	11,000	6,000	11,500	13,000	13.0%	14.5%	15.2%	14.8%	15.1%
Total	69,000	76,000	39,520	77,750	86,000	100.0%	100.0%	100.0%	100.0%	100.0%
Total										
Medicare	59,000	64,000	32,000	64,700	70,000	41.3%	41.6%	40.5%	41.1%	41.2%
Medicaid	3,000	3,000	1,570	3,050	3,400	2.1%	1.9%	2.0%	1.9%	2.0%
Managed care	66,000	69,500	36,200	71,600	76,000	46.2%	45.1%	45.8%	45.4%	44.7%
All other	15,000	17,500	9,300	18,200	20,600	10.5%	11.4%	11.8%	11.6%	12.1%
Total	143,000	154,000	79,070	157,550	170,000	100.0%	100.0%	100.0%	100.0%	100.0%

These are some of the key features of the worksheet:

- Total gross revenues segregated by inpatient and outpatient areas, with no price increase
- Total contractual dollars projected for the upcoming budget year
- Total contractual dollars as a percentage of gross revenue for prior years, projected current year, and upcoming budget year
- Net revenues projected for the current year and budgeted for the upcoming year

	Contractual Allowance Dollars					Contractual Adjustment, Percentage of Gross Revenues			
2000 Actual	2001 Budget	June 2001 Actual	2001 Projected	2002 Budget	2000 Actual	2001 Budget	June 2001 Actual	2001 Projected	2002 Budget
16,500	21,000	10,000	19,500	24,000	45.8%	55.3%	52.6%	50.6%	60.0%
1,500	1,500	800	1,500	1,800	75.0%	75.0%	76.2%	75.0%	75.0%
8,200	10,700	5,200	11,000	13,500	27.3%	34.0%	32.1%	33.7%	39.7%
1,200	2,000	900	1,700	2,000	20.0%	30.8%	27.3%	25.4%	26.3%
27,400	35,200	16,900	33,700	41,300	37.0%	45.1%	42.7%	42.2%	49.2%
12,000	14,500	7,300	15,000	19,000	52.2%	55.8%	56.2%	57.3%	63.3%
800	800	400	800	800	80.0%	80.0%	76.9%	76.2%	80.0%
7,000	8,500	4,000	8,700	10,000	19.4%	22.4%	20.0%	22.3%	23.8%
800	1,000	400	800	900	8.9%	9.1%	6.7%	7.0%	6.9%
20,600	24,800	12,100	25,300	30,700	29.9%	32.6%	30.6%	32.5%	35.7%
28,500	35,500	17,300	34,500	43,000	48.3%	55.5%	54.1%	53.3%	61.4%
2,300	2,300	1,200	2,300	2,600	76.7%	76.7%	76.4%	75.4%	76.5%
15,200	19,200	9,200	19,700	23,500	23.0%	27.6%	25.4%	27.5%	30.9%
2,000	3,000	1,300	2,500	2,900	13.3%	17.1%	14.0%	13.7%	14.1%
48,000	60,000	29,000	59,000	72,000	33.6%	39.0%	36.7%	37.4%	42.4%

This is a significant worksheet. A considerable amount of time is devoted to reviewing this worksheet both at the July 15 meeting with the finance administrators and then at the July 18 meeting when the finance administrators present it to the assembled administration.

July 14: Review Salary and Nonsalary Assumptions

Although the organization's reimbursement specialist is concentrating significant time and effort on the gross and net revenue calculations, a couple of other finance members are working on the expense side of the equation. At this administrative meeting, the only issues that are discussed involve projecting upcoming expense increases. This is somewhat similar to certain of the techniques used during the strategic financial planning meetings held in March (see Chapter Three). The finance administrators use this meeting to facilitate a series of discussions on four specific expense topics, to be able to complete the preliminary budget:

1. Full-time equivalent (FTE) level
2. Wage and salary increase or decrease
3. Fringe benefit level and increase or decrease
4. Controllable nonsalary expense change

Full-Time Equivalent Level. FTE level is always the most important part of the meeting. Health care is an extremely labor-intensive industry. Labor costs— defined as all salaries, wages, contracted labor and fringe benefits—make up between 45 and 55 percent of all expenses in a typical health care organization. On the hospital side of the industry, some providers have as much as 60 percent of their expenses tied up in labor costs, while others may spend as little as 38 percent on the same set of expenses.

The most important driver of labor costs is the amount of staff used. Labor costs are a product of pay rate times the number of people employed. Each factor has a significant impact on the total salary and fringe benefit costs. But of the two, only the number of employees is controllable by management. Pay rate is almost always a function of labor market conditions. As an employer, the health care organization has to pay the going rate in the marketplace for its employees, or else it will not be able to recruit or retain staff. Management has greater control over the number and mix of staff in every department of the organization.

Because labor costs are so substantial, it is of paramount importance that the organization attempt to properly size its workforce to maximize results. In health care, the challenge is to create the best possible patient experience coupled with excellent clinical outcomes without overspending for those services. This spending objective is continuously challenged by the clinical staff (spearheaded by the nursing administration) and often provoked by many of the organization's staff physicians.

Determining the right staff size is not easy. Health care, like other industries, has adopted benchmarking techniques in the arsenal of analysis tools. In health care, however, benchmarking FTEs is fraught with peril. As was already explored in Chapter Three, FTEs per adjusted patient day, the most common industry benchmark, is highly susceptible to manipulation and produces a poor benchmark.

TABLE 7.3. RHMC DIVISIONAL FTE SUMMARY FOR THE BUDGET YEAR ENDING DEC. 31, 2002.

	2001 Budget			2002 Budget			2002 Budget Versus 2001 Budget Increase (Decrease)
	Regular	Overtime	Total	Regular	Overtime	Total	
Patient care services (nursing)	480.4	14.8	495.2	484.4	16.8	501.2	6.0
Clinical services (ancillary services)	215.8	5.0	220.8	218.6	7.1	225.7	4.9
Medical administration	11.0	0.0	11.0	12.0	0.0	12.0	1.0
Financial management	105.4	2.0	107.4	104.7	2.0	106.7	(0.7)
Human resource management	23.7	0.0	23.7	25.0	0.0	25.0	1.3
Facilities management	86.0	2.9	88.9	87.0	4.3	91.3	2.4
Information systems management	60.1	2.0	62.1	66.0	3.0	69.0	6.9
Administrative services	14.0	0.0	14.0	13.0	0.0	13.0	(1.0)
Total	996.4	26.7	1,023.1	1,010.7	33.2	1,043.9	20.8

FTE and Salary Trends

Total FTEs		1,023.1	1,043.9
Overtime FTEs		26.7	33.2
Overtime FTEs as a percentage of total		2.6%	3.2%
Salaries, benefits, and contract labor as a percentage of net revenues		47.05%	50.53%
FTEs paid per adjusted patient day		4.17	4.00
Net revenue per paid (total) FTE		$91,193	$91,005

The alternative benchmark—salaries, wages, and fringe benefits as a percentage of net patient service revenues—is a better measure of productivity. To use it in the annual budget analysis, however, the dollar value of the projected FTEs must be converted into this percentage. This can be easily accomplished, and at RHMC the percentages associated with alternative models are always presented.

During this meeting, prior year trends of total FTEs; FTEs per adjusted patient day; and salaries, wages, and fringe benefits as a percentage of net patient service revenues are presented, along with the values associated with the current projected year and the upcoming budget year. These organization totals are supplemented by detailed departmental information. This allows the administrative reviewers to identify staffing trends within the various departments to make informed budgeting decisions. Table 7.3 displays the divisional FTE summary page used in the budgeting process at RHMC, backed up by department totals within the various divisions.

Wage and Salary Increases. Increases in wages and salaries are often not problematic for a health care organization to calculate. In a nonunion shop, the organization accesses benchmark information from the health care industry around its region as well as increases predicted for other industries within the region that may be competing for the same pool of employees. This information is available through national and local hospital associations and other labor organizations. The finance staff merely calculate the impact of two or three potential increases being proposed by the human resource division and report the projected results on the income statement to the administration.

In a union shop, the organization can easily perform this step if it is in the middle of a multiyear contract that does not expire in the upcoming budget year. It must use only the amounts approved in the contract, which are essentially done. Budgeting for the remaining nonunion employees in the organization (often only management) becomes relatively easy because it involves fewer people and results in a much lower impact on the budgeted income statement.

Ultimately, the salary increase can be a function of the operating margin resulting from all the volume, revenue, and other expense assumptions used in the budget. This is the case if the initial budgeted bottom line does not meet the targeted level set by the board. The two factors that are often used to bring it into balance are reduction of the proposed salary increase, or reduction in FTEs.

Fringe Benefit Level and Increase or Decrease. Fringe benefits has become a major expense category over the years with the rising significance of this tool for recruitment and retention of staff. As was recounted in Chapter One in reviewing the MRI pro forma, fringe benefits can now account for as much as an additional 30 percent of the actual salaries paid to the staff.

As shown in Table 7.4, the largest expense item within the fringe benefit category is health insurance expense. Like any other employer, RHMC is always evaluating it to minimize overall impact on the bottom line. Over the years, it has moved health insurance from an indemnity plan to a managed care plan. Several years ago the medical center also started to require its employees to pay for a portion of the health insurance premiums; in the current year, this amounts to 30 percent of the total. In its benchmarking analysis, RHMC has determined that the competition requires their employees to pay 20 to 50 percent of the premiums.

For the upcoming budget year, the human resource department is suggesting that the budget include an expense increase of 4 percent for the health insurance premium, on the basis of competitive bidding of its account. No increase in the employee-paid portion of the insurance premium is recommended because of competitive human resource issues in the region.

TABLE 7.4. RHMC FRINGE BENEFIT EXPENSES
FOR THE BUDGET YEAR ENDING DEC. 31, 2002.

	2001 Budget	2001 Projected	2002 Budget
Non-FICA benefit expenses			
Health insurance premium			
Employer cost	$3,200,000	$3,200,000	$3,300,000
Employee offset	(1,000,000)	(1,080,000)	(1,050,000)
Postemployment expenses			
Pension	1,000,000	980,000	1,050,000
Tax-deferred annuity employer match	500,000	480,000	525,000
Life insurance	130,000	140,000	145,000
Long-term disability	100,000	110,000	110,000
Short-term disability	200,000	200,000	205,000
Workers' compensation	300,000	290,000	300,000
Unemployment insurance	60,000	55,000	60,000
Tuition reimbursement	60,000	62,000	65,000
Other expenses	50,000	40,000	60,000
Total non-FICA benefit expenses	4,600,000	4,477,000	4,770,000
FICA expense	2,400,000	2,450,000	2,500,000
Total benefit expenses	$7,000,000	$6,927,000	$7,270,000

The other fringe benefit line items are basically status quo for the upcoming year. No contentious issues are on the radar screen.

Controllable Nonsalary Expense Change. Nonsalary expense constitutes considerably less than 50 percent of the total expenses for the organization because salaries and fringe benefits tend to make up more than half; noncontrollable nonsalary expenses can make up between 15 and 25 percent of the remainder. Noncontrollable nonsalary expenses are generally defined as interest and depreciation expense. Controllable nonsalary expenses therefore make up 25 to 35 percent of total expenses.

Controllable nonsalary expenses are categorized into eight parts. As stated earlier in this book, RHMC uses a publishing service that specializes in analyzing trends in health care costs, the *Rate Controls* newsletter. The analysis goes backward and forward three years. It is published in annual percentage increases or decreases. RHMC uses the published upcoming year percentages as a guide to budgeting. There are times when one or several administrators believe they can

TABLE 7.5. RHMC SALARY AND NONSALARY EXPENSE CHANGES, SUMMARY OF PROJECTED PRICE INCREASE FOR THE BUDGET YEAR ENDING DEC. 31, 2002.

| | National Indices (Percentages) as of Apr. 30, 2001 | | | | | |
| | Historical | | | Projected | | |
	1998	1998	2000	2001	2002	2003
Salaries and wages	2.5	3.5	4.3	4.6	4.7	4.8
Employee benefits	0.8	2.1	4.3	5.2	5.4	5.6
Professional fees	3.3	3.2	3.7	3.8	3.8	3.8
Supplies, medical and surgical	0.1	−0.9	2.9	3.2	3.0	3.0
Pharmaceuticals	20.3	1.2	3.1	3.5	3.7	3.9
Dietary	−0.9	0.2	2.3	3.0	2.8	2.5
Utilities	−2.6	−0.3	12.0	10.0	4.0	4.0
Insurance	3.6	3.2	5.1	2.0	2.0	2.0
Purchased services	4.2	4.0	4.0	4.2	4.2	4.2
Other expenses	1.6	2.7	3.4	3.2	3.1	3.1
Plant and equipment	2.1	2.3	1.9	1.8	1.7	1.7
Total hospital inflation	2.5	3.2	4.3	4.7	4.7	4.8

Source: Rate Controls: Trends in American Healthcare.

beat the published increases, through more aggressive negotiating skills or changing the mix of products or services currently being acquired. Table 7.5 is a summary of the methodology used by *Rate Controls* and employed by RHMC.

July 15: Review Gross Revenues and Contractual Adjustments and Validate Payor Mix

This is a meeting internal to the finance department and its administrators. The assumptions used by the financial analysts leading to the July 11 revenue and contractual adjustments summary, shown in Table 7.2, is reviewed with a fine-tooth comb. It is imperative that all the assumptions used be validated to the greatest extent possible. Although it is not possible to actually see the future, it is essential that the entire set of assumptions track from the past to the future using internal and external assessment tools.

During this meeting, the finance administrators grill the analysts to determine if there are any holes in the logic of the analysis. Because these finance bosses are going to present the outcomes to the rest of the administration in just a few days, they want to assure themselves that the information is solid and acceptable. In the case of RHMC, both the analysts and the administrators have been together for years, so all the questions are expected and the answers are already available. Had this not been the case, there is a good possibility that some questions would need to be further researched and answered outside the meeting—though within the next twenty-four hours, so that it is available for the meeting on July 18, three days hence.

July 18: Review 2000 Budgeted Income Statement, Determine Price Increase Targets, and Revise Salary and Nonsalary Assumptions

This is the big meeting of the year, when the executives and other administrators first see the projected and budgeted bottom line. This bottom line is based on the dozens of assumptions that have been discussed and debated over the past six weeks. These assumptions can be summarized as follows:

- Inpatient and outpatient volumes based on historical trends and future expectation of physician referral patterns
- Gross revenues based on these volumes with no price increase yet proposed
- Contractual adjustments based on best-guess Medicare, Medicaid, and managed care rates
- Salaries based on the number of employees and the proposed wage increase percentage
- Fringe benefit expenses based on the proposed employee health and welfare package, including the recommended medical plan and the amount of premium that the employees will be expected to pay
- Nonsalary expenses based on any changes over the current year and the projected rate of inflation for these expense items

The meeting immediately turns to the current year projected and budget year operating margin, as shown in Table 7.6. If the budget year margin amounts to the targeted 4 percent of net patient revenue, then the meeting is over, well short of its two-hour time limit. In the new century, this is not likely to be the case. A declining reimbursement rate and generally reduced inpatient admission resulting from utilization controls required by managed care health plans have made bottom line management much more difficult.

An article in the April 23, 2001, issue of *Modern Healthcare* titled "Still Struggling: Not-for-Profit Hospitals Post Small Increases in Margins, New Study Shows" indicates that 2000 was another tough year for nonprofit hospitals. "Although overall operating profitability rose slightly, to 3.7 percent from 3.3 percent in 1999, that wasn't enough to signal the beginning of a recovery," says Gregg

TABLE 7.6. RHMC PRELIMINARY BUDGETED STATEMENT OF OPERATIONS FOR THE BUDGET YEAR TO DATE ENDING DEC. 31, 2002 (JULY 18, 2001).

	2000 Actual	2001 Budget	June 2001 Actual	2001 Projected	2002 Budget	Percentage Change	
						2002 Budget Versus 2001 Budget	2002 Budget Versus 2001 Projected
Revenues							
Inpatient revenue	$ 74,000	$ 79,000	$ 38,500	$ 77,800	$ 84,000	6.3%	8.0%
Outpatient revenue	69,000	77,000	37,600	76,100	86,000	11.7%	13.0%
Total patient revenue	143,000	156,000	76,100	153,900	170,000	9.0%	10.5%
Less							
Contractual and other adjustments	(48,000)	(60,000)	(29,000)	(59,000)	(72,000)	20.0%	22.0%
Charity care	(2,200)	(2,700)	(1,300)	(2,500)	(3,000)	11.1%	20.0%
Net patient service revenue	92,800	93,300	45,800	92,400	95,000	1.8%	2.8%
Add							
Premium revenue	1,300	2,100	1,100	2,100	1,000	−52.4%	−52.4%
Investment income	5,500	5,000	3,500	6,000	5,000	0.0%	−16.7%
Other operating income	1,200	1,200	600	1,100	1,200	0.0%	9.1%
Total revenue	100,800	101,600	51,000	101,600	102,200	0.6%	0.6%
Expenses							
Salaries	34,000	35,500	18,000	36,500	39,000	9.9%	6.8%
Contract labor	1,500	1,400	400	800	1,200	−14.3%	50.0%
Fringe benefits	6,800	7,000	3,500	6,900	7,800	11.4%	13.0%
Total salaries and benefits	42,300	43,900	21,900	44,200	48,000	9.3%	8.6%
Bad debts	4,400	4,400	2,400	4,400	5,000	13.6%	13.6%
Patient care supplies	15,000	15,200	8,200	16,000	17,100	12.5%	6.9%
Professional and management fees	3,600	3,400	1,900	3,800	4,200	23.5%	10.5%
Purchased services	5,600	5,600	2,900	5,600	5,600	0.0%	0.0%
Operation of plant (including utilities)	2,500	2,700	1,300	2,600	2,800	3.7%	7.7%
Depreciation	10,500	11,000	5,600	10,500	11,500	4.5%	9.5%
Interest and financing expenses	7,600	7,400	3,700	7,400	7,200	−2.7%	−2.7%
Other	4,600	3,800	2,000	4,000	5,000	31.6%	25.0%
Total expenses	96,100	97,400	49,900	98,500	106,400	9.2%	8.0%
Operation margin	4,700	4,200	1,100	3,100	(4,200)	−200.0%	−235.5%
Nonoperating income							
Gain/(loss) on investments	600	1,200	800	1,400	1,000	−16.7%	−28.6%
Total nonoperating income	600	1,200	800	1,400	1,000	−16.7%	−28.6%
Net income	$ 5,300	$ 5,400	$ 1,900	$ 4,500	$ (3,200)	−159.3%	−171.1%
4% targeted operating margin					$ 3,800		
3% targeted operating margin					$ 2,850		
2% targeted operating margin					$ 1,900		

Source: Rate Controls: Trends in American Healthcare.

Bennett, president of Solucient, a health care information company. "I suspect that hospital operating margins are not on an upward swing. Cost increases (particularly for labor and drugs) and the reluctance of purchasers to pay more than they are now are ominous for the hospital industry" (Jaklevic, 2001, p. 36).

Thus, a gap between the initial budgeted bottom line and the target is likely at most health care institutions. This is true at RHMC. The initial 2002 budgeted operating margin presented by the finance administrator at this meeting is a $4.2 million loss. Meanwhile, the hospital needs an operating margin of $3.8 million to achieve the board mandated 4 percent target. This establishes a gap of $8 million that has to be closed.

This gap is large but not necessarily surprising to many of the administrators in the room. Many have sat through dozens of budget meetings in their time and seen an initial bottom line almost as bad as this. They are not highly disturbed (although they should be). There are, however, a number of factors that are extremely troubling. Administration must deal with continuing managed care cost pressure, the escalating nursing shortage, the continued increase in drug costs, and ongoing negative margin from the employed physician practices that the hospital owns.

Value of Price Increases. The remainder of the meeting is devoted to figuring out how to close the budget gap initially. Several techniques are used. The first decision is how many dollars the organization will net for every 1 percent increase in its listed prices. Because RHMC's primary payor mix is Medicare and managed care, it would initially appear that price increases have no impact on the bottom line. In fact, the administrators at RHMC are aware that this is not case. There are at least two reasons for this. First, not all managed care contracts are per diem–based. There may still be a number of contracts based on discount from gross charges. If so, a piece of any price increase is passed along to the managed care plan, depending on the particular level of discount that has been negotiated. Second, there are still payors reimbursing RHMC on gross charges. Even if it is only a small percentage, say 10 percent, this can still have a positive impact on the bottom line.

In the case of RHMC, analysis performed by the finance department indicates that every 1 percent increase is worth an incremental 25 cents on total dollars charged. This estimate is based on payor mix assumptions, level of managed care contracts paid on a percentage-of-charge basis, and percentage of payors still paying full charges. From this estimate, it is concluded that net revenue generated from a 1 percent price increase is $425,000 ($170 million total gross charges times 1 percent price increase times 25 percent net revenue realization).

Although the administrators now know the value of each percentage point increase, they still need some context to determine how much of an increase is acceptable to their community and the managed care payors. Although very few patients continue to pay for their health care out of pocket, there is continuing fascination with the health care organization's price list. Leading the region in high charges can create a public relations problem for any organization. Being in Illinois (as is true in other states as well), RHMC is required to report to a state agency a series of specific charges and a group of bundled procedure charges. These items are then published by the responsible state agency and available to anyone who wants a copy.

Like any other good finance department, RHMC's people review the output of this report to determine the level of charges compared to competitors. Finance staff members report the organization's position during this phase of the budget meeting. For the latest report year available, RHMC is directly in the middle of the pack for most of its charges, fifth among a total of nine competing organizations. With this knowledge, and some anecdotal information that some of the other organizations are raising their charges by the approximate level of health care inflation, the administration decides preliminarily to propose a price increase of 4 percent. Although this increases the gross revenues by $6.8 million ($170 million preincrease gross revenue times 4 percent average price increase), it will only net $1.7 million on the bottom line.

Budgeted Expense Reductions. With this 4 percent price increase set, the administrators are then able to determine how much additional expense has to be cut, or if there are any other revenue sources that could be considered. From the expense side, staffing level is once again the first item on the list to be discussed. Although this was discussed in depth only a week ago at the July 14 meeting, now that the preliminary bottom line is in play it is reviewed again to determine where cuts could possibly be made.

The best way to determine these cuts would be with appropriate productivity measures. RHMC is currently developing these productivity measures. There is a lot of work involved in developing, maintaining, and then tracking productivity. Once an organization makes the decision to do so, it is taking a step toward practicing better management. Productivity management is an art. It supplies the administrators and department managers with information they never had before. Managers believe they know the amount of time it takes their employees to perform individual tasks, however research conducted for cost accounting studies indicates that manager perception is never a good measure of actual time spent.

Productivity management techniques allow department managers to understand

- The tasks being performed
- Whether or not the tasks are value-added
- How long these tasks take

When all the tasks and their time frames are totaled up, the total minutes should indicate the number of staff members needed. If the organization sets its parameters between 90 and 110 percent of standard, then it is possible to scientifically determine which departments are overstaffed or understaffed.

Exhibit 7.1 indicates a list of possible cuts that were discussed by the RHMC administrators during this meeting. The initial outcomes are provisional and de-

EXHIBIT 7.1. RHMC "CLOSING THE GAP" ANALYSIS, 2002 BUDGET.

Operating margin, July 18 meeting		$4,200
4% net price increase		1,700
Improvement in investment income		1,000
Salary expense reductions, at $40,000 average per employee:		
10 FTEs	400	
20 FTEs	800	800
30 FTEs	1,200	
40 FTEs	1,600	
50 FTEs	2,000	
Fringe benefits: reduce additional benefits proposed in initial budget meeting of July 14:		
	200	
	300	300
	400	
	500	
Reduce bad debt expense through better collection efforts:		
	250	
	500	500
	750	
	1,000	
Reduce patient care supply expenses:		
	300	
	400	
	500	500
	600	
	700	
Reduce professional and management fees:		
Cut consulting fees	200	
	300	300
	400	
Reduce other expenses:		500
Revised operating margin		$1,400

pendent on subsequent requests of the department managers. The finance staff therefore issue departmental budgets with an aggregate total bottom line of $1.4 million. All the administrators are aware that additional decisions must be made after the managers return their budgets in about a month.

July 25: Issue 2001 Projected and 2002 Budgeted Worksheets to Department Managers

From all the decisions made in the previous budget meetings, the finance department is now ready to issue the following year's budget to the department managers. This is first time that most of the managers have an inkling of what is expected of them in the upcoming year. This submission is crucial to the level at which the manager can operate his or her department, now and in the coming year.

The first thing that the managers review is their staffing level. They are concerned whether administration has already made any cuts. In addition, because RHMC is a top-down budget organization, the managers are also aware that they cannot add any staff unless they can prove that they are not already appropriately staffed, and that an additional staff member will either improve net revenue production above the cost of the new FTE or decrease other departmental costs.

Of course, this is seldom the case. Instead, requests for most new FTEs are justified on the grounds of improved patient or physician satisfaction or a decrease in overwork.

The managers are also interested in the other revenue and expense assumptions made by the administration. Revenue-producing managers did have some input into the volumes, of course, but they want to know if their assumptions have been changed. In any event, the most important reason the administration issues this preliminary budget to the managers is so that they can review every line item and determine if the finance staff made any clerical or technical errors that require changing. After doing error checking, studying appropriate volumes, and reviewing all other nonsalary expense items, the managers are expected to return their budgets with any changes to their administrators by August 15.

Capital Budgeting (July)

Concurrent with the operating budget, the capital budget process continues. The finance department staff are now working overtime. They are trying to keep up with the mass of analysis materials coming into the department as well as the reams of material going out to department managers and administrators during the month.

Steps that need to be completed in the July capital budget process:

- July 11: Submit 2000 capital budgets by department managers back to the finance staff through capital budgeting software
- July 12–23: Review by finance staff of all capital proposals for completeness
- July 24–August 6: Capital budgets reviewed by proposal reviewers (facilities management, materials management, and information systems)

On July 11, the department managers are mandated to return all of their capital budget requests to the finance department with all required elements filled in. Over the two or three weeks that the managers have to complete their portion, they are expected to contact any individual who must obtain equipment within the department. Thus, for example, in a clinical department such as radiology the manager should speak to the physician in charge of the clinical aspects of the department to determine whether this physician is aware of (1) any new equipment that has come on the market that could improve patient outcomes or offer a new revenue stream to the organization or (2) any current department equipment that has become obsolete, is no longer state-of-the-art for diagnosis or treatment, or is harmful to the patient's care.

The physician may want the manager to submit a request for updated equipment during this capital budget process. This is in fact the appropriate time to do so. Here is a summary of the required elements of the electronic capital request form:

- Proposal name
- Proposal preparer's name, title, department, phone number
- Purchase information (vendor name, manufacturer, model number)
- Description of item
- Price of capital item
- Classification of item
- Executive summary: why should it be acquired?
- Detailed summary: why should it be acquired? (explanation and justification, using strategic plan elements)
- Pricing details
- Five-year pro forma profit-and-loss statement (if cost is over $100,000)

Managers need to fill in all the blanks of the electronic capital request form for their request to be appropriately considered; they have already been told that their proposal will be returned if they leave out any of these required elements.

Actually, this is exactly what the finance staff will be doing during the next project step. Between July 12 and July 23, the staff review all of the proposals to be sure that these elements are met. Acting in an advisory and consulting role, the finance representatives assigned to all these projects help the managers fill in any of the elements that have been left blank. They also advise the managers how they might be able to strengthen their proposals, where appropriate. Some managers do not write or justify proposals as well as others do. It is RHMC's practice to attempt to level the playing field in this regard. The task of the finance staff member responsible for the capital budget is to ensure that all the proposals that will be reviewed by administrators are complete so that the review process is as fair as possible.

Between July 24 and August 6, the proposal reviewers get their crack at each proposal. These reviewers come from three technical areas: facilities management, information systems management, and materials management. Each area is required to review every proposal to determine if any additional costs arise should the requested item become operational in the organization. At RHMC, the information management department is required to review every capital item that is powered by a microchip. They are attempting to determine if any nonstandard setups may be required or if the requested purchase requires information management expertise that is not currently available onsite.

The role of facilities management is similar. Almost every piece of requested capital equipment plugs into the wall. Most managers take the plug and the wall outlet for granted. However, each one adds power requirements, and they add up, sometimes resulting in the need for facilities management to acquire new power distribution equipment (at substantial cost). It is their job to know all the energy flowing through the organization. Therefore it is absolutely necessary for them to perform their review before the evaluators see the proposals. The facilities management review may increase the cost of the proposed item. It is good to know this at the time the evaluators evaluate, not afterward.

Materials management ultimately has to issue the purchase order for all approved capital items. Therefore, its review ensures that all the data elements that they require have already been included in the proposal.

Regulatory and Legal Environment

Still, routine and capital budgets are not the only aspects of operation that are being managed during the month of July. Administrators of the various divisions (clinical, operations, and financial) have been spending time making sure that they and their staff are performing all of their duties in compliance with the many laws and regulations governing operation of a health care facility.

Like every other industry in America, health care is heavily regulated. Not only is the industry governed by state, federal, and local laws, it is also subject to additional regulations, formal rulings, and interpretations. In addition to being governed by several common sets of regulations, each industry segment has specific rules that it needs to follow.

As with all things, the highest level of authority is law, passed by legislative bodies. Health care laws are extensive and tend to cover a variety of areas within the industry. Federal laws, which must be followed, are passed by Congress and signed by the president. To properly follow the laws, providers seek guidance through regulations issued by the government agency that has the responsibility for each program. In health care, the appropriate federal agency is The Center for Medicare and Medicaid Services (CMS), formerly known as the Health Care Financing Administration (HCFA), which is charged with administering the Medicare program through the authority of the Department of Health and Human Services (DHHS).

Medicare and Medicaid Fraud and Abuse

As we explored the Medicare and Medicaid programs in Chapter Five, it was evident that these are highly technical programs. The technical specifications create huge holes that are occasionally taken advantage of by unscrupulous individuals. Although not dealing only with the inherently unscrupulous, the laws were designed to ensure that bad or crooked providers are punished.

The framers of the Medicare and Medicaid programs were concerned that the government pay only for applicable services that should have been appropriately rendered under the law. Historically, they were aware that other government programs had, over the years, been billed for goods or services not rendered or received. On occasion, bills had been inflated above the rate agreed to. Because of this, at the conclusion of the process the Social Security Act of 1965 contained several provisions to combat this problem:

- Criminal penalties, applicable to persons convicted of committing specified fraudulent acts:
    Filing of false claims
    Misrepresentation of the qualification of an institution
    Solicitation, receipt, or offering of kickbacks, bribes, or rebates
- Civil money penalties, applicable to persons determined by the secretary of HHS to have committed these acts:
    Filing fraudulent claims under the programs
    Charging beneficiaries for services in violation of any agreement entered into with the HHS secretary
- Exclusion from Medicare and Medicaid program participation for those providers and practitioners who are convicted of crimes involving:
    Health programs established under the Social Security Act
    Patient abuse or neglect

There is special language surrounding much of these regulations, owing to great concern that providers would attempt to illegally profit from Medicare and Medicaid by submitting inappropriate or bogus claims. To combat this, the Social Security Act authorizing the programs created express provisions against any individual who knowingly and willfully submits a false claim to the government (in this case, the Medicare or Medicaid program).

Kickbacks, Bribes, and Rebates. In addition, the laws spend a considerable amount of time and effort in detailing efforts to prevent kickbacks, bribes, and rebates. The government was particularly concerned with the possibility that individuals would conspire with others to illegally obtain Medicare and Medicaid money. These laws penalize individuals who knowingly and willfully solicit or receive any remuneration (including any kickback, bribe, or rebate) directly or indirectly, overtly or covertly, in cash or in kind, in return for

- Referring an individual to a person for furnishing or arranging furnishing of any item or service for which payment may be made in whole or in part under Medicare
- Purchasing, leasing, ordering, or arranging for or recommending purchasing, leasing, or ordering any good, facility, service, or item for which payment may be made in whole or in part under Medicare

If convicted of these offenses, the individual is guilty of a felony and fined or imprisoned for not more than five years, or both.

Further, the law penalizes individuals who knowingly and willfully offer or pay any remuneration (including any kickback, bribe, or rebate) directly or indirectly, overtly or covertly, in cash or in kind to any person to induce someone to

- Refer an individual to a provider for furnishing or arranging for furnishing of any item or service for which payment may be made in whole or in part under Medicare
- Purchase, lease, order, or arrange for or recommend purchasing, leasing, or ordering any good, facility, service, or item for which payment may be made in whole or in part under Medicare

If convicted of these offenses, the individual will be guilty of a felony and fined or imprisoned for not more than five years, or both.

These are just a few of the many laws and regulations that providers are required to observe if they want to continue to participate in the Medicare program and stay out of jail. A number of other laws are currently on the books and used by the government to enforce compliance:

- HIPAA, enacted in 1996, which has a number of fraud and abuse provisions built into it
- False Claims Act, which was enacted in 1863 to combat fraudulent claims billed for services to the federal government during the Civil War. This statute was much in use by the OIG during the late 1990s, as it attempted to combat fraudulent health care claims resulting from services billed for Medicare beneficiaries

Office of Inspector General Work Plan. Indeed, the OIG has been extremely busy in its attempt to eliminate health care fraud in both billing and nonbilling issues. It is easy to determine which areas of potential fraud and abuse the office is targeting in any given year, since OIG publishes its annual work plan on the Internet (http://www.hhs.gov/progorg/oig). Table 7.7 displays selected items from the OIG's 2001 plan.

As can be seen, the OIG is involved in many types of review and audit. The office is focused on more than just the billing and claims processing issues highlighted in Chapter Five. Their vision, as "guardians of the public trust," is to ensure effective and efficient HHS programs and operations by minimizing fraud, waste, and abuse (DHHS, 2001). In addition to pure billing issues, OIG gets involved in PPS rate formulation to ensure reasonableness. It also monitors utilization patterns to determine if providers are "gaming the system" illegally to improve their Medicare or Medicaid reimbursement.

Other Regulatory and Business Compliance Issues

In addition to the highly complex and punitive requirements of Medicare fraud and abuse rules and regulations, RHMC is also responsible for following normal business compliance:

- Occupational Health and Safety Administration laws
- All labor department rules and regulations
- State health department rules
- Tax or tax-exempt rules and regulations

Furthermore, as a health care provider, RHMC needs to comply with a whole series of supplementary rules and regulations designed specifically for the industry, including the following:

- Special state requirements pertaining to licensing as a health care facility
- Private insurance requirements, usually administered by the state insurance commissioner

- Special requirements by the federal government for participation in programs such as Medicare, Medicaid and CHAMPUS
  Eligibility
  Payment
  Utilization review
  Quality (which takes the form of accreditation)
  Fraud and abuse (as represented by the OIG's work plan)

Meeting all of these areas of compliance requires management and employee vigilance. This book has already highlighted some of these areas and the types of technique and methodology that enhance the organization's financial performance, such as Medicare and Medicaid payment issues in Chapter Five and fraud and abuse issues in this chapter.

Corporate Compliance

Good managers expect to exceed many of the basic practices that are spelled out in the previous section. Ultimately, the organization is responsible for ensuring that there are no deviations from rules necessary to maintain licensure or accreditation. As we have seen, failure to do so can lead to fines for the organization or individuals. Furthermore, it can lead to jail time for the individual offenders. These facts alone should be deterrent enough to ensure that neither the organization nor its employees engage in any hanky-panky.

Yet, given all of the various rules, regulations, and interpretations that health care providers are required to follow, it has become an ongoing process to identify and monitor compliance. Until the government became more diligent in its enforcement efforts in the early and mid-1990s, providers did not devote a great deal of time, money, or energy to compliance. This started to change when the OIG began extensive Medicare cost report audits of selected academic medical centers around the nation. This brought enforcement attention to the industry at large because of the visibility of the targeted institutions. These audits not only resulted in publicity for the government's efforts but also wound up collecting millions of dollars in fines, which were turned back to the treasury.

That was just the beginning. Larger and better-funded government efforts followed. Most of these were billing audits, some of which were highlighted in Chapter Five. Still, the industry was now on notice; it needed to clean up its act. In 1996, the government issued a Model Laboratory Compliance Plan. This was followed in 1997 with a Model Hospital Compliance Plan. Although providers did not have to follow these model plans explicitly, the mere existence of a plan

TABLE 7.7. DHHS OFFICE OF INSPECTOR GENERAL, FISCAL YEAR 2001 WORK PLAN, SELECTED AREAS OF REVIEW, EXCLUDING BILLING AND CLAIMS PROCESSING.

Area of Concern	Issue
Hospitals	
One-day hospital stays	Evaluating the reasonableness of Medicare inpatient hospital payments for beneficiaries discharged after spending only one day in a hospital. The review will concentrate on the adequacy of existing controls to detect and deny unauthorized care.
Outpatient prospective payment system	Reviewing implementation of the new PPS for care provided to Medicare beneficiaries by hospital outpatient departments. Also, evaluating the effectiveness of internal controls intended to ensure that services are adequately documented, properly coded, and medically necessary.
Home health	
Physician involvement in approving home health care	Reviewing the extent of physician involvement in approving and monitoring home care for Medicare beneficiaries. Reviewing the frequency with which physicians examine home care patients, and identifying obstacles to physician involvement in monitoring their patients.
Home health PPS controls	Monitoring the implementation of the new PPS used to pay home health agencies for providing care to Medicare beneficiaries. Also, evaluating the adequacy of controls intended to ensure that services are provided only to homebound individuals and are adequately documented, properly coded, and medically necessary.
Skilled nursing home care	
Role of the nursing home director	Examining how the role of the nursing home medical director has been interpreted and implemented and how the medical director affects quality of care.
Quality assessment and assurance committees	Examining the role and effectiveness of quality assessment and assurance committees in ensuring quality of care in nursing homes.
Physicians	
Advanced beneficiary notices (ABN)	Examining the use of advance notices to Medicare beneficiaries and their financial impact on beneficiaries and providers. Physicians must provide advance notices before they provide services that they know or believe Medicare does not consider medically necessary or that Medicare will not reimburse.
Reassignment of physician benefits	Evaluating the practice of allowing physicians to reassign their billing numbers to clinics. This practice shifts the accountability and liability for billing abuses away from the physician to the clinic. Past reassignment abuses will be examined to determine specific vulnerabilities.

Source: Health Care Financing Administration Projects, Work Plan, Fiscal Year 2001. Office of Inspector General, Department of Health and Human Services. (http://www.dhhs.gov/progorg/oig/wrpln/2001/wp2001.pdf)

at a provider's site could obviate more severe government-imposed penalties if some errors were uncovered. This was important because the government was now taking the position that seemingly unintentional errors, often clerical in nature, were being considered as fraud and abuse and were being threatened with prosecution as such.

Ridgeland Heights Medical Center, like most of its competitors and peers, always believed that it followed all the required rules and regulations. Administrators believed they knew the rules and had systems in place to ensure compliance. Yet, this new persistence by the government to make sure the rules were followed convinced RHMC administrators that they needed to observe them with even more diligence and rigor.

To this end, RHMC has developed a major corporate compliance policy. Its purpose is to (1) ensure that all RHMC employees are aware of and follow all the laws, regulations, and policies affecting their duties; and (2) ensure that all employees recognize the organization's values and reflect them in their actions.

The organization and its administration always believed in doing the right thing, but this new initiative codified policies and further reinforced and established new procedures toward compliance standards. The plan states that the organization is committed to conducting its business in a manner that facilitates quality, efficiency, honesty, integrity, respect, and full compliance with applicable laws and regulations. In addition, it expresses ongoing commitment to ensure that its affairs are conducted in accordance with both the letter and the spirit of laws and regulations and its own policies and practices. The plan requires employees to maintain standards of behavior that are lawful and ethical.

Key Features of Compliance Plan

- Designation of specific RHMC officials responsible for directing the effort to enforce compliance
- Identification of a corporate compliance code of conduct, including an educational and training plan for dissemination of the code
- Incorporation of standards and policies that guide RHMC employees and other third parties affiliated with the organization in regard to their conduct
- Coordinated education and training for RHMC employees and other third parties affiliated with RHMC in regard to their conduct
- Publication and uniform mechanisms for employees and other third parties affiliated with RHMC to raise questions and receive appropriate guidance concerning their conduct
- Provision of a framework for specific compliance areas, such as billing and collection activities

- Publication process for employees to report possible compliance issues and development of a procedure for investigating and resolving reports of possible compliance matters
- Formulation of corrective action plans to address any compliance problems that are identified
- Development of a plan to monitor the organization's overall compliance efforts

Accreditation Issues

Health care organizations have more to worry about than just criminal and civil penalties if they fail to comply with applicable laws, regulations, and policies. Many have also chosen to participate "voluntarily" in accreditation programs.

Major U.S. Health Care Accrediting Organizations

- Joint Commission on Accreditation of Healthcare Organizations (JCAHO)
    American Hospital Association (AHA)
    American Medical Association (AMA)
    American Osteopathic Association (AOA)
    American Dental Association (ADA)
    American College of Surgeons (ACS)
- Accreditation Association for Ambulatory Health Care (AAAHC)
- College of American Pathologists (CAP)
- National Committee for Quality Assurance (NCQA; HMOs)

There are significant practices that should be followed to be considered in compliance with the accrediting organization's rules, and reasons these health care providers have chosen to be involved in accreditation.

First, accreditation by the JCAHO automatically deems the provider eligible to participate in the Medicare and Medicaid programs and qualified to bill for and receive reimbursement from the government payors.

Second, there are marketing advantages available to organizations that have been accredited. Being able to advertise the accreditation allows a health care provider to imply or express a higher standard of care, if it so chooses.

Third, the ability to contract with MCOs is enhanced with acceptance by a reputable accrediting organization. Another way to say this is that organizations not accredited probably are not able to contract with any MCO to provide care to the health plan's enrollees. Because of this, it is extremely difficult to act as a health care provider without accreditation.

The largest accrediting body in America is the JCAHO. It evaluates and accredits more than eighteen thousand health care organizations and programs. As can be seen in the list, the Joint Commission is an amalgam of five major health care provider associations. Since 1951, it has developed professionally based standards and evaluated the compliance of health care organizations against these benchmarks. As is evident in the next list (http://www.jcaho.org/about_jc/jcinfo.htm), the Joint Commission's evaluation and accreditation services are extensive and cover the entire spectrum of health care provider organizations:

JCAHO Evaluation and Accreditation Services

- General, psychiatric, children's, and rehabilitation hospitals
- Health care networks, including health plans, integrated delivery networks, and preferred provider organizations
- Home care organizations, including those that provide home health services, personal care and support services, home infusion and other pharmacy services, durable medical equipment services, and hospice services
- Nursing home and other long-term care facilities, including subacute care programs, dementia programs, and long-term care pharmacies
- Behavioral health care organizations, including those that provide mental health, chemical dependency, mental retardation, and development disabilities services for patients of various ages in various organized service settings; and managed behavioral health care organizations
- Ambulatory care providers, including outpatient surgery facilities, rehabilitation centers, infusion center, group practices, and others
- Clinical laboratories

The Joint Commission has had its ups and downs over the years. Its biggest triumph was in being deemed the accrediting body of choice by the federal government for the Medicare and Medicaid programs in 1966. However, in recent years some providers have challenged some of the Joint Commission's practices and procedures. JCAHO has attempted to evolve over the years, trying to lead its provider organizations into newer quality management techniques. Although the controversy may not quiet down anytime soon, the ongoing debate seems destined to strengthen overall provider quality simply by keeping it constantly on the administration's front burner.

The other three organizations listed earlier along with the JCAHO's five constituents have the same goals. The last organization on the list, the National Committee for Quality Assurance (NCQA), does not accredit health care providers. Instead, it certifies health plans or MCOs that act as third-party payors to millions of insured enrollees. The NCQA is a private, nonprofit organization dedicated to assessing and reporting on the quality of managed care plans.

The NCQA is relatively new. It began accrediting MCOs in 1991 in response to the need for standardized and objective information about the quality of these organizations. Since then, it has expanded the range of organizations that it certifies to include managed behavior health care organizations, credentials verification organizations, and physician organizations.

Like the JCAHO programs, the NCQA accreditation program is voluntary. Regardless of the motivation of the providers and health plans for participating, these accreditation programs enable the industry to properly claim a basis for quality care.

Patient Satisfaction Issues

There is one more major issue not directly related to the finance function that can have a significant impact on the health care organization's bottom line. Because health care organizations really do care about offering very good service to their customers, over the years many have attempted to understand patient satisfaction, though they were not always able to effectively measure it. Recently, a few major national patient satisfaction firms have sprung up to offer an assessment mechanism for health care providers.

These organizations permit the provider to have each patient within various service categories (such as inpatient, emergency department, or ambulatory surgery) to evaluate her satisfaction level. More important, because these patient satisfaction firms have many clients, it is possible to compare each provider against a peer group and determine its own ranking. This is critical because it allows the provider to set certain goals, not only for improvement against prior scores but also against the peer group.

At RHMC, the organization has developed criteria so the level of patient satisfaction is part of the annual incentive compensation model. By incorporating it into the incentive compensation formula, the organization is putting its money where its mouth is, making the point to employees and the community that it takes patient satisfaction seriously. The RHMC administration believes that the community and physicians will notice a high level of patient satisfaction. It is believed that physicians are as a consequence more willing to refer, and patients are more willing to come, to an institution that has an objective record of excellent patient service. It appears that this has been borne out over the past few years because RHMC has had a lesser reduction in its admissions than some of its competitors have. Patient satisfaction ranks as one of the differentiators.

CHAPTER EIGHT

AUGUST

Margaret McGregor, RHMC's vice president of patient care services and nursing, is having a pleasant morning, reviewing the improved patient outcome scores that have just been delivered. She is aware that some of the improvement is the result of an increased level of care management provided to patients and physicians. The changes were aimed at standardizing care through enhanced consumption and utilization controls. But she has a nagging feeling that something is missing. So she picks up the phone and calls the one person who might know the answer.

"Hi, Sam, it's Maggie. How are you this morning?"

"Maggie, I'm fine. It sure is a pretty morning. I was just looking out the window and wondering how we could extend this weather year round. Of course, if we could then we'd be like San Diego and everybody would want to live here," Sam says. "Anyway, I digress. What's up this morning?"

"Well, I was wondering about something. I was just looking over patient outcome results and they're very encouraging, but I also noticed that there's no cost data on the reports. I can't tell if these improvements cost us money or saved us anything."

"You're right. When we initiated the care management program before you started here, we didn't have a cost accounting system. Because of that, we couldn't produce a baseline analysis. Therefore, we can't tell how much we've improved. We can, however, tell you how much each patient is costing us now. We can tell you the length of stay of each patient. We can even develop analyses allowing you to compare our physicians' resource consumption and costs against each other or against regional or national benchmarks and create trend lines over time."

"Sam, that sounds really good. I know that would help us a lot as we keep trying to improve our clinical outcomes and our cost base. With that kind of information, my nursing directors and their staff will be able to focus on areas that require the most improvement."

"That's great. I'm aware that the biggest bang for the buck would be to identify utilization patterns by individual physician, determine the average, and try to bring those physicians that are outside the norm back in line. We have great opportunities to save money for the organization while still increasing the patient satisfaction scores."

"So how come you didn't tell me about all this great stuff before?"

"Mags, that's a real good question. You need to understand that I've been trying to get the nursing division to accept and use this information for the last few years. They have just shown no inclination to use it. That's why I'm really pleased that you're here now. I know that you've used data like this before and that you know the value of it. So I'm thrilled that you're asking for it now."

"Yeah, yeah, yeah—but next time, I expect you to come to me with something like this first, OK?"

The dog days of summer. Hot days. Even hotter nights. As the temperatures soar into the triple digits, extraordinary numbers of city and suburban dwellers have gone fishin'. They take their companions, their kids, their dogs, and sometimes their turtles and leave town. They leave behind whatever work didn't get done. It's a theme at this time of year. The pace slows down to a delightful crawl. Margaritas and moonlight meet. Daytime is extended as daylight is magnified.

As hot as it is outside, it is even hotter inside the four walls of Ridgeland Heights Medical Center. August is the month that final decisions are made on the operating and capital budgets. For the finance staff, no vacations are scheduled and no vacations are allowed. They are busy crunching numbers and supporting both the department managers and the administration, helping them improve some of their budget presentations late in the game. They are in an all-out blitz to ensure that all the deadlines in a month of meetings are met. And so it goes. . . .

Capital Budget (August)

Now that August has arrived, the role of RHMC's administrators in the capital budget process takes center stage. Prior to this month, a lot of preliminary work has been performed. The department managers have prepared all of their capital requests, with input from the medical directors where appropriate. The finance staff have reviewed each proposal for completeness and consistency to allow them all an equal chance of success during the administrator's evaluation phase. Finally, facilities management, materials management, and information systems management examined the proposal to ensure that the proposals included any extra information that could potentially affect their areas. The proposals are complete, clean, and ready to be judged on their merits.

These are the steps that need to be completed in the August capital budget process:

- August 11: Detailed discussion of all proposals over $100,000 and training of all proposal evaluators
- August 12: Discussion of all pool proposals with the pool evaluators

- August 12–15: Evaluate proposals online
- August 22–25: Various pool consensus meetings with pool evaluators
- August 25: Consensus meeting for all proposals over $100,000
- August 26–28: Revision of ratings, if necessary, on the reviewer's desktop

August 11: Detailed Discussion and Training for All Proposals over $100,000

The meeting of August 11 is highly anticipated by the administrators. This is the first time they see the entire list of capital items being requested for acquisition in the year 2002. Prior to this, each administrator has seen only the capital requests from his or her division. The primary purpose of this meeting is to allow each administrator to present a verbal detailed story about the capital items being requested from that division and see the competing items requested from all other divisions. In effect, each administrator is given an opportunity to champion items for that division. The secondary purpose of the meeting is to train each administrator in using software for analysis.

In this meeting, it has already been determined that the dollar cutoff point for major project evaluation is $100,000. This decision was made by the finance administrator within the past three weeks, but only after the entire list of requested capital items was assembled. The dollar cutoff number is not fixed but can vary from year to year. It depends on the total number and dollar value of capital items being requested. Essentially, experience has shown that the evaluators can effectively review no more than forty to forty-five projects in detail. If they are asked to do more, they lose effectiveness and the objectivity of the criteria-based capital budget process is diminished.

In the case of the 2002 RHMC capital budget, the requested items were stratified into dollar categories as shown in Table 8.1. Capital items are defined as equipment or building items that cost at least $2,500 and have a useful life greater than one year.

Table 8.1 shows that 194 capital items were requested in total. Looking at the items from lowest to highest dollar values, it is clear that to avoid exceeding the limit of forty to forty-five items, the 2002 capital budget cutoff should be at $100,000. This dollar limit can change each year; it is entirely dependent on the dollar value and number of requests. There can also be finer stratification of the requests; the stratification jumps can be whatever makes sense to the organization. Although RHMC used $25,000, other organizations might use $10,000 or even $100,000. All items under the $100,000 cutoff level are evaluated in a somewhat different manner. They are grouped into six pools and evaluated separately by a small team of expert users and administrators.

TABLE 8.1. RHMC SUMMARY OF 2002 CAPITAL BUDGET, BY NUMBER OF REQUESTS.

Value of Requests	Number of Requests	Backward Accumulation of Requests	Total Value of Requests
$2,500–$24,999	78	194	$ 800,000
$25,000–$49,999	42	116	1,400,000
$50,000–$74,999	19	74	1,200,000
$75,000–$99,999	15	55	1,300,000
$100,000–$125,000	18	40	2,000,000
$125,000–$199,999	12	22	2,400,000
$200,000–$249,999	7	10	3,200,000
Over $250,000	3	3	4,000,000
Total requests	194		$16,300,000

During the first part of the meeting, the proposal evaluators (administrators) are trained on how to use the software. They are advised to set aside about two hours of concurrent time so that they can perform their review in one sitting. This is because they are being asked to score each proposal against all the others by ten criteria.

The methodology they are trained on works like this:

• The evaluators are reminded that their review is based on the ten strategic plan criteria, with which they are refamiliarized:

Strategic Plan Criteria

1. Community health promotion
2. Facility quality
3. Image and reputation
4. Information and decision support
5. Market share
6. Operating efficiency
7. Patient and family satisfaction
8. Patient outcomes
9. Physician outcomes
10. Physician satisfaction

The evaluators are told to review all proposals in total, one time, before doing any scoring. This allows them to get an overall feel for the entire mix of proposals before them.

• Then they are told to go back to review and score each proposal on just the first strategic plan criterion, in this case community health promotion.

• The key concept in the scoring, they are told, is to determine, after reading all proposals, which of the forty they consider best meet the criteria. This proposal is awarded one thousand points on a scale of 0 to 1,000. The other thirty-nine proposals are then judged against this "best" proposal. The evaluators are strongly encouraged to give out zeroes where a proposal does not have any features that meet the criteria. Thus, for example, using this methodology an evaluator may decide that one of the other proposals is only 10 percent as effective in meeting the community health promotion criterion. The evaluator then awards the second proposal one hundred points for this criterion.

• After completing the scoring for all the proposals on the first criteria, they are told to go back to the second strategic plan criteria and continue the process, and so on until they finish all ten criteria.

This system is extremely efficient and relatively fast. Using a desktop PC and the requisite software creates an amazingly compact process. In fact, one of the administrators has been known to complete the forty-item list, with its ten criteria, in forty-five minutes. The average time among the group is about ninety minutes. Remember, this means that each RHMC administrator spends only an hour and a half a year allocating as much as $10 million. Not bad, and far superior to the previous smoke-filled backroom process.

The software enhances the process in several ways. First, each detailed proposal is just a mouse click away if the administrator needs to research any specific aspect. Particularly important in this regard are the justifications within any of the criteria that the department managers have claimed; the software summarizes them on one easy-to-read screen. Second, the software actually leads the administrator through the process, forcing him to complete the first strategic plan criteria before allowing him to move on to the second. This therefore enforces discipline in the process. Last, the software encourages the manager to complete a screen for any additional information that she may deem important to making her case. This screen is always available to the evaluator with a single mouse click.

The administrators are given one additional piece of information during this meeting that is critical to fully understanding the criteria-based capital budget. Although these administrators serve as evaluators for each proposal and cumulatively their scores are totaled and ranked, high to low, there is still one additional concept that significantly affects the final total.

It turns out that the ten criteria are not evenly weighted at 10 percent each. Instead, this process mandates that the CEO gets to weigh the ten criteria, to decide which are more important to the organization's well-being and which are less important. At RHMC, this weighing was kept secret from the evaluators so that these same administrators would not be allowed to game the system by trying to overjustify the highly weighted criteria in their own division's requests. The only two people who know this weighing are the CEO and the finance staff member assigned to inputting it into the computer.

This is all explained to the administrators before they and their colleagues begin to attempt to verbally sway each other. Now that they know what they will be evaluating over the next few days in the privacy of their own offices, each evaluator can better formulate questions during the second part of the meeting they are all attending.

August 12: Discussion of All Pool Proposals with the Pool Evaluators

There has been a lot written about the main capital budget process for all requests over $100,000. A significant amount of information is requested and then evaluated for equipment and projects above this threshold. Yet as we saw in Table 8.1, there are many other requested projects under the threshold. The criteria-based capital budgeting process is streamlined and does not generally involve all the administrators, yet it still meets the objective of using strategic plan criteria in making yes-or-no decisions.

There is a reason for the streamlined process. It follows the classic 80/20 principle of finance, which expresses that in almost every case the top 20 percent of a process accounts for 80 percent of the value, while conversely, the bottom 80 percent of a process accounts for only 20 percent of the value. The principle works to a large extent in this case. Twenty percent of the 194 requests means 39 proposals should be reviewed. In this case if we round up to forty cases that just happen to meet the $100,000 threshold, we can see again in Table 8.1 that these proposals have a dollar value of $11.6 million. This is 71.2 percent of the 194 cases, which is fairly close to proving the 80/20 principle ($11.6 million divided by $16.3 million equals 71.2 percent).

The process for all requests under $100,000 divides all the items into five categories: clinical equipment, facilities construction and renovation projects, information systems, market development, and office equipment. Small specialty groups are assembled to review the requested items in their categories. Each group develops a smaller set of criteria related to the strategic plan. They use these criteria to rate and score the requests.

The groups are made up of directors and managers with significant responsibility for the areas in question. Table 8.2 shows the representative groups responsible for pool evaluation.

TABLE 8.2. RHMC POOL EVALUATORS.

Pool	Evaluators
Clinical equipment	Vice president, patient care services; directors of nursing; director of clinical services
Facilities and construction	Director of facilities, manager of environmental services
Information services	Chief information officer, manager of hardware services, manager of application services
Market development	Chief strategy officer, director of external communications
Office equipment	Finance administrator, materials manager

At the first meeting, the finance facilitator explains the role of each group, how it operates, and how much money is available for funding. They then review all of the requested proposals for the first time. The review consists of detailed discussion of each item and how it relates to the decision criteria set by the group. If there are any questions that cannot be answered at this meeting about any of the proposals, a small additional amount of time is set aside to get the answer. At the end of the meeting, the group is instructed as follows.:

- Think about what they have just discussed.
- Get answers to any open questions.
- Return between August 22 and 25 to make final decisions on the requests.

Funding Availability

The amount of money available to both the over-$100,000 items and the under-$100,000 items is determined by taking the initial total funding determined by the finance administrator and allocating it among the categories. For example, after the organization decided to fund its capital at 100 percent of depreciation expense, it then needs to determine the allocation between the over and under groups. At RHMC, they look at the dollar level of requests between those over and under $100,000 and use the percentage ratios between the two. Again, if we examine Table 8.1, we see that RHMC will fund 71.2 percent of its depreciation expense for the over-$100,000 requests and 28.8 percent for those under $100,000.

This funding limitation sets up constraints for the organization and justifies the need for this type of capital budgeting process. Table 8.3 summarizes the differences between the capital requests and capital available by category.

TABLE 8.3. RHMC 2002 PROPOSED CAPITAL BUDGET, FUNDING SUMMARY.

	Total Requested	Total Funded		
		Total	Criteria-Based	Non-Criteria-Based
Main strategic	$11,600	$8,184	$3,184	$5,000
Clinical equipment	1,800	1,270	870	400
Facilities and construction	1,500	1,058	258	800
Information services	900	635	635	0
Market development	300	212	212	0
Office equipment	200	141	141	0
Total	$16,300	$11,500	$5,300	$6,200

First, it is obvious that some department managers are not approved for all the capital they requested. The organization's funding level is $11.5 million. The capital requests are $16.3 million. That's a gap of $4.8 million. The organization can approve only 70.5 percent of its requests.

Non-Criteria-Based Capital Funding

A counterintuitive concept inherent in this criteria-based capital budgeting system is the non-criteria aspect built into the process. At its heart, this concept expresses that not all capital acquisitions need to or are even able to formally meet strategic plan criteria and therefore need a safety valve for approval. In addition, there are capital items that might compete well in the main process, but because the administration as a whole agrees that these items need to be purchased no matter what, they are deemed eligible for automatic approval.

Examples of RHMC non-criteria-based capital items are HIPAA-mandated information system upgrades and fixes and information system infrastructure upgrades to support HIPAA fixes. In addition, the administration has determined that it is in the organization's best interest to approve construction of a new emergency department and renovation of one of their medical/surgical nursing units. These items alone amount to $4.8 million in capital. This amount is therefore deducted from the total amount available to be funded, thereby reducing the amounts available for those criteria-based projects that need to compete against each other.

August 12–15: Evaluate Proposals Online

Finally, between August 12 and 15 the administrators (proposal evaluators) get their opportunity to score each of the proposals against all others using the ten strategic plan criteria. This is done on the evaluator's PC, which is attached to a local area network (LAN) so that all the scoring is linked and aggregated by the software. This results in a streamlined and efficient outcome at the end of the process. They follow the rules set down at the meeting of August 11 and are given three days in which to find a two-hour time block to get it done. The finance division has two staff members available during these three days to come over to any evaluator's office in the event of a question or problem with the concepts or the software. At RHMC, over these three days, no problems are encountered.

August 22–25: Various Pool Consensus Meetings with Pool Evaluators

Between August 22 and 25, the pool evaluators get together again to make final recommendations on their category requests. If there are no controversies, they are done. If however, no consensus has been reached, each group has one more chance to settle on their recommended list over the following week. In essence, these meetings are held to give any of the pool evaluators one more chance to lobby for their own proposal or champion any other. These meetings are usually short and conclusive.

August 25: Consensus Meeting for All Proposals over $100,000

This is the day that many of the administrators have been waiting for. It is when they learn if the capital requested by their division has made the cut of the criteria-based capital budgeting system. All of the previous process has been important, but it was also a prelude to this. The power of the criteria-based capital budget now becomes evident.

At this meeting, a list for the 2002 recommended and nonrecommended capital items is presented. It is the culmination of the administrator's rating and the CEO's weighing of the ten strategic plan criteria. The initial output from the licensed software is called the weighted value score (WVS). It is literally the administrators' judged priority ratings multiplied by the CEO's priority weighting. This output, when arrayed from the highest WVS to the lowest, is a clear indication of which requested capital items meet the administrators' concept of strategic plan importance.

But this array is not the final list of recommended projects. The final step required to produce the best outcome is to divide each of the weighted value scores by its cost. This produces a benefit-to-cost ratio that can then be ranked. The higher the result, the more likely the capital request will be approved. This simple mathematical equation allows the administration to put the requested capital expenditures into context. For example, there could be a request for an item that has a high WVS but also high cost. The result can easily move it down the list, lower than an item with a lower WVS but much lower cost.

These rankings allow the administration to *make rational decisions using objective criteria and techniques,* something that was not possible before at RHMC. The rankings are machine-generated from their own consensus inputs. Still, they are not required to use them, all or in part, if they so choose. As a group, they can decide not to fund a machine-recommended item in favor of one that did not initially make the cut. An administrator may try to lobby for a project that missed the cut. However, the odds are stacked against a change because everyone went through the process and if a substitution is made, one of the other recommended projects will have to be cut.

It is a zero-sum game. The funding is set and will not be increased. So when the software ranked the projects, it drew the cutoff point above the funding limit. Replacement requires substitution. Because of this, arguments are eliminated in the meeting. Everyone has participated and is aware of the process. They understand that they have met criteria and that the decision is completely defensible to the losers.

RHMC, in fact, experienced an intended consequence of the process that was quite positive for the organization. During last year's capital budget, the organization's chief operating officer (COO) requested a CT scanner costing $800,000. Based on the final WVS and benefit-to-cost ratio, this project did not make the cut. Still, the COO felt strongly that this was an important project and needed to be funded. This was because the request was initiated by the medical director for the radiology service, a powerful and politically connected individual.

In the past, the influence of the requester and the project champion meant this argument would have prevailed over the strategic plan importance. However, because of the new process, the COO decided to go back to the radiologist and explain the situation, the objectivity of the process, and the desire of the group not to override the criteria outcome. Lo and behold, the radiologist backed off on his request and decided to come back the following year with a request for an even more enhanced scanner. This was a major success for this year's process. Next year will take care of itself.

As the meeting progresses, the finance administrator can make changes to any of the inputs online and in real time through the software. Because the results are being projected on a screen in the front of the room, the results of revised assumptions can be analyzed and reviewed immediately. The software reoptimizes the results instantaneously. This also enhances the value of the process, where the assembled brain trust can pursue its desired results.

At the end of this meeting, the capital budget has been set based on established funding levels and strategic plan criteria, or else there is a clear need to bring back certain additional information on some of the projects, if so desired. If this is so, the administrators have to perform one more set of evaluations to finalize their ratings. If it is not necessary, the 2002 capital budget is done.

August 26–28: Revise Ratings, if Necessary, on the Reviewer's Desktop

These next three days are necessary only if there was any kind of dispute at the August 25 meeting involving an administrator's pet project, or if additional information is requested during the meeting. It is really used as a fail-safe device, allowing the capital budget to have extra time built into the process. Although the capital budget software allows the administrators to immediately see the results of any changes to funding level, they might need some additional data to make an informed decision. If this is so, that information is transmitted electronically into the networked software for all the administrators to see and react to online, possibly by changing their evaluation scoring.

If this is done, the group meets again early next month to perform one final review of the capital budget requests to finalize it.

Operating Budget

Although the finance staff members are hard at work on the capital budget, the beginning of August is a time when they are able to take a breather on the operating budget. The department managers and their bosses, the administrators, are doing almost all of the work this month. They are reviewing the operating budgets that have been in their hands since July 25. The main role of the finance staff during this time is to be available to answer any questions the managers have. They also continue to hold small formal classes on how the managers can best do their budgets. Still, for the most part, August finds the finance staff devoting most of their time to the capital budget.

August 15: Department Managers Need to Return Their Operating Budget Worksheets to Their Vice Presidents

By August 15, the managers have had the operating budget worksheets in their hands for three weeks. They were expected to review the full-time equivalent employees (FTEs) and salary levels, the volume assumptions, and the nonsalary line items to determine if there were any clerical or technical errors made by the finance staff in preparing the budget. If there were any errors of this sort, they are expected to make a note of it on the budget so that it can be corrected when it is returned to finance.

After the error check is complete, the managers have an opportunity to request additional resources for the department. This is problematic. Health care at the beginning of the twenty-first century is an industry under considerable financial pressure. Because of reimbursement limitations, additional resources are not easily granted. The best way to ensure that a request for additional staff is approved is to demonstrate that net revenue will exceed the cost of the position. Proof is the problem. It's easy for a manager to say that additional volume and revenues will accumulate if another staff member is added. It is much harder to prove because for the most part this is tantamount to telling the future.

In Chapter One, the validity of volume assumptions was discussed at length in the MRI pro forma section. The administrators, who have dozens of years of cumulative experience, have heard all kinds of stories from managers about how this added FTE or that added FTE would allow them to earn significant additional revenue for the organization. But it doesn't always happen, and then the organization loses money on the assumption. The addition of MRI service was an example of the organization taking a chance on proven medical technology where they thought there was a good chance of meeting the pro forma volume.

Similarly, revenue-producing department managers are currently deciding where they too may have an opportunity to expand their department services. For example, the radiology department manager may decide that there is an opportunity to expand CT scan service. They know there is an absolute capacity level to their one-and-only CT scanner. They also know that they are currently open for two full shifts, from 6:30 in the morning until 10:30 at night. Finally, there is currently a two-week waiting list for outpatient testing. Because of these facts, the department manager decides that it would be appropriate to request a second CT scanner as well as three additional FTEs to run the new machine. Once again, because of the magnitude of this purchase, a pro forma analysis is prepared to determine if the net revenues will exceed the additional expenses, including staffing, additional fringe benefits, supplies, and depreciation on the new equipment.

Smaller projects involving revenue-producing departments need similar analysis. For example, the physical therapy department may have been built to accommodate a far greater volume of patients than is currently being served. However, if RHMC has just recruited a new orthopedic surgeon, it may be presumed that the need for additional therapies will commence soon. In this case, the request for a new physical therapist in the department is almost certain to be accepted.

But it may not be so easy if the physical therapy manager can show no particular event that increases revenues. Still, the manager believes that additional staff will bring additional people to the organization for service. This is the "if we build it, they will come" theory of management. It almost never works and will be rejected out of hand by the RHMC administrator. If, however, this manager does her homework and writes a marketing plan that includes specific actions to be taken to recruit physicians, health plans, and individual patients, there is a better chance for the extra FTE(s) to be accepted.

Nevertheless, if it is difficult for a revenue-department manager to add new staff, it is even harder to do so for a nonrevenue manager. Nonrevenue-producing departments find it very difficult to justify additional staff as a result of additional workload because it is always so hard to prove. Later in this chapter, we look at cost analysis and decision making. In this section, let us discuss how to measure workload. This is an important discussion that, if performed correctly, can truly help to justify additional staff.

The most likely method for a nonrevenue-producing manager to justify additional staff is to claim cost reduction in other areas of the department. Yet it is usually rejected because this is almost never verifiable. Like the volume argument used by the revenue-producing manager, the proof is elusive. Because this argument usually fails, the nonrevenue manager does not have many good justifications remaining for additional staff.

Nonsalary expenses are the other line items the managers review for accuracy. They determine whether the supplies, purchased services, and all other services reflect the current year's reality and the upcoming budget year projection. They do this using some financial analysis techniques, but mostly it is determined by gut feel. Because they know what they are spending this year using the financial reports shown by finance, the managers can speculate on next year's expenses. It is easy for many managers to recognize whether any of their large expense items have been lost through clerical error. If these nonsalary expenses appear correct, then they are ready to accept the budget and move it on to their administrator for further review.

August 18–28: Review of the Proposed Operating Budget by the Divisional Vice Presidents and Then Return to Finance

During this ten-day period, each administrator receives a budget package that has been reviewed and accepted by each of his or her department managers. Each administrator's role is to aggregate all the department budgets and determine how the total volumes, revenues, and expenses equate to the current year budget and the current year projection and how they relate to the original following year budget proposed at the July 18 meeting.

Their role is to understand the budget assumption of each one of their departments. They are required to present and defend any request that deviates from the July 18 budget, particularly if it reduces the bottom line. Here are some actions of this sort:

Department Manager Actions That Decrease the Budgeted Bottom Line

- Volume reduction
- Gross revenue reduction owing to price decrease (to conform with market forces)
- Expense increase, characterized by
  FTE increase
  Salary increase above the organization's established average
  Supply cost increase because of additional consumption above the current average

Administrators also need to be prepared to speak up at the September 9 administrative budget meeting if the budgeted bottom line once again fails to meet the board's established targets. They need to bring contingency plans and expense items they can "give up" if, as is almost certain, additional expenses have to be cut.

The administrators also understand that their role is tenuous. They need to walk a fine line between supporting the perceived needs of their managers (whose job it is to run daily operation of the department) and the board goals (which mandate specific bottom-line requirements). They use their experience and training in attempting to achieve these goals.

Budget Variance Analysis

While managers, directors, and vice presidents are performing all this work to present the best budgeted bottom line for the upcoming year, the current year is taking place. During the year, the administration constantly monitors not only its actual financial results but also how those results compare to the current year budget. That is really the whole point of the budget; it is a plan developed by management and approved by the board, and it is meant to be followed. Deviation from the budgeted results should be explained to understand why variances occurred. Then action should commence to bring the actual performance back into conformance with the budget, particularly if performance is negative.

Accounting and finance track and report budget variance diligently. In general, variance is not inherently bad or good. It is just a deviation from the expected. Yet budget variance is a concept that many managers have a hard time accepting.

Budgets are not effective without appropriate feedback mechanisms. Feedback allows the managers to review the variance between actual operational results (including volume, revenues, and expenses) and expected (budgeted) results. All budget variances should be explainable. The concept of explainable variance should not be foreign to the clinical manager, who probably has a scientific background and should understand the concept of deviation from the norm. An explainable variance is one that results from a specific event different from the expected event.

For example, let's say that a water main on the second floor of RHMC broke in the month of August. The resulting flooding caused water damage to six rooms on the first floor. Ignoring any potential insurance claim, the cost to fix the damage was $10,000 and was charged to the facilities department. The manager of the department is disturbed because this $10,000 charge has put him over budget by $9,000 for the month. He is concerned that he will be singled out for criticism when the monthly financial statement is distributed because of the negative budget expense variance.

This should not be the case, and it is not so at RHMC. The administrators understand the concept of explainable variance. So long as a manager can appropriately explain significant negative or positive variance, she will not be maligned or disparaged. In the previous case, the administrator is reminded of the reason for the overage when she reviews the monthly variance analysis report required to be completed by all managers (see Exhibit 8.1).

This variance report allows the manager to record reasons for positive or negative difference in net revenue, salary expense, and nonsalary expense. The purpose of the report is to require the managers to research and discuss variance with their administrators. It allows both individuals to know their businesses better. In addition, the finance administrator uses these reports to explain their variances to the finance committee. It is the best way to get and maintain a complete record of activities that deviate from the financial performance expected when the budget was developed in previous years.

Although the paper method of budget variance has been in place for several years, the RHMC administrators are currently installing a new financial decision support system that allows administrators to easily monitor their managers: through exception reporting and alert management. The system is a user-friendly operating and capital budgeting product and also a tool that automatically alerts department managers and their managers to any deviation from the established exception parameters set by the administration (say, plus or minus 5 or 10 percent). The system automatically alerts, through e-mail notification, the appropriate manager and his or her vice president, as well as the hospital president, of the variance. The manager is required to respond to the e-mail with rationale and

EXHIBIT 8.1. MONTHLY DEPARTMENTAL "KNOW YOUR BUSINESS" REPORT.

Use this form to provide information if your actual operating margin for the month was ±10 percent of budget.

Department _____

Cost Center Number _____ Month _____

Operating margin variance: _____ percent $ _____

In the space below, identify the major factors contributing to the variance.

Account	Amount ($)	Amount (%)	Explanation of Variance
Net Revenue			
Salary Expenses			
Nonsalary Expenses			

This form is due to your vice president no later than the last business day of each month for the previous month's profit-and-loss statement.

justification for the variance, as well as a corrective action plan, if required. This response is logged and automatically routed to higher-level administrators. This system instills a much greater level of accountability throughout the organization (Healthcare Insights, EnteleTRAC decision support software system; www/healthcareinsightllc.com).

Budget Variance Parameters

A key element of the variance report is the parameters set by the organization, triggering the need for an explanation. The organization's culture has a great deal to do with the parameter levels. For example, RHMC uses a 10 percent level; this means it does not question revenue and expense variances that fall within the 90 to 110 percent range around the budget. Other organizations may be tighter or looser with the parameter range.

Regardless of the range, it is important for the organization to enforce variance analysis. This allows administrators to maintain an understanding of the financial record of departments. Those with consistent problems maintaining positive variance from their budgeted margin should be monitored closely. If necessary, the organization needs to consider replacing any manager who does not contribute positively to budgeted organizational results.

Flexible Budgeting

Flexible budgeting is another aspect related to budgeting and budget variance reporting. A flexible budget is one adjusted for change in volume. The budget used by RHMC is not flexible but static. Static budgets "are not adjusted or altered, regardless of changes in volume or other conditions during the budget period," as Horngren and Foster put it in their legendary textbook, *Cost Accounting: A Managerial Emphasis* (1987, p. 181). This is why RHMC department managers have been using the variance report in Figure 8.3 to explain whether their variances are related to volume or whether they are positive or negative for the original budget. The organization's new budgeting and monitoring system automatically flexes the budget according to the selected volume statistic chosen for each department.

An organization that uses a flexible budget already flexes the budget column in the monthly departmental financial report to factor out any volume variance. The flexible budget is "based on a knowledge of how revenue and costs should behave over a range of activities" (Horngren and Foster, 1987, p. 181). Because RHMC does not yet use a flexible budget, we do not discuss it in detail. However, many health care organizations use flexible budgeting rather than static budgeting; it is a cultural and software system preference that can be changed by the CEO, COO, or CFO.

Cost Accounting and Analysis

Cost accounting in health care has had an interesting and rich existence since 1966, when Medicare and Medicaid were created. Prior to these programs, the health care industry was smaller and less sophisticated. There was a perception at that time that because of the relatively charitable nature of the industry, accurate costing of organizational activity was unnecessary and unwarranted. Many nonprofit organizations did not care as much about their bottom line. Remarkable as it seems today, they often had donors who agreed to fund any bottom-line losses at the end of each year. These losses were usually moderate and reflected a time when less dramatic care was furnished to patients. A hospital's mission then was more convalescent, less intensive.

The advent of Medicare made health care into a big industry. All of a sudden, money flowed freely. With this came the need for better accounting of organizational revenues and costs. In fact, the Social Security Act that brought Medicare into existence mandated annual filing of a cost report for each organization treating Medicare patients. As reported in some detail earlier in Chapter Four, the MCR mandated a cost accounting methodology for the industry called the ratio of cost to charges (RCC). The RCC was developed by allocating the organization's indirect (or overhead) costs to revenue-producing cost centers according to a step-down methodology. Because of the relative ease of this methodology, much of the industry accepted RCC as its cost accounting system. Unfortunately, the system is not totally accurate for developing or determining the actual cost of doing business at the unit-of-service level.

The RCC costing method is faulty because it does not meet the general requirements needed for a good cost accounting methodology. Cost accounting is a financial management technique that requires costs to be separated into meaningful categories to allow identification. These are the relevant cost components:

- Direct costs: those directly attributable to the operating or revenue-producing department in question
- Indirect costs: also called overhead costs, not directly attributable to an operating department
- Variable costs: those varying (increasing or decreasing) with change in volume
- Fixed costs: those that do not vary with an increase or decrease in volume

The RCC and step-down methods of cost accounting do not do a reliable job of separating the components with relative accuracy. In fact, although these methods purport to at least separate direct from indirect component, they do not do so at the unit-of-service level and they do not attempt to separate the variable from the fixed component.

Consequently, if a health care organization wants to "know" the cost of producing any service, it must adopt different and better techniques to do so. The list just below elaborates on why the organization would want to have a good idea of the component parts of its costs at the unit-of-service level. Each objective of a cost accounting system is important in its own right. The cumulative effect of the objectives makes it an organizational imperative to be able to perform reasonably accurate cost accounting. Cost accounting separates costs into meaningful categories, allowing managers to

- Measure the effects of change in intensity and case mix
- Evaluate and measure performance against a plan
- Acquire the information required to manage resources efficiently
- Identify those costs that can be converted from fixed to variable
- Identify inefficient functions and demonstrate the nature of the problem, such as price, volume, or practice

There Is No Such Thing as "True" Cost!

While reviewing established cost accounting techniques, it is important to discuss some reasons why there is no "true" cost in cost accounting. Many people—among them administrators, department managers, and physicians—believe that the cost accounting figures presented by the finance staff are an accurate and objective portrayal of cost components. The problem is that this is just not true. Developing costs at the unit-of-service level involves assumptions. In any finance or accounting concept, the first time an assumption is used, complete accuracy is lost. The best that can be said of cost accounting is that it is representative of the cost picture.

To understand why unit cost can never be completely true or accurate, let's look at the example of a reasonably common test done at a hospital, a CT of the abdomen. This is a digital diagnostic test ordered by physicians to rule out or determine whether a medical problem exists in the patient's abdomen. As we'll see, there are assumptions used to determine the direct and indirect (overhead) costs at the unit level. To ascertain costs at the unit level, the financial analyst has to first determine the direct costs. In the case of a CT of the abdomen, costs of staffing and nonsalaries have to be determined.

For staffing, there are at least three ways to determine unit costs:

1. Time and motion studies
2. Department manager time studies
3. Department manager perception

TABLE 8.4. CT SCANNING DEPARTMENT, LIST OF TESTS PERFORMED.

Test	Technician Time
CT of the head	30 minutes
CT of the chest	45 minutes
CT of the abdomen	30 minutes
CT of the pelvis	45 minutes
CT of the spine	60 minutes

In all three, several assumptions are used. The biggest one regards the amount of time it takes each employee to perform each of the various jobs within the department. Table 8.4 shows an example of the tests performed in the CT scanning department and the technician time that has been determined as required to perform each test.

To develop what is called *microcosting* within each department, it is important to have a list of all the services performed. The direct departmental costs are then split between staffing and nonstaffing costs. All of these direct costs are then segregated into their various component parts. In the case of staffing at RHMC, this is done through use of time logs kept by the staff and reviewed by the department manager over the course of a four-week period. In the case of supply costs, actual invoices are used wherever possible.

Table 8.5 is a summary of the direct cost inputs for the CT of the abdomen. The direct costs for the test are assembled and split between variable and fixed components. In this case, there were no direct fixed costs, just direct variable costs. A computer model is then used to allocate all of the direct departmental costs across all the tests.

Allocation of direct staffing costs entails several additional cost components not already included in the time log, such as fringe benefits and nonproductive time. In fact, nonproductive time doubles or triples the actual direct cost of performing a test. Nonproductive time is often categorized as stand-by time, which is when the technician is standing around, waiting for the next patient to present herself for treatment. Other nonproductive time includes paid breaks and holidays, sick time, and vacation time. All of these costs are encountered in the CT scanning department (also known as a cost center), and they all need to be allocated back to individual tests.

After the computer model completes its direct cost allocation at the unit level, it allocates indirect costs to revenue-producing departments through a statistical methodology based on usage. Here are common statistical allocation bases for developing indirect cost centers:

TABLE 8.5. DEVELOPMENT OF PROCEDURE-LEVEL UNIT COSTS, CT OF THE ABDOMEN: INPUTS.

Direct Variable Costs **Labor Costs**	**Pay Rate**	**Average Test Time (in Minutes)**	**Total Cost**
Senior radiology technician	$17.90	30	$8.95

Nonlabor costs	**Unit Cost**	**Quantity**	**Total Cost**
Film	$1.59	11	$17.49
Contrast media	$40.44	1	$40.44

Other	**Total Departmental Cost**	**Annual Tests Performed**	**Total Cost**
Equipment depreciation	$200,000	5,000	$40.00
Equipment service contract (on CT scanning machine)	$50,000	5,000	$10.00
Total direct variable cost inputs			$116.88

Department and Statistical Basis

Building depreciation	Departmental square feet
Employee benefits	FTEs
Human resources	FTEs
Information services	Total expenses
Plant operations	Departmental square feet
Environmental services (housekeeping)	Departmental square feet
Cafeteria	FTEs
Administration	Total expenses
Financial services management	Total expenses
Materials management	Supply expenses
Laundry and linen	Laundry pounds
Patient accounting	Inpatient and outpatient units of service
Medical records	Inpatient and outpatient units of service
Planning and marketing	Total revenues

Medical staff	Total revenues
Central transportation	Adult admissions
Food services	Adult patient days
Community services	Total revenues
All other overhead	Total expenses
Bad debt	Total revenues

This allocation scheme deposits these indirect costs into a revenue-producing department, awaiting a mechanism to further allocate the costs down to the unit-of-service or procedure level. Costs are assigned at the procedure level through an allocation based either on departmental revenue or volume.

Furthermore, one final assumption is used to determine unit costs. The 80/20 rule suggests the number of service or procedure codes to study. In this case, the rule theorizes that 80 percent of the departmental costs are used by only 20 percent of the departmental tests performed. As previously reported in Chapter Seven, this rule applies to many resource-based subjects. Therefore the RHMC department manager needs only to analyze the top 20 percent of the tests in the department, not 100 percent, to feel confident in the costing outcomes. A computer matrix allocates the unstudied procedures on the basis of gross charges.

After all the allocations are done, the computerized cost accounting system produces a detailed analysis of the unit cost for each test. It allocates all the costs between fixed and variable, direct and indirect because each component acts differently in the course of departmental business. Exhibit 8.2 represents the output of the cost allocation process for CT of the abdomen. It is interesting to note that the variable salary output is $31.67, compared to input costs of $8.95. The difference represents those stand-by and nonproductive costs mentioned earlier. In this case, the fully allocated salary is 3.5 times the direct salary. That alone should raise some questions about the productivity level in the department.

It is also interesting to note that total costs at $249.55 are 87.8 percent greater than direct costs at $132.91. This means that the indirect cost markup for CT of the abdomen is 87.8 percent. This is another area that managers and administrators can review for cost-saving opportunities. It may mean that overhead costs are too high.

In summary, it is now obvious that a considerable number of assumptions are used to develop cost accounting standards at the procedure or unit level. Thus, cost accounting is useful to understanding an organization's cost components within the various revenue-producing procedures performed, but the costs that are developed are not true or genuinely accurate. They are reasonable and can be consistently applied.

EXHIBIT 8.2. DEVELOPMENT OF PROCEDURE-LEVEL UNIT COSTS, CT OF THE ABDOMEN: OUTPUTS.

Direct Costs		Indirect Costs	
Fixed costs		Fixed portion	$63.21
Salaries	$0.16		
Nonsalary	2.17		
Total fixed costs	2.33		
Variable costs		Variable portion	41.16
Salaries	31.67		
Nonsalary	46.42		
Equipment service contract	12.49		
Total variable costs	90.58		
Equipment depreciation	40.00	Equipment depreciation	8.93
Building depreciation	0	Building depreciation	3.34
Total direct expenses	$132.91	Total indirect expenses	116.64
		Total direct expenses	132.91
		CT of the abdomen total unit costs	$249.55

RHMC uses these cost accounting standards to produce a number of reports and analyses that aid in understanding departmental financial performance. They are used to determine which departments are making or losing money (winners and losers). Because the costs are developed at the procedure level, winners and losers can be aggregated in many ways:

- Diagnostic-related groups
- ICD-9-CM clinical diagnostic codes
- Nursing and ancillary departments
- Charge codes
- Physicians
- Payors
- Patients
- Service area
- Zip code
- Age
- Sex

Cost accounting leads to decision making. If used properly, it becomes an important tool in the administration's management arsenal. Winners can be rewarded and enhanced; losers can be disbanded. Loss leaders can be established and endured as they are developed by intent. Cost accounting is an art that acts like a science. In this case, the artist can paint with a broad brush.

August Finance Committee Special Agenda Items

In August, the finance committee has two special items to consider.

Review Next Year's Budget Assumptions

At the August finance committee, the finance administrator presents an abbreviated list of budget assumptions for the administration to formally present at the October meeting. It is still too early to propose a preliminary budgeted profit-and-loss statement, but this list allows the administration to introduce some of its preliminary thinking on the upcoming year. By doing so, the administration is able to gauge the mood and thinking of the finance committee. If there is some apparent disagreement in the direction being taken, it permits the administration to change its focus over the next few weeks prior to the October meeting.

Table 8.6 shows the budget assumptions submitted to the finance committee at the August meeting. The assumptions are strictly volume-related because no revenue or expense assumptions are ready. The assumptions include an abbreviated explanation for volume changes. This helps management begin its discussion with the board members about the direction in which they believe the organization is heading.

Annual Materials Management and Inventory Level Review

Once a year, RHMC management presents a report to the finance committee on the status of the organization's materials management goals and accomplishments. The report highlights the various efforts taken and achieved by the department in the areas of purchasing and receiving and central sterile supply, processing, and distribution. The report is presented in this format order:

- Trends in supply expenses per day
- Revenue enhancements
- Expense reductions
- Operational efficiencies

TABLE 8.6. RHMC 2002 BUDGET ASSUMPTIONS, AUG. 2001.

	2000 Actual	2001 Budget	2001 Projected	2002 Budget	Percentage Variance, 2002 Budget Versus 2001 Projected
Acute care					
Adult admissions	8,100	8,760	9,023	9,787	8.47%
Average length of stay	3.89	4.05	4.05	4.20	3.72%
Adult patient days	31,500	35,496	36,561	41,131	12.50%
Skilled nursing facility					
Number of admissions	800	840	850	900	5.88%
Average length of stay	11.00	10.00	9.50	8.30	−12.63%
Patient days	8,800	8,400	8,075	7,470	−7.49%
Newborns					
Admissions	1,950	2,145	2,165	2,382	10.00%
Average length of stay	2.00	2.00	2.00	2.00	0.00%
Patient days	3,900	4,290	4,330	4,763	10.00%
Total inpatients					
Admissions	10,850	11,745	12,038	13,069	8.56%
Average length of stay	4.07	4.10	4.07	4.08	0.39%
Patient days	44,200	48,186	48,966	53,364	8.98%
Outpatient visits	167,150	181,000	194,400	210,000	8.02%

Notes: The 2002 budget is being prepared at this time to be presented for approval in October. This information summarizes the volume assumptions being considered for this budget. The variances are based on the explanations noted here.

Explanation of variances:

(1) Maternity admissions increase 10 percent because of newly expanded unit and recruitment of four obstetricians.

(2) Psychiatric admissions increase 20 percent from addition of several new psychiatrists on staff.

(3) Medical and surgical admissions increase 4 percent owing to additional affiliation of several primary care physicians.

(4) Outpatient visits increase 8.0 percent based on prior year trends and continued emphasis on physician and consumer marketing.

FIGURE 8.1. RHMC SUPPLY COSTS PER ADJUSTED
PATIENT DAY, 1996–1998.

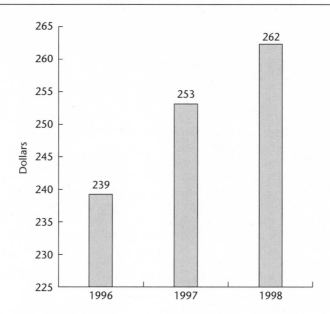

A summarized version of the report is presented to the finance committee. It has the gist of the important concepts to be communicated and understood by the finance committee to further their governance role. The finance committee usually needs to take no action on the information it receives so long as the report does not contain information showing problems with inventory level or the supply expense per adjusted patient day (see Figure 8.1).

CHAPTER NINE

SEPTEMBER

"Damn it, Barnes, you've screwed me up again," Frank Jacobs screams over a telephone line bristling with static and distortion.

Sam has but a moment to react. It is early in the morning, and he has not yet had his first cup of coffee. Recognizing the voice on the other end of the phone as one of his usual complainers, Sam responds, "Oh, come on, Frank, what did I do now?"

"Listen, Barnes, you can't fool me. I know you were personally responsible for signing that managed care contract that cheated me out of a whole lot of revenue," says Jacobs, one of the leading orthopedic surgeons on the Ridgeland Heights Medical Center staff.

"Now, Frank, really, you and I have talked about this before. You know that although I did sign that agreement, I did not do it unilaterally. The contract was discussed with the board of the IPA [independent practice association] as well as an advisory group of your colleagues on our PHO [physician hospital organization]. They all felt it was in the best interest of the hospital, and of all the physicians in the IPA, to sign this contract rather than lose all the business generated by it."

"Horsepuckey, Barnes. I just know that the hospital will benefit from this contract a lot more than the doctors. You are fully conflicted in your role of lead negotiator for the hospital and the IPA."

Sam Barnes is getting steamed, but he decides to keep his cool.

"Frank, I'm really sorry you feel like that, but it just isn't true. I know you were around here when the PHO was formed ten years ago so that the hospital and physicians who chose to join the IPA—like yourself—could jointly present themselves in a united way to the managed care companies. In fact, over those ten years, we have jointly contracted with over fifty MCOs. Your representatives on the IPA monitor these negotiations. Frank, I'm not out to get you. It's in the best interest of the hospital to get you the best deal that can be made."

"Barnes, you're full of it. The rates you're negotiating are killing my office income. I can hardly afford to keep my whole staff together and still maintain my lifestyle anymore. I know you're driving the rates down every time you accept a lower reimbursement."

"No, Frank, I'm not! I know you believe that, but our acceptance of the lower rates is not causing the rates to plummet. This is an industrywide phenomenon. The payment structure has changed over the last several years, and we're not immune. In fact, you should be thanking me rather than harassing me. We've actually held the line a lot longer than many of the PHOs around the area. I'm sorry your income is going down. But I also know that you need to look at the management of your office practice. It's probably the best way you have right now to try to maintain your income. There are many ways you can economize without hurting your quality of care and patient satisfaction."

"Barnes, thanks for the advice, but I'll pass. Your advice on behalf of my business is already killing me. I'll figure out what's in my best interest by myself," Jacobs blurts out as he slams down the receiver.

The first part of September is always an interesting time of year in the northern region of the United States. Almost ideal weather conditions predominate. Cool Canadian air wafts down out of the north, mixing with the warm breezes traveling up from the Gulf of Mexico. This is the best time of the year to live in this part of the country. Temperatures are in the high seventies during the day, the low sixties at night.

But with Labor Day fast approaching, the end of the unofficial summer season is near. The roadways around the densely populated region are already beginning to get more congested. The grocery stores and shopping malls are getting busier, while the swimming pools are preparing to close. It is a season of melancholy for many. The end of summer means the distant winter season is not too far away. It's time for many to put away their toys and return to the real working world.

Of course, at the RHMC finance offices, real work never went away. The summer was one of their two busy seasons, with budget preparation dominating the effort. Other tasks also needed to be done. For instance, this month the CEO requested additional financial analysis of the physician practices owned by the organization. There was concern that the practices were not contributing to the overall bottom line of the organization and were operating negative to budget. The multifaceted analysis was designed to highlight the financial condition of the practices as well as the impact that the practices have on the hospital's bottom line. The finance department was preparing to give the CEO a detailed analysis by the end of the month.

Operating Budget

Meanwhile, September is the month in which the heavy technical work that the finance staff perform on the operating budget is completed. Subsequent work is more clerical in nature. There is only this one additional short stretch for the finance staff to stimulate their enthusiasm. The efforts in September look like this:

- September 9: Validate or adjust budget assumptions and semifinal budget approval by the administrators
- September 17: Final review and approval of the operating budget and review of the human resource committee package

- September 30–October 14: Prepare first draft through final copy of the 2000 budget for the finance committee

Right around the Labor Day weekend, the finance staff work being performed on the operating budget revs up again. After the vice presidents complete their operating budget review on August 28, it is returned to the finance division for processing. The finance staff have only eleven days to crunch the volumes, revenues, and expenses submitted by the department managers into an understandable set of reports. At the September 9 meeting, the administrators validate or adjust the assumptions submitted by the department managers. Therefore they need the best description and summary of the submitted financial data that they can get to make the best budgeting decisions for the organization.

For the finance staff to give their best summary of the data, once again they perform significant analyses at the level of detailed department line items. This is done to determine whether the changes requested by the managers make sense in the overall scheme and scope of the operating budget. The manager's job during August is to

- Review the FTEs and salary levels
- Review volume assumptions and nonsalary line items for any clerical or technical errors made by the finance staff in preparing the budget
- Request any additional resources for the department, whether staffing or nonsalary

The finance staff's job is to review the manager's changes for objectivity and purpose. If a mistake was previously made, this is now the time to correct it. It is imperative that any mistakes be corrected before final decisions are made. They are much more difficult to correct, from a political standpoint, after final administrative approval is granted. Because this is the version that ultimately goes to the finance committee, no CEO or chief financial officer wants to make any changes and admit to a mistake if at all possible.

An even worse time to find a mistake is after the budget is approved by the board of directors. The approved board budget is the formal direction of the health care organization and cannot be changed administratively. Going back to the board for subsequent approval is the only way to change the current year's budget. No administrator wants to take a weak story back to the board. Therefore, common or small mistakes must be absorbed by the division responsible. It is to everyone's advantage to catch any errors at this point in the process.

The outcome of this work by the finance staff will be a presentation to the executive and administrative staff on the upcoming year's budgeted profit and loss statement. This is done at the September 9 meeting.

September 9: Validate or Adjust Budget Assumptions and Semifinal Budget Approval by the Administrators

September 9 is another big meeting date for the finance and nonfinance administrators. Once again, there is trepidation as each enters the room to learn the financial fate of the upcoming year: How much money will we still have to cut? How many employees have to be eliminated to balance the budget? Who will remain to take care of the patients, the facility, and electronic backbone of the computerized medicine now being practiced?

This particular budget meeting is often the hardest one of the year. This is where most of the final decisions are made. It becomes all the more difficult when department managers request big expense increases without any offsetting net revenue. During this particular budget process, ten additional FTEs were requested in the areas of facilities management, information services, planning, and marketing.

In addition, the clinical services division requested two additional FTEs for its rapidly growing MRI and CT scanning departments. Diagnostic services, particularly high-tech imaging services, is an extremely fast growing segment of the organization's business. The physicians are fully aware of the value of these diagnostic devices. Thus the diagnostic imaging manager is planning to add late afternoon and evening shifts for both services and needs a technician in each area. These two FTEs will be approved because the incremental revenue far outpaces the expenses of the additional staff and supplies.

The other positions are more problematic and not so automatic. In fact, the only other two positions that are approved at this meeting belong to the information services department. They are granted two additional network specialists, responsible for maintaining the LAN and the devices attached to it. This means they are the installation and troubleshooting team for more than one thousand personal computers, three hundred local printers, and all the network hardware and system software. As RHMC places more pieces of software on the network, the problems multiply, and more attention is required by the information services staff. Because these problems are visible to administrators, it is easy for the information services administrator to get approval for these new jobs.

At this meeting, the finance administrator presents the modified preliminary budgeted statement of operations, which is based on (1) the changes suggested at the July 18 meeting and (2) changes requested by the department managers (see Table 9.1). In both cases, the changes include a 4 percent price increase and suggested improvements in investment income.

There are two issues surrounding the change in investment income. First, RHMC reports its investment income above the operating margin line in its GAAP-audited financial statement. Therefore, any improvements to investment

TABLE 9.1. RHMC PRELIMINARY BUDGETED STATEMENT OF OPERATIONS FOR THE BUDGET YEAR ENDING DEC. 31, 2002 (PREPARED SEPT. 9, 2001) (IN THOUSANDS OF DOLLARS).

	2000 Actual	2001 Budget	2001 Projected	2002 Budget (7/18/01)	2002 Budget (Administrators 9/9/01)	2002 Budget (Managers 9/9/01)	Percentage Change 2002 Budget Versus 2001 Budget	2002 Budget Versus 2001 Projected
Revenues								
Inpatient revenue	74,000	79,000	77,800	84,000	87,360	87,360	10.6	12.3
Outpatient revenue	69,000	77,000	76,100	86,000	89,440	89,440	16.2	17.5
Total patient revenue	143,000	156,000	153,900	170,000	176,800	176,800	13.3	14.9
Less								
Contractual and other adjustments	(48,000)	(60,000)	(59,000)	(72,000)	(77,100)	(77,100)	28.5	30.7
Charity care	(2,200)	(2,700)	(2,500)	(3,000)	(3,000)	(3,000)	11.1	20.0
Net patient service revenue	92,800	93,300	92,400	95,000	96,700	96,700	3.6	4.7
Add								
Premium revenue	1,300	2,100	2,100	1,000	1,000	1,000	−52.4	−52.4
Investment income	5,500	5,000	6,000	5,000	6,000	6,000	20.0	0.0
Other operating income	1,200	1,200	1,100	1,200	1,200	1,200	0.0	9.1
Total revenue	100,800	101,600	101,600	102,200	104,900	104,900	3.2	3.2
Expenses								
Salaries	34,000	35,500	36,500	39,000	38,200	38,600	7.6	4.7
Contract labor	1,500	1,400	800	1,200	1,200	1,200	−14.3	50.0
Fringe benefits	6,800	7,000	6,900	7,800	7,500	7,600	7.1	8.7
Total salaries and benefits	42,300	43,900	44,200	48,000	46,900	47,400	6.8	6.1
Bad debts	4,400	4,400	4,400	5,000	4,500	4,500	2.3	2.3
Patient care supplies	15,000	15,200	16,000	17,100	16,600	16,900	9.2	3.8
Professional and management fees	3,600	3,400	3,800	4,200	3,900	4,000	14.7	2.6
Purchased services	5,600	5,600	5,600	5,600	5,600	5,600	0.0	0.0
Operation of plant (including utilities)	2,500	2,700	2,600	2,800	2,800	2,800	3.7	7.7
Depreciation	10,500	11,000	10,500	11,500	11,500	11,500	4.5	9.5
Interest and financing expenses	7,600	7,400	7,400	7,200	7,200	7,200	−2.7	−2.7
Other	4,600	3,800	4,000	5,000	4,500	4,700	18.4	12.5
Total expenses	96,100	97,400	98,500	106,400	103,500	104,600	6.3	5.1
Operation margin	4,700	4,200	3,100	(4,200)	1,400	300	−66.7	−54.8
Nonoperating income								
Gain/(loss) on investments	600	1,200	1,400	1,000	1,000	1,000	−16.7	−28.6
Total nonoperating income	600	1,200	1,400	1,000	1,000	1,000	−16.7	−28.6
Net income	5,300	5,400	4,500	(3,200)	2,400	1,300	−55.6	−46.7
4% targeted operating margin				$3,800	$3,868	$3,868		
3% targeted operating margin				$2,850	$2,901	$2,901		
2% targeted operating margin				$1,900	$1,934	$1,934		

income helps to improve the operating margin target. However, reporting the investment income above the line is somewhat controversial. In many organizations, an increase or decrease in investment income is not considered an appropriate change to the operating margin.

Second, in attempting to improve investment income, RHMC needs to change the investment strategy to favor somewhat riskier positions. Because past results do not guarantee future outcomes, this is one of the bigger gambles in the budget package. In fact, it is possible that the finance committee, the investment committee, or the board of directors will reject this recommendation as too radical.

Some other expense changes involve reducing

- Some additional fringe benefit increases initially proposed by the human resource administrator
- Bad-debt expenses through better collection efforts
- Patient care supply expenses
- Consulting fees

According to the budget compiled by the finance staff, the budgeted operating margin, after all requested changes are processed, would be $300,000, or 0.3 percent. This is still considerably below the original 4.0 percent mandated by the board. Therefore, the administrators must now do the job they are paid to do: make final determinations on how to achieve the budgeted target.

To aid in this effort, the finance staff once again present the closing-the-gap analysis from the July meeting (see Exhibit 7.1). The administrators are reminded of the cost-reduction opportunities they already used and the level at which they used them. They must decide if they want to make further cuts in any of these line items, or announce whether they have any additional ideas. The finance administrator also reminds them that the radiology manager brought the only revenue enhancements above and beyond the original budgeted volume targets. Because there is little additional net revenue being proposed, expense reduction is the only remaining area that can be used to reach the budget target.

After some discussion, the administrators agree to make a further series of cuts to the proposed 2002 budget (see Exhibit 9.1).

The biggest reductions come from staffing. Instead of the original cut of twenty FTEs proposed at the July 18 meeting, they agree on a total cut of thirty-eight. It is interesting to note that although the administrators have agreed to cut this many, the overall FTE count will decrease by only 17.2 because the department managers had already requested an additional 20.8 FTEs in July. So the impact of the thirty-eight cuts is not so severe as originally proposed. It is also agreed

EXHIBIT 9.1. RHMC FINAL CLOSING-THE-GAP ANALYSIS, 2002 BUDGET.

Operating margin, July 18 meeting	$(4,200)
4% net price increase	1,700
Improvement in investment income	1,000
Salary expense reductions, 38 FTEs at $40,000 average per employee	1,520
Fringe benefits: reduce additional benefits proposed in initial budget meeting of July 14:	500
Reduce bad-debt expense through better collection efforts	1,000
Reduce patient care supply expenses	500
Reduce professional and management fees, by cutting consulting fees	400
Reduce other expenses	500
Final set of changes since July 18 budgeted income statement	7,120
Revised operating margin	$2,920

that these FTEs not be cut proportionally or across the board, as often happens. Instead, for this budget cycle the revenue-producing departments will absorb a cut of only 25 percent, while the nonrevenue areas will disproportionately take 75 percent of the cut. It is the responsibility of the finance staff to develop the formula for this before the September 17 meeting.

One additional decision was made at this meeting. As all the administrators struggled to determine other places to cut expenses to meet the 4 percent operating margin target, the CEO decided that no additional cut should be made beyond the 3 percent level for the second year in a row. He reasoned that the organization needed additional time to implement service enhancements to offset the negative net revenue changes wrought by the changes imposed by the Medicare Balanced Budget Act reductions, coupled with increasing and continuing intransigence on the part of managed care companies to negotiate reimbursement rates in good faith.

Therefore the chief executive was willing to support a measure at the level of the finance committee and board to change the 4 percent operating margin target to 3 percent for the second time in two years. He fully reserved the right to move this target level back up to 4 percent for the 2003 budget year, depending on circumstances.

With these changes, the budget was essentially completed. The finance staff still needed to crunch the numbers one more time to make sure all the changes did indeed add up to the 3 percent operating margin. They would have eight days in which to do so as well as recommend the number of staff members to be cut, by division.

September 17: Final Review and Approval of the Operating Budget and Review of the Human Resource Committee Package

At the September 17 meeting, the administrators are presented with the final version of the 2002 operating budget (see Table 9.2). Through a series of columns, the table shows the progression of changes made to bring it home. This version, without the intermediate columns, is to be presented to the finance committee for approval at their October meeting.

The administrators are also presented with the finance-produced list of FTE cuts by division. It is the responsibility of the division heads to determine how to implement the cuts required by the list. They will employ a number of techniques to make these determinations, including these possibilities:

- Eliminate all vacant positions (the number one answer of all time for administrators)
- Cut the level of overtime
- Replace FTEs with part-time employees
- Replace part-time employees with as-needed employees (known as PRNs)
- Eliminate currently filled positions (layoffs)

These are hard decisions to make, but always necessary. The vice presidents are also responsible for deciding which departments within their division need to make the cuts. Fairness is not always involved at this point. The cuts may be made proportionally or disproportionally. But they must be made since there will be no budget dollars available to support these positions in the new year.

At this meeting, the human resource committee package is presented, following preparation by the finance staff with the assistance of the human resource staff, before it goes to the board. It includes a narrative of the human resource decisions that are being proposed by the administration, such as the actual, projected, and budgeted staffing levels by dollars and FTEs; details of the fringe benefit package; and discussion of the wage and salary levels. These include minimum and maximum pay scales across various job classifications and the going market rate pay scales around the region. This allows the entire administrative staff to see what the board sees and gain any additional understanding of the subject at this time.

TABLE 9.2. RHMC PRELIMINARY BUDGETED STATEMENT OF OPERATIONS FOR THE BUDGET YEAR TO DATE ENDING DEC. 31, 2002 (PREPARED SEPT. 17, 2001) (IN THOUSANDS OF DOLLARS).

	2001 Budget	2001 Projected	2002 Budget (7/18/01)	2002 Budget (Administrators 9/9/01)	2002 Budget (Managers 9/9/01)	2002 Budget (9/17/01)	Percentage Change 2002 Budget Versus 2001 Budget	Percentage Change 2002 Budget Versus 2001 Projected
Revenues								
Inpatient revenue	79,000	77,800	84,000	87,360	87,360	87,360	10.58	12.29
Outpatient revenue	77,000	76,100	86,000	89,440	89,440	89,440	16.16	17.53
Total patient revenue	156,000	153,900	170,000	176,800	176,800	176,800	13.33	14.88
Less								
Contractual and other adjustments	(60,000)	(59,000)	(72,000)	(77,100)	(77,100)	(77,100)	28.50	30.68
Charity care	(2,700)	(2,500)	(3,000)	(3,000)	(3,000)	(3,000)	11.11	20.00
Net patient service revenue	93,300	92,400	95,000	96,700	96,700	96,700	3.64	4.65
Add								
Premium revenue	2,100	2,100	1,000	1,000	1,000	1,000	−52.38	−52.38
Investment income	5,000	6,000	5,000	6,000	6,000	6,000	20.00	0.00
Other operating income	1,200	1,100	1,200	1,200	1,200	1,200	0.00	9.09
Total revenue	101,600	101,600	102,200	104,900	104,900	104,900	3.25	3.25
Expenses								
Salaries	35,500	36,500	39,000	38,200	38,600	37,480	5.58	2.68
Contract labor	1,400	800	1,200	1,200	1,200	1,200	−14.29	50.00
Fringe benefits	7,000	6,900	7,800	7,500	7,600	7,300	4.29	5.80
Total salaries and benefits	43,900	44,200	48,000	46,900	47,400	45,980	4.74	4.03
Bad debts	4,400	4,400	5,000	4,500	4,500	4,000	−9.09	−9.09
Patient care supplies	15,200	16,000	17,100	16,600	16,900	16,600	9.21	3.75
Professional and management fees	3,400	3,800	4,200	3,900	4,000	3,800	11.76	0.00
Purchased services	5,600	5,600	5,600	5,600	5,600	5,600	0.00	0.00
Operation of plant (including utilities)	2,700	2,600	2,800	2,800	2,800	2,800	3.70	7.69
Depreciation	11,000	10,500	11,500	11,500	11,500	11,500	4.55	9.52
Interest and financing expenses	7,400	7,400	7,200	7,200	7,200	7,200	−2.70	−2.70
Other	3,800	4,000	5,000	4,500	4,700	4,500	18.42	12.50
Total expenses	97,400	98,500	106,400	103,500	104,600	101,980	4.70	3.53
Operation margin	4,200	3,100	(4,200)	1,400	300	2,920	−30.48	−5.81
Nonoperating income								
Gain/(loss) on investments	1,200	1,400	1,000	1,000	1,000	1,000	−16.67	−28.57
Total nonoperating income	1,200	1,400	1,000	1,000	1,000	1,000	−16.67	−28.57
Net income	5,400	4,500	(3,200)	2,400	1,300	3,920	−27.41	−12.8
4% targeted operating margin			$3,800	$3,868	$3,868	$3,868		
3% targeted operating margin			$2,850	$2,901	$2,901	$2,901		
2% targeted operating margin			$1,900	$1,934	$1,934	$1,934		

September 18–October 14: Prepare First Draft Through Final Copy of the 2000 Budget for the Finance Committee

Over the next four-week period, the finance staff are heavily involved in preparing, and the finance administrators are heavily occupied in reviewing, the budget reports for the human resource committee, the finance committee, and the board of directors meetings. These reports are between sixteen and thirty pages in length and contain varying degrees of detailed information. Preparing and reconciling the schedules for volume, revenue, staffing level (FTEs), and staffing dollars is a tense and intense chore. It takes an individual with a high level of commitment, organization, and perfectionism to lead this effort. RHMC is fortunate to have an accounting director with such drive and skill to do so.

The budget drafts are prepared on schedule so that effective review can be performed. As the date of each presentation draws closer and closer and the draft copies get cleaner and cleaner, the final implications of the budget packages are revealed.

Operating Budget System of the Near Future

In subsequent years, it is expected that much of this paper pushing between department managers and finance staff during the budget process will be eliminated by using computers and networks. The steps in the process may not change, but a lot of the manual steps performed by the finance staff can actually be done through the work that is already required of the department managers and vice presidents. A considerable amount of work typically flows back and forth between the finance department and the department managers in manual mode; there are ways to improve this process.

Computers are already capable of streamlining the budget process. RHMC plans to install specialized budgeting software in the following year. The organization will be able to use this software to enhance its budget process because it has already invested in construction of a computerized LAN. By going to the expense of installing the computer infrastructure (wiring, cabling wall outlets, and the various computer closets needed for coordination), all the PCs at the organization are hooked up to a common computer (server). Because of this linkage, all the PCs can talk to each other without having to access any outside communications service, such as the phone company. Here are some of the functions available to the organization and its staff because of the LAN linkage:

- An internal electronic mail system (e-mail)
- External e-mail with a firewall to maintain overall system security
- Internet access, with the firewall attached

- A common calendar program, which enables any eligible staff member to request a meeting with one or more staff members electronically
- The heavily developed financial and clinical decision support system and data warehouse, available to all management staff, with certain capabilities:
    Operating budgeting
    Capital budgeting
    Monitoring and alert management systems

The near future will bring electronic capabilities to the budgeting process. These new capabilities will allow the finance staff and department managers to conduct their business online. In a nutshell, the finance staff will be able to send the budget out electronically over the LAN instead of on paper. The managers can then perform their analysis online and send changes back over the wires. Because the changes are already in a digital format, the finance staff will no longer have to reenter the data. Instead they can devote their efforts to analyzing the department managers' justifications and analysis of the requested changes. This is much better use of the analyst's time and energy. Then, the decision support system will enhance the organization's knowledge base by automatically notifying the managers and their bosses of any variance from established parameters. RHMC has purchased a reasonably low-priced system that does perform all these functions and is excited about the installation over the course of the following year.

Capital Budget (September)

The September 4 meeting to discuss the results of the main strategic capital budget evaluation and final administrative approval of the 2002 capital budget is necessary only if the administrators were unable to come to a final decision during the meeting on August 25. If there were still open issues present at the end of that meeting and additional evaluation scoring was performed over the preceding week, then the administrators use this meeting to finalize the budget. This approval is required because the finance staff need to budget depreciation expense on the operating budget; to do so, staff must know the capital assets that will be acquired in the coming year.

In this particular year, the RHMC administrators were able to complete their review and come to a consensus at the prior meeting. This was due in large part to the new process and software used by the organization to produce a much more efficient and effective outcome. Because of the early conclusion, the finance staff are able to determine the depreciation expense for the operating budget in record time.

Cash Budget

Once a year, at the conclusion of the capital and operating budget phases, the finance department staff prepare a cash budget. This is a necessary step that allows the organization to determine how to optimize the value of the cash being generated by its operations. Consider these facts:

- Excess cash can be kept in an interest-bearing checking account at a rate equal to 350 basis points below the prime lending rate; in this case, RHMC could perhaps receive 5 percent interest income on its excess cash (100 basis points is equal to 1 percent)
- It can be invested on a short-term basis (defined as twelve to eighteen months) for approximately 5.5 percent to 6 percent in a set of low-risk intermediate-term bonds
- It can be invested on a moderate-risk, longer-term basis in a mix of fixed instruments (bonds) and equities (stocks); a moderate risk portfolio would consist of a mix of 65 percent stocks and 35 percent bonds, whose previous ten-year average return has been 11.3 percent annually (determined from analysis performed by the organization's investment consultants)

If the board has an appetite for a moderate risk strategy that offers greater-than-average return on their investments, it becomes imperative to invest the maximum amount of excess cash in the higher-earning alternative. To do so, however, the organization has to have a clear understanding of its stream of receipts and disbursements, preferably on a weekly basis (see Table 9.3). This allows them to remove the optimum amount of cash from the checking account so that it can be invested in the longer-term, higher-earning assets.

At the conclusion of the annual budget process, the finance staff prepare a fifty-two-week cash budget that attempts to forecast the receipts and disbursements represented by the income statement revenues and expenses. Table 9.3 shows an eight-week set of the 2002 cash budget prepared by the finance staff. The most problematic line in this budget is patient cash receipts. It is the most difficult line to forecast because of the problem with the industry's third-party payors (Medicare, Medicaid, managed care plans), many of whom—particularly the nongovernment managed care plans—have varying definitions of what a clean claim is. A claim is clean if it should be paid within a narrowly defined time period. However, many of the major health care provider segments have had their share of trouble collecting promptly on these clean claims. This makes it difficult to prepare a reasonable cash budget. Still, it is achievable assuming that

TABLE 9.3. RHMC 2002 CASH BUDGET, SELECTED WEEKS.

	Actual March 4–8	Actual March 11–15	Actual March 18–22
Cash receipts			
Patient receipts	2,400,000	1,400,000	2,100,000
Other operating receipts	30,000	40,000	30,000
Miscellaneous items	5,000	3,000	8,000
Total receipts	2,435,000	1,443,000	2,138,000
Cash disbursements			
Trade vendors payable	1,100,000	1,150,000	1,800,000
Self-insured health care payments	0	60,000	0
Debt payments	0	0	0
Miscellaneous items	5,000	5,000	4,000
Total accounts payable and other	5,000	65,000	4,000
Transfers to payroll	850,000	250,000	800,000
Payroll taxes	450,000	40,000	0
Other payroll transfers	100,000	2,000	100,000
Total payroll disbursements	1,400,000	292,000	900,000
Total cash disbursements	2,505,000	1,507,000	2,704,000
Net activities	(70,000)	(64,000)	(566,000)
Cash balance, beginning	4,000,000	3,930,000	3,866,000
Cash balance, ending	3,930,000	3,866,000	3,300,000

cash receipts are collected evenly throughout the year. The method that RHMC uses to budget receipts takes three steps:

1. The finance staff spread the annual budgeted net revenue across the twelve monthly time periods according to days in the month (for example, January is allocated 31/365th of the net revenue, February is allocated 28/365, and so on).
2. The staff split the months into seven-day weeks and apply a proportional amount of the monthly receipts to each week.
3. The weeks are reviewed to detect any anomalies, such as whether a holiday falls within the week (those weeks are adjusted accordingly).

The caveat in budgeting cash receipts is that a change in the accounts receivable can wreak havoc on the forecast. The initial cash budget should proph-

Actual March 25–29	Forecast April 1–5	Forecast April 8–12	Forecast April 15–19	Forecast April 22–26
2,100,000	2,109,000	2,109,000	2,109,000	2,109,000
40,000	35,000	35,000	35,000	35,000
3,000	0	0	0	0
2,143,000	2,144,000	2,144,000	2,144,000	2,144,000
1,500,000	1,025,000	1,025,000	1,025,000	1,025,000
170,000	0	0	0	80,000
0	0	0	0	0
5,000	0	0	0	0
175,000	0	0	0	80,000
260,000	841,500	268,500	841,500	268,500
500,000	444,000	43,400	444,000	43,400
2,000	105,000	0	105,000	0
762,000	1,390,500	311,900	1,390,500	311,900
2,437,000	2,415,500	1,336,900	2,415,500	1,416,900
(294,000)	(271,500)	807,100	(271,500)	727,100
3,300,000	3,006,000	2,734,500	3,541,600	3,270,100
3,006,000	2,734,500	3,541,600	3,270,100	3,997,200

esy collection of 100 percent of budgeted net revenue. If this does not happen, the cash budget could fail, leading to two problems:

1. A shortfall to pay required disbursements, such as payroll and trade vendor payables
2. A need to borrow funds at a rate higher than is being earned by the invested funds

It is important to remember that a budget—whether operating, capital, or cash—is nothing more than a forecast based on a set of assumptions for future activities. Because the cash budget can have so much potential negative impact if the forecast is not reasonable, it is imperative to update these budgets weekly. This allows close monitoring of actual cash balances, which leads to better ability to move the cash into its most appropriate asset category. Still, it is extremely important to note that forecasts can never be accurate because it is not possible to foretell the future with certainty.

The RHMC board has requested that the administration maximize its investment income, wherever possible, without resorting to a risky investment strategy. One way this can be accomplished is by keeping checking account balances as close to zero as possible without going into an overdraft position ("going negative"). Table 9.3 shows a $4 million actual opening balance for the week ending March 8, 2002. Eight weeks later, the projected balance is still $3,997,200.

Given this information, it appears that if the organization wants to maintain a balance closer to zero, it could transfer, let's say, $3 million out of the checking account and into its stock portfolio. This would still leave it with a $1 million cash cushion in its checking account. Unfortunately, RHMC would overdraft its checking account if it transferred the $3 million according to this weekly forecast because the forecast for the week ending April 5 shows an ending balance of $2,734,500. If the $3 million had been transferred prior to that date, the ending balance would have therefore been a negative $265,500. Not good!

The moral of the story is that cash balances fluctuate with normal organizational activity; the organization has to look at the lowest weekly cash balance when forecasting checking account balances if it does not want to overdraft. The organization should also negotiate a line of credit, at a favorable interest rate, with its bank to cover a situation where there could be an overdraft. In this case, the finance administrator would not be so concerned about a short-term overdraft. Hence cash budgeting can have great value to an organization if it has a desire to maximize cash assets, comfort in the forecasting, and available overdraft protection or a line of credit.

Physician Practice Management Issues

Physician practice is a major segment of the health care industry. As we saw in Chapter One, physician practices accounted for $269 billion a year in 1999, encompassing almost 20 percent of the industry's financial outlays. Although they also make up 20 percent of the industry, the impact of physicians and their office practice on the process of health care is enormous.

In every important way, physicians affect most of the health care costs generated in this country. They personally control the $269 billion of their own pure office revenues; they also have a great deal of control over the expenses generated in the $390 billion hospital segment of the industry. It is important to note that most clinical hospital expenses are originated by physician orders. Thus the costs of every hospital inpatient case are the result of the type and quantity of diagnostic test, therapy, drug, and supplies ordered by the physician. Still, the manner in which physicians manage their own office practice is often an indicator of how frugal or profligate they are in managing the resources of other health care organizations with which they are affiliated.

Physician Office Management

There is an art to (and many variables in) running a successful physician's office practice. One of the biggest is the size of the practice, ranging from a solo practitioner's office to a building housing a four-hundred-physician multispecialty clinic. Regardless of size, there are still a number of basic financial characteristics that all physician office practices must adhere to. Here is a list of the fundamental ways a physician office practice can optimize its financial condition:

Revenue Enhancement

- Improve documentation to bill for and support higher-reimbursement procedures
- Improve patient throughput
- Retain ancillary revenues in the office setting

Expense Reduction

- Trim the payroll through use of benchmarks and levels of support staff
- Hold down supply costs through lower usage and less costly items
- Maximize automation of clinical and financial records
- Reduce malpractice premiums
- Cut office space costs; consider time sharing

Unfortunately, over the last several years it has become obvious to many physicians and physician groups that they are no longer capable of optimizing their own financial condition. The rapid rise of managed care plans dealt a crippling blow to many a physician's old back office. Managed care plans mandated dozens of new requirements, some for billing but mostly for referrals. Primary care physicians (PCPs) who signed up with a managed care plan are required to get preapproval for all treatment modalities that take place outside the physician's office (except for the large United Healthcare plan). This has caused an avalanche of paperwork, with concomitant cost that was unknown in prior eras.

Specialists are not immune to this phenomenon. First, they are the recipients of referrals requested by the PCP and processed by the health plan. Therefore the specialist's staff have to be sure that each managed care patient being treated has the required approval for payment. This is an onerous task; health plans do not always process their approvals expeditiously, yet the patients must be seen promptly, which creates a potential conflict between the physician and his patient. Second, they too need to request further referrals from the PCP if they want to perform additional tests or treatments on the patient beyond the original referral.

There are other medical practice issues that physicians have to deal with in the current era of health care:

- Fraud and abuse, particularly related to Medicare rules and regulations under what are called the Stark II laws, as characterized by:
  Billing issues
  Documentation issues
  Corporate structure of the practice
- Cash flow, owing to the long time it takes some health plans to pay capitation premium and other insurance claims
- The need for capital to fund acquisition of efficiency-producing and revenue-enhancing information technology, such as electronic medical records systems
- Consumers who are demanding new tests, treatments, and drugs under the influence of print ads, televisions ads, and the omnipresence of the Internet
- If a small practice (fewer than five physicians), the need for capital to continue to compete for managed care contracts against the much larger groups that are being courted by the large consolidated managed health care plans

Into the breach, in the early and middle 1990s, rode the physician practice management company (PPMC). This form of business had many corporate structures. There are for-profit and nonprofit, hospital-based, equity-based, and academic medical center–based PPMCs. Their mandate was to operate the physician office practice in a professional, businesslike manner. It was the PPMCs' conviction that many solo and multispecialty practice settings operated with little financial focus, or ability to manage these issues. Therefore these PPMCs sold physician practices, both solo and multispecialty, on their ability to optimize revenue enhancement and cost-reduction strategies. They became popular in the early and middle 1990s as a vehicle to improve the financial condition within the physician office setting.

Wall Street became enchanted with PPMCs in the early 1990s. They enjoyed exceptional growth in the equity-based market. The market capitalization for PPMCs increased from under $1 billion in 1993 to $12 billion three years later. At the same time, the number of publicly traded PPMCs increased from three in 1990 to over twenty-five in 1996—an explosion in a nascent industry.

In 1997, there appeared to be no limit to this industry's size. Doctors were selling themselves to PPMCs by the thousands. The PPMCs targeted medium- and large-sized groups for acquisition. They were on a roll. Although they had not yet proved that they could invigorate the financial condition of physician practices, they were able to acquire many vulnerable groups because of a hard-to-refuse come-on: "Come be a part of us and we will make you very rich through the increase in our stock price." Because equity- or stock-based companies always sell at a premium to their underlying value, equity-based PPMCs could offer physicians stock in the PPMC that was ten, fifteen, twenty, maybe thirty times the value of the practice. It made multimillionaires of some physicians in early-adopter practices.

The come-ons were relentless. Every independent physician or physician group was talking about its future in relation to PPMCs. They were hoping to be courted by, or they were making an initial overture to, a PPMC. Or they were talking about rejecting it if extended an offer because of cultural differences or the simple desire to stay independent. Equity-based PPMCs grew exponentially, fueled more by their tremendous acquisition binge than by improved earnings from practice improvement.

Meanwhile, this phenomenon did not go unnoticed by the hospital and health systems side of the industry. They were worried. There are historical linkages between hospitals and their affiliated doctors. In most not-for-profit hospital or health system settings, physicians maintain independent status while gaining the privilege of using the hospital for those specific services for which they were granted credentials. Hospitals have a financial interest in granting these credentials. After all, it is these privileged physicians who refer patients to the hospital for inpatient and outpatient services. Physicians can become privileged in any of several categories, each of which confers its own rights and responsibilities. (Exhibit 9.2 is a listing of the categories of RHMC's medical staff and some of the privileges afforded to them.) These categories create linkage between the health care organization and the individual medical staff members.

Anything that disrupts these linkages is viewed as an obstacle by the hospital. Thus, hospitals attempted to counter the trends of "their" physicians' selling or aligning themselves with equity-based PPMCs. One step that many hospitals and health systems took was to organize the equivalent of their own PPMC. Called a management services organization (MSO), they would offer to purchase the physicians' practice or manage it while the physician retained control.

It was extremely important to the hospitals that they maintain linkage, particularly in the era of expanding managed care. They knew that being able to strike a bargain on managed care contracts was enhanced if a single negotiator could speak for the hospital and physician providers. It gave a small amount of leverage

EXHIBIT 9.2. RHMC CATEGORIES OF MEDICAL STAFF.

Provisional staff: newly appointed to the staff; this is essentially a one-year probation period.

Courtesy staff: physicians whose practice is exclusively office-based but who seek membership to use hospital services or specialists or participate in hospital-based MCOs. They will be credentialed but not privileged to admit or treat patients within the inpatient or outpatient hospital setting. (Some hospitals may allow a limited number of patient admissions.)

Associate staff: three-year term after completion of provisional status. It is available to staff members who have:

    (1) Demonstrated increasing need for the hospital facilities through satis-faction of their respective utilization criteria

    (2) Shown an active interest in the affairs of the hospital

    (3) Demonstrated through their professional work qualities of maturity and responsibility to indicate that they are likely to become eligible for promotion to active staff.

Consulting staff: physicians whose work is not primarily at this hospital but who are exceptionally qualified and experienced in their specialty. Their appointment to the consulting staff shall be determined by their potential for contributing service to the hospital and the community. They shall not have admitting privileges, shall be exempt from all utilization criteria policies, and shall not have the right to vote or hold office.

Active staff: physicians who have completed associate staff and have satisfied or-ganizational bylaw requirements that qualify them to conduct the business of the medical staff. They are entitled to admit patients to the hospital, vote on all mem-bers, and hold elected office.

against the health plans, in contrast to the hospitals and physicians coming to the contract table separately. In addition, single-signature contracting keeps hospitals and their physicians on the same side, allowing both entities to maintain a con-tract with the same MCO. It was therefore in the interest of RHMC to do its best to create a strong affiliation with its many primary care and multispecialty physi-cians on its staff.

RHMC did this in two ways.

First, it encouraged its affiliated (credentialed) physicians to form an inde-pendent practice association (IPA). This gave the physicians a legal base from which to negotiate as a single unit with the managed care companies. Any physi-cian who became a member of the IPA gave it the authority to negotiate rates for him or her and the practice. So long as the IPA board approved a deal, the indi-vidual physicians in the IPA had to accept it.

Second, although RHMC had no control over the IPA (which was 100 percent physician-owned and -operated), it was now able to work with the IPA to develop a fifty-fifty physician hospital organization (PHO). This allowed the unified physician organization and the hospital to negotiate deals with health plans.

The Management Services Organization

Meanwhile, RHMC took one additional giant step. Like other health care organizations in the country, it set up an MSO to

- Offer back-office services to independent physicians who felt the need to outsource these efforts
- Offer management services for PCPs employed by the health care organization

The rationale for MSO formation was to allow RHMC to have some control over the patient referral pattern within its primary and secondary service areas. Employed physicians refer 100 percent of their non-office-based clinical services back to RHMC. It also created for RHMC a growing physician practice, giving it some additional leverage with the managed care companies.

The MSO was another operating company within the overall RHMC corporate structure. Its creation was costly to RHMC, involving as it did setup of a back office operation consisting of billers and collectors, physician office managers, and administrative personnel. These individuals were responsible for operating the physician's offices, from hiring all the office personnel (including nurses) to procuring the supplies and making the office facility meet high standards. The point of the MSO was to allow the physicians to concentrate on the clinical issues pertaining to their patients and not worry about office management and cash generation.

One of the biggest features of most MSOs was the responsibility to negotiate all the managed care contracts. In the case of the RHMC MSO, this was not applicable because every member of the MSO was also a member of the IPA. Thus the IPA through the PHO was the negotiating muscle for the MSO.

There were several areas in which the MSO was particularly effective, notably managing the office staff (which included hiring, firing, supervising, and reviewing nursing and clerical staff). A key responsibility of the clerical staff was to process the primary care physician's (PCP's) referral for any other medical or surgical service. This could include referrals to specialist physicians, hospitals, or home health agencies.

Referral Issues. Making referrals for other medical and surgical services encompassed some difficulty in the late 1990s in the United States. The most important piece of information that the physician's clerical staff need is the patient's insurance carrier and plan. This allows the clerk to determine the exact benefits applicable to the patient. It permits the PCP to know which specialist physician or hospital the patient can be referred to. This is possible because each and every insurance plan has a particular provider panel attached to it. Insurance companies allow only a contracted PCP to refer to other physicians in the panel associated with the insurance plan being paid for by the individual employers.

Billing and Collection Issues. Another service that the MSO offers is billing and collecting. There are specific rules and regulations that physician billers and billing services must follow. Some of the rules and regulations are the result of laws written for the Medicare and Medicaid programs. Others are the result of contractual stipulations agreed to between the organization and all the managed care companies with which it has decided to do business. The rules involve all phases of the operation. Some of the main rules that need to be followed:

- Determination of patient third-party status (capitation or fee-for-service)
- Amount of the copay that needs to be collected from the patient
- Second opinion
- Referral
- Preauthorization of services
- Coordination of benefits
- Fraud and abuse regulations (compliance issues)

It is extremely difficult to perform all the required steps properly and not run afoul of contract stipulations or the law. It is akin to juggling a set of rare china dishes without breaking any of them. Proper identification of the patient during the check-in period is critical to the success of the billing process. Determining the third-party payor's requirements then becomes essential to speedy billing and collection of the account if it is a fee-for-service type contract. If the patient is capitated, no bill for collection is sent, to payor or patient.

The rapid increase in managed care volume in many physician offices set off a rush by some physicians to acquire the tools to manage these additional new requirements. As mentioned earlier in this chapter, there was a great need to acquire state-of-the-art information technology to enhance the ability to bill and collect patient accounts from Medicare, Medicaid, and managed care payors efficiently. Some of these information systems included "edits" within the programming to identify and flag gaps in information required to be submitted with bills based on the payor. This was useful to the billers; they could avoid having to manually review every bill against a payor's contract.

But there was one enormous downside to acquisition of these new information technology billing and collecting tools: they are very expensive. The cost of a system varies with the size of the practice, the number of patients treated, the number of members capitated, and the number of physician sites being connected. There are several information system vendors catering to the physician office practice market, and their products come in a variety of shapes, sizes, and costs.

Here are some of the popular features and functions of a PPM billing and collecting system (Worley and Ciotti, 1997):

- Electronic charting
- Voice recognition (still unproven)
- Optical imaging
- Office scheduling
- Managed care contract billing and contract compliance

These features and functions aid the physician and office staff in optimizing their billing and collections. They should also help in clinical practice. However, given the current health care reimbursement climate, the problem is deciding what mechanism to use to finance acquisition of a system. Many practices in the 1990s turned to PPMCs for help. In 2001, a variety of physician practices are turning to application service providers (ASPs) to offer continuously updated software at a monthly rental in place of the PPMC alternative (Conn, 2001). We will review the ASP concept in the next chapter.

Patient Throughput

An important concept in PPM involves patient throughput. This is defined as the number of patients a physician can see in a defined time period, usually stated in hours or days. Put another way, patient throughput concerns the amount of time a physician spends treating his or her patients. This is best explained using an example.

Let's say that a physician currently treats, on average, twenty-one patients a day over a standard seven-hour day. This means the physician is treating three patients per hour. That is, the physician is seeing, on average, one patient every twenty minutes. There are two important concepts inherent in this example.

First, in regard to the physician seeing a patient every twenty minutes, it is critical to understand all of the work that the physician needs to perform during this time period. First and foremost, the physician needs to put hands on the patient. When a patient enters a doctor's office, he wants the physician to physically poke and prod. This gives the patient comfort that the physician is doing her job.

It is this spending of time that is the physician's most valuable commodity. But because of the nature of twenty-first-century practice, the physician needs to perform many more functions than just sitting with the patient while making a
diagnosis and devising a treatment plan, as this list suggests.

Steps Taken by a Physician During an Office Visit

- Examine the patient!
- Fully document all the relevant signs and symptoms of the patient to allow the
  physician coder and biller to accurately produce a bill that stands up to
  scrutiny by a federal government or managed care auditor.
- Review the patient's chart from prior periods to ascertain if any previous illness or injury is connected to the current medical problem; if so, review the
  previous treatment patterns for success or failure.
- Create any referral notes and paperwork that may be needed so that the patient can move on to a higher level of care, if warranted.
- Write up any prescription that the patient may need.
- Explain to the patient any particular instructions that need to be given for
  home care.

Now, consider the patient. Does he think that twenty minutes is enough time
for the care rendered? Does he want more? Does he think that the physician is
able to do an effective job in that time period? The answer to most of these questions is NO! Patients are demanding and often aware that the physician is on a
short time schedule. It's always been this way, hasn't it? Well, of course, the physician has always had an appointment book. The biggest difference is that back
then, in the Marcus Welby 1950s and 1960s, physicians often booked patients
into thirty- and forty-five-minute time slots. Nowadays, the twenty-minute time
slot just described is too long!

These days most PCPs (the Marcus Welbys of this era) schedule four patients
an hour—one patient every fifteen minutes. In fact, some physicians book patients every ten or twelve minutes apart (five or six patients per hour) to maximize
their revenues.

Improving patient throughput in a physician's office was a sure-fire way for
the PPMC to increase the physician's revenue, so long as there was pent-up demand for the physician's services. It was one of the first things looked at by a
PPMC that was performing due diligence in the event of a practice acquisition.
The PPMC could immediately ascertain if the practice had throughput of 2.0,
2.5, 3.0, and so on patients per hour. It was easy math to determine immediate
improvement.

The equation seems too easy—like pushing the speed-up button on the assembly line to produce more cars, thus generating more revenue. Unfortunately, in the late 1990s theory could rarely be turned into practice. The main reason is that most physicians who have been in practice for a few years have developed a practice pattern with which they are comfortable. Altering this pattern is akin to changing a successful baseball player's batting style or a golfer's swing. Yes, it's possible, but only after a lot of hard work and effort. And she has to want to change.

The method used by most PPMCs was to develop an incentive compensation arrangement. This gave the physician a financial incentive for meeting productivity goals. Thus, she might be able to earn between 10 and 50 percent over base compensation for producing patient throughput in various levels above an agreed-upon standard. For example, over the course of a year, the physician and the PPMC may have agreed on a base salary of $110,000 with a stipulation that the physician would see 6,174 patients (28 patients per day times 4.5 days per week times 49 weeks). However if the physician sees two more patients per day on average, she can earn 15 percent of her base salary; seeing four more patients per day, the incentive rises to 30 percent of base salary.

This is just one physician compensation method attempting to raise physician throughput. There are dozens more, some quite esoteric. Many books, articles, and seminars around the country concentrate on these methods and should be referred to for advanced discussion in this area.

Although PPMCs emerged because of the rise of managed care and the reduction in physician income, when push came to shove many physicians chose not to alter their practice patterns even with the carrot of the incentive compensation being waved in front of them. Thus physicians did not always increase their incomes because there were few, if any, improvements in patient throughput and the PPMCs did not generate the kind of revenue that they expected.

The concept of improving patient throughput as a driver to physician financial success, and lack of success with it, became a beacon in the industry. Physicians began to rebel against throughput guidelines. Other physicians who had not yet signed on with PPMCs as employees, but might have been considering it, stopped. In effect, in 1997 and 1998 the PPMCs ran out of physician practices to acquire. Through 1993 to 1996, the only thing fueling PPMCs growth was acquisition, not bottom-line improvement. Thus when acquisition dried up, so did a good part of the industry. In fact, the beginning of the end of the PPMC model of the 1990s is evident in Figure 9.1, which shows the obvious and significant reduction of physician mergers and acquisitions (which had been primarily PPMC-based) in 1999.

FIGURE 9.1. PHYSICIAN MERGERS AND ACQUISITIONS, 1995–1999.

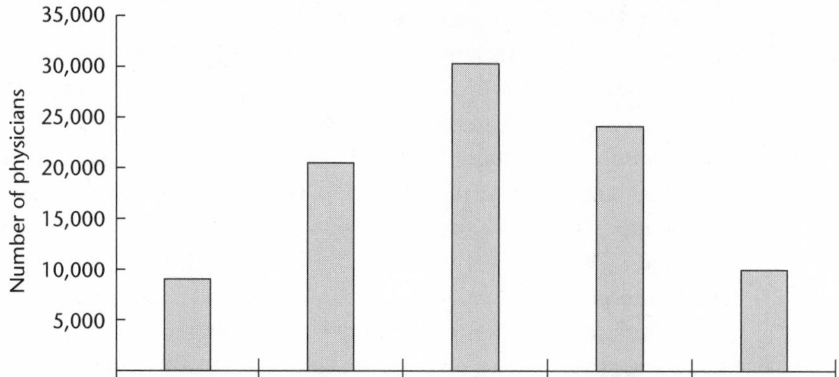

	1995	1996	1997	1998	1999
☐ Number of physicians	8,830	20,290	30,060	23,880	9,750

Source: Data from Irving Levin Associates, 2000.

The Equity-Based Physician Practice Management Company

Take the case of the two largest equity-based PPMCs, MedPartners and PhyCor. In 1995, MedPartners was trading at a stock price of $17. By 1996, its highest stock price was $32. In late 1998, its price, which had been tumbling since late 1997, hit a low of just under $2 a share. Similarly, PhyCor started out trading at just over $3 a share in early 1992. Throughout 1993, 1994, and 1995, it experienced a steadily rising stock price until it hit its peak in late 1996 with a stock price of $40 a share. Subsequently, it suffered a precipitous drop in its stock price, back down to $4 a share.

PPMCs fell out of such favor that MedPartners abandoned its commitment to physician practices in November 1998 in favor of pharmacy benefit management and therapeutic services. In a news release dated November 11, 1998, Mac Crawford, the company's president and chief executive officer, said that "we believe that it is in the best interest of our shareholders and our affiliated physicians to divest our PPM operations because it allows MedPartners to exit an industry that is viewed unfavorably by the investment community as presently configured."

Phycor hung on somewhat longer. It continued to sell and service its traditional PPMC model, which it had established in 1988, through 2000. But like MedPartners, it did not ultimately survive as a PPMC company. It lost $444 million in 1999 and $608 million in 2000 despite continuing efforts to sell off under-performing assets; it was left to contemplate filing for Chapter 11 bankruptcy protection or going out of business completely (Versel, 2001).

Thus went the meteoric rise and subsequent fall of the equity-based PPMCs. But the future is not yet told for this segment of the industry. Consider that there are still many physicians under contract to several other smaller PPMCs. In addition, the underlying issues that gave rise to PPMCs still exist. Managed care continues to dominate many parts of the country. Physician earnings are still affected by managed care rates and there is still opportunity for expense reduction and revenue enhancement in physician office practices. In fact, "physicians still need someone to help them with the myriad of tasks a PPM performs: administrative and marketing support, staff management, access to capital, contracting with insurers, offering the latest in business software and information systems technology and upgrades, running employee benefit plans, organizing disease management programs, helping groups interface with patients and so on" (Heimoff, 2000, p. 30).

In addition, the most successful type of PPMC currently operating is the single specialty PPM, which is able to deal with the problems and issues surrounding specific specialties rather than having to worry about compensation models and productivity issues across multispecialty groups. The PPM of the future will have to continue to evolve, or else there is a chance it could cease to exist, even as a concept.

The Hospital-Owned PPMC

Still, not all PPMCs are alike. Even with the turmoil in the equity-based PPMC industry, there are still segments of the industry that have not been so heavily tarnished: "Good PPMCs—defined mostly as single-specialty and hospital-based PPMCs—are suffering from a backlash caused by a few companies' problems, but they will survive any industry shakeout because they still provide the money and management skills most physicians lack" (Cook, 1998, p. 2). In fact, although many hospital-owned PPMCs continue to operate into the new millennium with renewed purpose and greater financial returns, "several well-known systems . . . have announced that they are divesting their practices" (Tschida, 2000, p. 84).

Like many of the equity-based PPMCs, those sponsored by hospitals did not produce good financial results during the middle and late 1990s. In fact, according to the Center for Healthcare Industry Performance Studies, hospitals were more likely to lose money on physician practice acquisition than equity-based PPMCs were. This was the conclusion of a survey conducted between 1994 and 1996 of more than 1,200 physicians and 460 practice acquisitions (Cleverly, Knott, and Dye, 1998). In fact, this conclusion was supported by a study conducted by the Medical Group Management Association, which reported that health systems in 1997 lost an average of $79,000 per employed physician (Tschida, 2000).

TABLE 9.4. RHMC PHYSICIAN DEVELOPMENT, KEY SUCCESS FACTORS FOR THE MONTH AND YEAR TO DATE ENDED SEPT. 31, 2001.

Month					
Prior Year	Actual	Budget	Percentage Prior Year	Variance Budget	Factor
					Employed physicians
					Total number of capitated lives
360	380	370	5.6%	2.7%	Office visits, new patients
1820	1870	1900	2.7%	−1.6%	Office visits, established patients
2,180	2,250	2,270	3.2%	−0.9%	Office visits, total
4.57	4.75	4.8	3.9%	−1.0%	Patient satisfaction rating (scale = 1 to 5)
					Accounts receivable
					A/R balance (in thousands)
					Days net revenues in A/R
					Total hospital activity
180	200	190	11.1%	5.3%	Patient days
32	35	36	9.4%	−2.8%	Inpatient admissions
310	330	350	6.5%	−5.7%	Outpatient services
−190	−150	−140	−21.1%	7.1%	Physician practice operating margins
450	520	490	15.6%	6.1%	Total gross revenues (in thousands)
265	320	300	20.8%	6.7%	Total net revenues (in thousands)
					Incremental contribution margin (in thousands)
160	180	200	12.5%	−10.0%	Net revenues minus incremental expenses
(30)	30	60	−200.0%	−50.0%	Total physician contribution to the corporation (in thousands)

There tend to be a number of reasons for these conclusions. Hospitals generally pay higher salaries to employed physicians than do other firms that may offer equity (stock) as an added inducement. They do this because they believe there are opportunities to raise practice revenue or decrease costs to make the practice more profitable. Also, there are substantial opportunities for additional revenue as employed physicians may legally make appropriate referrals back to the hospital.

	Year to Date			
Prior Year	Actual	Budget	Percentage Prior Year	Variance Budget
2,000	2,400	2,200	20.0%	9.1%
4,000	4,100	4,200	2.5%	−2.4%
18,000	22,000	22,000	22.2%	0.0%
22,000	26,100	26,200	18.6%	−0.4%
4.65	4.78	4.8	2.8%	−0.4%
350	450	0	28.6%	n/a
42.0	41.0	40.0	−2.4%	2.5%
2,000	2,100	2,200	5.0%	−4.5%
380	400	420	5.3%	−4.8%
3,000	3,400	3,600	13.3%	−5.6%
(2,400)	(2,000)	(1,800)	−16.7%	11.1%
5,000	6,000	5,800	20.0%	3.4%
3,000	3,600	3,500	20.0%	2.9%
1,800	2,100	2,300	16.7%	−8.7%
(600)	100	500	−116.7%	−80.0%

The high practice losses did not deter many hospitals that had the opportunity to establish a PPMC. As stated earlier in the chapter, these hospital-owned PPMCs met the criteria of keeping control of some of the organization's best doctors rather than losing them to an outside influence, and in some cases establishing a new practice in an underserved part of the service area, thereby generating new referral revenue.

Still, hospital organizations did not go out of their way to create physician practice losses in the PPMC. Most of them had every intention of making the business segment profitable. Many of the losses experienced by hospital-based PPMCs could be construed as start-up losses over the first few years of their existence. In fact, steep investment costs and pressure to pay high physician salaries led many hospital-owned physician practices into the red.

Some hospitals reported decreasing losses during the late 1990s. This was the situation being experienced at RHMC. When it entered the PPMC business in the mid-1990s, the center expected to lose money in the early years of the practice and budgeted accordingly. Although practice acquisition was a major thrust of the plan, in their market they were not many physician practices wanting to be acquired. RHMC turned instead to developing its own physician practices, hiring relatively young PCPs who agreed to be employed. RHMC then acquired office space for these physicians in those parts of the service area that RHMC wanted to seed.

The biggest problem with a new physician practice is that it takes a long time to mature. Depending on the area, it could take from three to five years (that is, to bring in enough revenue to offset the total practice costs, which include the physician's salary). Developing a volume and revenue base involves becoming known in the community and applying for certification by the several managed care plans that allow medical insurance coverage in the area. This brings the physician into the managed care plan's pamphlet of eligible providers, thus permitting a managed care member to access the physician. The cycle could take a year or longer.

The start-up costs during this cycle tend to be high. The two largest are (1) the salary of the physician, who is sitting around waiting for the next patient to come through the door; and (2) the office rent, a fixed cost that must be amortized by patient volume. Almost all the other costs are variable and thus relatively easily absorbed in a low-volume environment. Still, although the losses are real, they can be somewhat offset by the volume of patients who are referred to the hospital for required testing, when appropriate.

RHMC has developed a monthly board report that shows a summary financial review of the physician practices. It includes the profit or loss on the office practice itself as well as the incremental revenue generated by the hospital on the services provided through referral by the office practice. Table 9.4 shows an example of this report. Although the finance committee of the board continues to be dissatisfied with the direct losses generated by the physician practices, the members are well aware of their value in extending the health care organization's reach into the deepest corners of the service area. In addition, the committee's dissatisfaction is somewhat ameliorated by the last line on the report, which shows an overall positive physician financial contribution to the organization.

In addition, the board is aware that the direct losses suffered by the physician practices are slowly decreasing. Over the few years that the practices have been in existence, their managers have quickly learned the reasons for the losses and have taken steps to improve the problems. RHMC's problems are similar to those described in a 1998 article in *Medical Group Management Journal* on the subject (Bohlmann, 1998). In summary, these are the factors contributing to practice losses:

- Reduced physician productivity (throughput)
- Decreased collection rate
- Expansion problems
- Managed care contract negotiation issues
- Centralization of ancillary department revenue
- New costs, such as computer and facility upgrades
- Occupancy issues
- Level of physician compensation

RHMC management and staff assigned to the physician practice have made significant improvement in many of these areas, as the direct losses experienced by the organization are moving toward break-even. This tends to be the case in other hospital-owned physician practices around the country. The RHMC finance committee and board continue to support the efforts in regard to their hospital-owned PPMC, but they also demand improvement.

In summary, the rise of the PPMC in this country has produced some interesting and everlasting changes to the health care industry. Physicians are the dominant group of health care practitioners in the United States, by virtue of their education, experience, and licensure. Only they can prescribe medical testing, order inpatient hospital admissions, order drugs and medical supplies, and prescribe all other medical or surgical referrals. The 1990s have brought upheaval to established physician practices, particularly the dramatic oversight function by managed care companies. This story is far from over. It is likely that physicians, as a group, will attempt to reexert the control they have historically enjoyed as leaders of the health care community.

CHAPTER TEN

OCTOBER

It is 7:30 in the morning. Josephine Morton, RHMC's vice president of information services and chief information officer (CIO), has just arrived at her office. She has a big day ahead of her and is trying to brace herself for it. Heading for her first cup of coffee of the morning, she runs into Sam, coming out of his office down the hall.

"Hey, Jo, slow down!"

"Oh, sorry, Sam, I've got a lot on my mind today. We're rolling out the final phase of the electronic nurse charting system. I'm on my way to a nursing floor right now to see how it's working in action."

"Final phase, today? That's fantastic. I thought we'd never get there," offers the always optimistic Sam.

"Yeah, I'll tell you, this has been a heck of a year. Between HIPAA planning and replacing several modules of our information system during the past several months, I think the organization owes me about two months of sleep."

"I know how you feel. I often feel that way during certain phases of the budget process. Still, I know the job you've been through is quite a bit bigger and longer than the annual budget."

"Speaking of the budget, between the main hospital computer module replacements and the HIPAA project, we've spent even more money than the very large budget that was approved by the board," notes the suddenly worried CIO. "How are you going to handle that?"

"That's a good question. I've thought a lot about how to present the final dollar amounts to the board. First of all, we've been keeping them informed all along. Whenever there was a break between the budget and the actual expenses, we've let them know and asked for subsequent approval. They haven't always been happy, but they usually understand why there have been budget variances, particularly capital budget breaks. You know, most of our finance committee members are CEOs, and they've faced these issues first hand at their own companies."

"Well, I know I've prepared some analysis for you and the finance committee. So that's good to hear."

"I'll tell you, Jo, the toughest part of the increased budget that we needed to explain was the tremendous cost of upgrading the computer infrastructure. It was hard to describe the need to spend several million dollars to replace all the wires behind the walls and build dozens of computer closets to help in controlling the flood of digital data as it flows across those wires. The way we were able to make them understand it was to explain how we send and receive e-mail across the local area network that you have set up."

"That's a good way to do it. I'm glad to hear that the finance committee has accepted the budget changes. I gotta go now. I need to get to that nursing floor to see the new system in action."

"OK, but let me ask you to try and not have any more budget breaks. It gets harder and harder to deal with them."

October dawns gorgeous, as usual. The leading edge of the trees that populate the remaining forests of northern Illinois is beginning the turn from bright green to flaming orange and red. The temperature, reaching the high sixties at noon and the mid-forties at night, is likewise perfect. The brisk autumn air invigorates the region. Productivity is high, and that's useful because October is traditionally a month when hospital beds fill up with various illnesses and injuries.

At RHMC, October is always a transitional month because of the proposed budget presentation to the finance committee in the middle part of the month and the board of directors a few days later. At the beginning of October, the anxiety always begins to build as the dates approach.

The finance staff are working constantly to clean up the presentation package, giving particular care to explain any discrepancies that emerged. These discrepancies must be evaluated and clarified. At RHMC, because of the process of the previous five months that systematically weeded out anomalies, there are rarely any discrepancies to cause the finance staff to recommend a change in the budget before presentation to the finance committee.

At the same time, the finance staff are making heavy use of computers to perform the budget work. The computer technology enhances the staff's performance in generating, calculating, and evaluating the operating and capital budgets. In fact, the finance staff would need to double or triple in size if the computers suddenly disappeared.

Information Systems Implications for Health Care Financial Management

Throughout this book, it has been shown that much of the process and practice performed by the finance staff is facilitated by use of information technology (IT). In fact, in essence the staff members all have a computer keyboard attached to the end of their arms. Just as a carpenter has a hammer, the finance and accounting staff have their spreadsheet programs. The accounting profession was invented in 1492, when an Italian named Pacioli invented double-entry bookkeeping using a

FIGURE 10.1. TRADITIONAL (ESTIMATED) IT SPENDING AS A PERCENTAGE OF OPERATING COSTS.

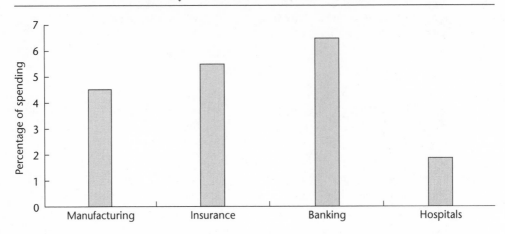

quill pen. The current practice is somewhat more advanced (though still double-entry). In the early 2000s, quills are a bit too slow to keep up with the pace of change in the health care industry.

It may be obvious that all industries have adopted IT as a cost-reduction and labor saving tool, but uses for IT in health care have a distinctly patient-oriented focus. General ledger and payroll programs are the most basic pieces of software in any industry and thus are not at issue here. They work the same in health care as in any other industry. It is the other programs that produce value in health care and health care finance.

The essential function of information systems management is to get the right information to the right user at the right time to support effective decision making. The improvements contemplated for health care IT are generally predicated on improved patient care and involve moving previously unavailable information to the clinical practitioner at the patient point of service. The practitioner might be a physician, a nurse, a physical therapist, or a dietician. It could also be a massage therapist, an acupuncturist, a pharmacist, or a psychologist. In every case, the need to know what happened to the patient prior to the current visit is critical to effective and cost-efficient care.

Health care IT functions are extensive. There is critical need in areas such as clinical operation, financial operations and analysis, facility management and planning, and marketing development. Yet the health care industry has been behind the curve in IT spending. Figure 10.1 is a chart of IT spending within health care and other industries.

This failure to invest in IT has hurt the industry by holding it back from making some of the major productivity strides achieved in other industries. For example, the auto industry is a leader in automated production processes. Banking, which specializes in the movement of money in both global and local marketplaces, could not exist without major advances in IT. After all, the proliferation of automated teller machines allowed banks to reduce their labor costs while improving service to customers who needed more than the basics.

So health care is late to the IT table. But it started to close the gap in IT spending in the late 1990s. Many health care chief executives and their boards have been gaining understanding of the organizational needs and capabilities of IT. They have accepted the need to move beyond the 2.0 to 2.5 percent average spending on IT. Figure 10.2 is an indication of the sort of costs involved. Each item has an expense history. For example, over the past few years the cost of computer hardware has plummeted. Computer users now have hardware that is thousands of times faster, with the ability to store and hold much greater amounts of data, than just a few decades ago. On the other hand, the cost of IT personnel has increased much more quickly than the rate of normal inflation as a result of the demand for personnel who can write programs and fix glitches that arise in the course of operations.

Like most of its industry counterparts, RHMC has researched its future IT needs. It does this formally through an IT strategic plan, updated annually. The goals of the plan:

- Determine the organization's needs
- Review its current capabilities
- Ascertain how to close the gap between need and capability

The IT plan starts with a review of the strategic initiatives that the organization is attempting to achieve, in accordance with the main strategic plan. These are the strategic initiatives that the IT plan must focus on.

Strategic Initiatives

- Providing superior health care to all the clients of the system, and improving the health status of the community
- Integrating physicians into the health delivery system, and expanding the primary care physician network
- Managing health care delivery across the continuum
- Reducing cost per unit of health care service by increasing utilization and efficiency

FIGURE 10.2. POTENTIAL IT SPENDING IN HEALTH CARE.

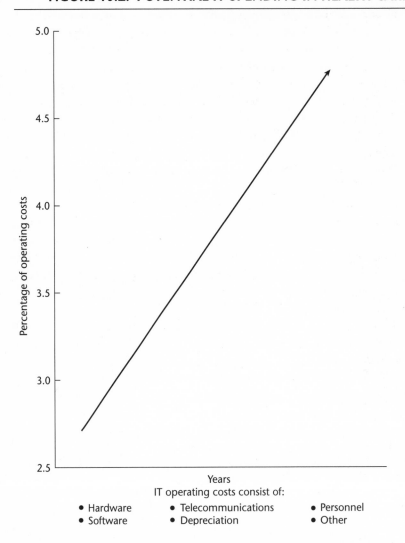

Information Technology Strategic Plan Initiatives

Each of the four strategic organizational initiatives shown in the list has to be aligned with specific IT needs that are not currently being addressed. At RHMC, this led to determining that there should be a concentration in four key areas:

1. Build systems to support enhanced clinical process management and data access.
2. Integrate data and reporting to support enhanced decision making.
3. Build the IT infrastructure and delivery capabilities.
4. Become HIPAA-compliant.

In the late 1990s, the Y2K issue absorbed a great deal of RHMC's personnel and capital resources for two years. Because of this, many other needs that were identified during the IT strategic plan still awaited accomplishment.

Build Systems to Support Enhanced Clinical Process Management and Data Access

When RHMC upgraded its computer systems for Y2K compliance, it still did not install many of the new and improved clinical applications that can generate significant improvements:

- Physician satisfaction through timely results reporting
- Patient satisfaction, thanks to the physician's ability to give better diagnostic and therapeutic service and thereby treat the patient in a timely manner, allowing the patient to be discharged sooner (which should also improve bottom line)
- Employee satisfaction from the capacity of technology to help clinicians (nurses, technicians, therapists) record their observations (charting) into the clinical systems and have immediate access to their notes and those others in a format that enhances good clinical decision making
- Clinical data access for all levels of management; in addition to access by the actual caregivers, new clinical technologies allow RHMC management and administration to access summarized clinical information (not at the level of the individual patient) for the purpose of improving the quality of care being performed as well as reducing costs, where appropriate

Given these projected improvements, RHMC was eager to implement clinical applications. Also, as is seen later in this chapter, many projected financial implications for clinical application are favorable as well.

Integrate Data and Reporting to Support Enhanced Decision Making

The second IT strategic initiative—integrating data and reporting to support enhanced decision making—is extremely important to the organization. Without effective reporting and analysis systems, it is not easy for administrators to maintain proper control over their managers or for managers to gain proper understanding of their department operations.

Turning data into useful information is critical to the financial and clinical health of RHMC. Several areas of decision support allow managers to optimize the resources of their departments at all times; anything less than this type of commitment leads to inefficiency, ineffectiveness, and inappropriateness.

Effective Decision Support System Needed by the Health Care Organization

- Five-year strategic financial planning
- One-year operating and capital budgeting (exception basis development)
- Net revenue contract management monitoring and analysis
- Labor productivity management monitoring and analysis (with benchmarking capabilities)
- Cost accounting development and analysis
- Flexible monitoring and alerting system (with ratio analysis and benchmarking capabilities)

Build the IT Infrastructure and Delivery Capabilities

RMHC made a great commitment to improving its infrastructure and delivery capabilities during Y2K upgrades. As we see later, in Exhibit 10.1, the organization spent $4.85 million over a three-year period to upgrade a number of infrastructure areas for operation of the enhanced hardware and software. Still, this is an area that is never finished. As technology gets increasingly faster, smaller, and more reliable, the organization's technology infrastructure has to be continuously upgraded.

HIPAA Implementation Issues

In the meantime, while contemplating IT spending for all these items, like every other hospital in the United States RHMC is now faced with implementing a variety of new systems, both computerized and administrative, to comply with the Health Insurance Portability and Accountability Act of 1996. Though signed into law in 1996, as of 2001 not all provisions have been finalized. Reality, however, is closing in on those parts of the legislation that directly affect health care providers, payors, and a variety of vendors with which they do business.

HIPAA is a federal law in five parts:

- Title I: Health Insurance Access, Portability, and Renewal
- Title II: Preventing Healthcare Fraud and Abuse, and Administrative Simplification
- Title III: Tax-Related Provisions
- Title IV: Group Health Plan Requirements
- Title V: Revenue Offsets

For purposes of this book, we are only concerned with Title II, Subtitle F, which refers to six major elements of administrative simplification. These are the provisions:

1. Electronic transaction standards
2. Security
3. Unique health identifiers
4. Standard code sets
5. Privacy
6. Electronic signature standards

Each standard instigates significant changes to how business is done in the health care industry. In summary, the objectives of the administrative simplification provisions are as follows:

- Enhance the quality of patient care by improving clinical data access and information availability for caregiver decision making
- Improve health information security for Internet-based technology
- Protect the privacy and security of patient health care information
- Set standards for patients, providers, insurers, and employers
- Reduce health care administrative overhead costs (estimated at 26 cents of every health care dollar spent)
- Reduce health care fraud and abuse (estimated at 11 cents of every health care dollar spent)

The federal government and those affected in the health care industry have been on a long and winding road, from the time the law was signed to the middle of 2001. As you can see in Table 10.1, most of the various standards still do not have a final publication. In fact, although four standards were initially published in 1998 and a fifth was published in 1999, only two have a final publication date, neither of which requires implementation before October 16, 2002.

TABLE 10.1. TENTATIVE HIPAA ADMINISTRATIVE SIMPLIFICATION SCHEDULE, WEBSITE INFORMATION, AS OF FEB. 28, 2001.

Notices of Proposed Rule Making (NPRM) Already Published

Standard	NPRM Publication Date	Expected Final Rule Published	Expected Date Compliance Required*
Transactions and code sets	May 5, 1998	Published Aug. 17, 2000 (other than first report of injury and health claims attachments)	Oct. 16, 2002* (other than first report of injury and health claims attachments)
National provider identifier	May 5, 1998		
National employer identifier	June 16, 1998		
Security	Aug. 12, 1998		
Privacy	Nov. 3, 1999	Published Dec. 28, 2000	Apr. 14, 2003

NPRMs in Development

National health plan identifier			
Claims attachments			
Enforcement			
National individual identifier	On hold	On hold	On hold

*Standards are required to be implemented generally within two years of the effective date of the final rule. (The effective date of the final rule is generally sixty days after publication.) However, the effective date for national provider identification is likely to be delayed a few months to allow enough time for HHS to develop the system for implementing the identifier. (http://aspe.hhs.gov/adminsimp/pubsched.htm)

The law requires many groups to comply with the provisions of HIPAA law. These provisions apply to any organization that transmits, maintains, or stores electronic "covered" (also called protected health information, or PHI) patient and payment information. Therefore these provisions apply to

- Qualified health plans:
  ERISA plans
  Medicare
  Medicaid

- Other covered entities:
  All clearinghouses (if they are used to translate or convert data)
  Pharmacies
  Providers (including physicians)
  Employers

Covered patient information is defined as demographic, treatment, and payment information that is or will be stored electronically or on paper. Because all or almost all patient information is entered into a billing or registration system, all health care organizations (and many of their outsourced suppliers) need to apply HIPAA privacy standards to all patient information at all points in the chain of service. In particular, this means that all of the collection agencies with which the hospital contracts must certify that they also comply with the HIPAA standards. This is to be done through a "chain of trust" agreement.

In any event, by the middle of 2001 two of the original administrative simplification elements were in play. As you can see from Table 10.1, these were the transaction and code set standards (which must be implemented by October 16, 2002) and privacy standards (which must be implemented by April 14, 2003). From the table, it is clear that the government is unsure when the remaining standards will be published. There are tens of thousands of comments to sift through from the three standards that already have had their notice of proposed rule making.

The transaction and code set standards were designed to offer the health care industry uniform standards for conducting business through electronic means and apply to use of eight electronic sets mandated by HIPAA. It is important that all HIPAA-mandated organizations work hard to achieve compliance by the October 2002 date because there are penalties for noncompliance.

The civil monetary penalties for violating transaction standards are $100 per person per violation and up to $25,000 per person per violation of a single standard for a calendar year. The penalties for known misuse of individually identifiable health information can be up to $250,000 fine (civil) and ten years' imprisonment (criminal). Thus it is in the best interest of the organization to get it right within the time frames listed. It should be noted that clearinghouses and health plans must comply with the transaction and code set standards by October 16, 2002; providers are not required to use electronic transactions, but if they choose to they must also comply with the October 16, 2002, deadline.

Both of these standards require hospitals, health plans, physician groups, and others to make substantial changes in their paper medical records and their computer systems that contain demographic, insurance, or clinical information. In addition, the new privacy rule requires compliance in a number of areas, such as development of comprehensive and enforceable privacy policy and procedures, development of sanction guidelines for violation of privacy policy, offering mandatory training to employees regarding privacy policy, requiring all employees to sign a confidentiality agreement, and formalizing specific processes to manage access to the organization's computer systems.

Although HIPAA is still almost a year away at RHMC, the organization has already put most of the compliance features in place and continues toward completion, with a HIPAA steering committee facilitating the effort. In addition, RHMC plans to be ready to bill electronically on October 16, 2002, because the center believes that the electronic features will perform as advertised, making it much easier to verify and validate insurance coverage, bill, follow up, and collect outstanding accounts receivable from health plans. Tracking of clean claims can be done automatically and systematically, which should allow RHMC to eliminate some staff from back-end processing.

Thus RHMC is well on its way toward complying with the first two major HIPAA standards. There is still a substantial amount of work to be done, but the center has every intention of doing it. The administration also plans to be ready for any new standard that is finally published by the federal government.

Selection of a New Health Care Information System

HIPAA was initially intended to establish registration and billing standards within the health care industry, and to ensure privacy, confidentiality, and security for the information in these and other records that contain demographic, insurance, and clinical data. HIPAA did not relate to improved clinical information. Yet the opportunities to improve many of the clinical features and functions were enormous. So back in mid-2000, RHMC administration decided to enlist the aid of a computer consultant who would help them select the best possible system for their needs. They chose to interview a few consulting candidates to select the one best fit for their culture and needs. They were aware that consultants who help in IT selection processes could be expensive if allowed to perform extensive and unnecessary services. Instead, they chose a consultant to assist them with a narrow scope of work (Berger and Ciotti, 1993):

1. Creating the initial list of vendors suitable for RHMC's size

2. Helping to prepare the request for price quotation (RPQ), a twenty-page document that asks the vendor for a defined set of information and allows the consultant and organization to gain an understanding of those IT vendors being queried without creating an unmanageable and virtually useless set of information (Gibson, Berger, and Ciotti, 1992)

3. Summarizing the information contained in the RPQs returned by the vendors

4. Facilitating a focused yet streamlined selection process (staff of RHMC performed much of the analysis work related to software applications with which they would be involved, such as evaluating the features, functions, and ease of use and applying objective scoring criteria to determine the selection)

Features and Functions of the Selected IT System

After extensive negotiations, RHMC and the selected vendor got down to the troublesome implementation stage, in which time constraints were imposed to get the newly purchased system operational so that the organization could achieve some of its efficiency and effectiveness goals and upgrade the organization's IT capabilities as expressed by the strategic plan and its initiatives. Because of the time it took to select a system, negotiate the contract, and perform significant upgrades to the IT infrastructure, the organization wanted to go live with the system within twelve months of the contract signing date. Each department manager was therefore asked to review the features and functions of the vendors' systems and be sure about those most critical to improving and expanding operations in the first implementation phase.

Because the organization's baseline systems had been replaced in 1999 thanks to Y2K concerns, the big issues now facing RHMC were primarily clinical. The additional features and functions that RHMC would be gaining with its new system acquisition included the following:

- Patient integration
  Integrated scheduling and registration
  Enterprisewide master patient index
- Physician support
  Integrated clinical and administrative information access
- Clinical data integration
  Nurse charting
  Clinical point-of-care applications
  Clinical data repository
  Clinical outcomes measurement system
  Electronic medical record implementation
  Disease management analysis and reporting
  Encounter reporting

FIGURE 10.3. APPLICATION AREAS CONSIDERED MOST IMPORTANT OVER NEXT TWO YEARS (2001 RESULTS VERSUS 2000 RESULTS).

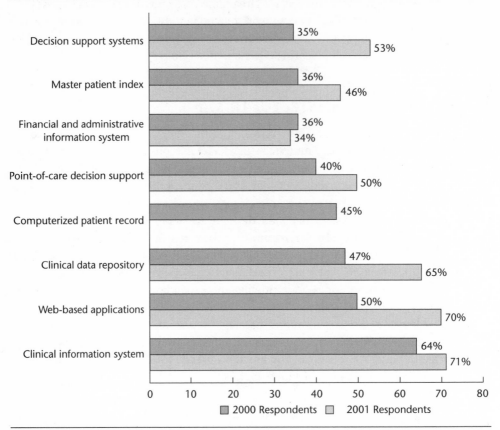

Source: 12th Annual Health Care Information and Management Systems Society (HIMSS) Leadership Survey, sponsored by Superior Consulting and Dell Computer, Mar. 2001.

RHMC's wish list was consistent with surveys conducted to determine the application areas considered most important to be available and installed by hospital or health systems over the next two years. A summary of one of the most widely cited surveys indicates that clinical systems are hot. Figure 10.3 clearly indicates that four of the top five applications are clinical in nature.

Furthermore, all of these clinical upgrades require significant improvements to the IT infrastructure:

- LAN upgrade (wiring, data closets, integration hardware)
- Additional staff support (more FTEs in applications and hardware support, and network engineering)
- Additional capability for multiple, complex project execution

Much of what RHMC planned was consistent with various surveys taken during 2000 and 2001. In general, for a majority of integrated delivery systems and hospitals, upgrading the IT infrastructure and patient-focused information were the priorities. In descending order, health care IT directors considered these items as most important in fulfilling their organization's mission:

1. Upgrading security and becoming HIPAA-compliant
2. Deploying Internet technologies
3. Improving the information systems department's cost effectiveness
4. Upgrading network infrastructure
5. Upgrading inpatient clinical systems
6. Implementing electronic data interchange and HIPAA compliance
7. Integrating systems in a multivendor environment
8. Implementing a computerized patient record system (12th Annual Health-care Information and Management Systems Society (HIMSS) Leadership Survey, sponsored by Superior Consulting and Dell Computer)

Financial Implications for RHMC

The work described here is extremely costly. In fact, it easily exceeds the 2.0 to 2.5 percent of average organizational spending on IT mentioned earlier in the chapter. Exhibit 10.1 shows the extent of RHMC's spending over the three-year period between 1999 and 2001.

This appears to be a significant amount of money for an organization of its size. Yet, it has been absolutely necessary, and RHMC was far from unique. Some of the cost is specifically related to last century's Y2K problem. Many organizations spent millions to achieve compliance with Y2K, and that did not include the cost of upgrading their systems to enhance features and functionality. Now health care organizations are facing the cost of HIPAA compliance.

According to a study performed by First Consulting Group for the American Hospital Association in March 2001, the cost that the hospital industry faces to comply with just the HIPAA privacy rules is estimated to be $4.0 to $22.5 billion. This is an aggregation of the costs for the minimum necessary use regulations, business associate contracting, and state law preemption (First Consulting Group, 2001).

EXHIBIT 10.1. RHMC INFORMATION TECHNOLOGY CAPITAL EXPENSES FOR COMPUTER INSTALLATION, 1999–2001.

Application software (financial and operational)	
General ledger	$ 60,000
Accounts payable	60,000
Payroll and personnel	60,000
Medical records abstracting	60,000
Medical records coding	60,000
Enterprise medical records	150,000
Patient accounting, billing, collections	90,000
Patient registration	60,000
Automated scheduling	30,000
Data repository	90,000
Subtotal financial and operational software	720,000
Application software (clinical)	
Order entry and results reporting	90,000
Radiology	90,000
Pharmacy	60,000
Automated nurse charting	90,000
Subtotal clinical software	330,000
Hardware	
Computer servers	800,000
Network	600,000
Peripherals:	
PCs (800 units)	1,600,000
Laser printers (200 units)	200,000
Miscellaneous	100,000
Subtotal hardware	3,300,000
Network infrastructure	
Architect and engineering fees	400,000
Network closets, cabling, electrical, outlets	4,000,000
Expansion of computer room	200,000
Renovation for additional classrooms	250,000
Subtotal network infrastructure	4,850,000
Other hardware and software costs	
Interface engine	250,000
Interface programming (12 systems)	200,000
Conversions (8 systems)	100,000
Subtotal other hardware and software costs	550,000
Vendor implementation fees	
Implementation fees to vendors (13 systems)	600,000
Travel expenses, for implementation and training	100,000
Subtotal vendor implementation fees	1,800,000
Implementation fees for RHMC	
Information technology staff	400,000
Consultants	400,000
Implementation team*	400,000
User training*	400,000
Subtotal RHMC implementation fees	1,600,000
TOTAL HEALTH INFORMATION SYSTEM IMPLEMENTATION COSTS	$13,150,000

*Cost transferred to IT system conversion budget to represent the time spent by RHMC staff working on the new computer system implementation.

RHMC is currently in the process of determining its cost of HIPAA privacy compliance. It will do whatever is necessary to fully comply with the regulations. The organization is also confident that improvements in efficiency and reduction in accounts receivable thanks to electronic eligibility, billing, and payment features will offset some of the costs of the compliance.

How Improvements to Clinical Systems Benefit RHMC's Financial Outcomes

As stated earlier in this chapter, the biggest benefits that RHMC expects to obtain from its upgraded information system are in the clinical services area. New software modules for nursing and ancillary department staff are expected to generate service and patient satisfaction improvement. The modules are expected to automate some of the clinician's documentation, freeing up more time for clinical analysis. The clinicians who will be using the system in the ordinary course of the day:

- Physicians
- Nurses
- Physical therapists
- Speech therapists
- Occupational therapists
- Cardiac services personnel, such as cardiac catheterization, cardiac rehabilitation, and other cardiology
- Respiratory therapists
- Pharmacists
- Pastoral caregivers
- Dieticians

Basically, any clinician who currently is required to document the service or education component of a patient's encounter can perform this documentation online. The benefits of online documentation (charting) are significant:

• Easier locating of inpatient unit chart. This is the case because clinicians who can document online from any computer no longer have to spend time locating the patient's paper chart. This is a time saver.

• Improved chart review capabilities. The computers will be located at several areas around the inpatient floors, in the patient's room and in every outpatient setting. This allows not only input capability but also clinician review of previous clinical notes as far back as has been input into the computer. It also permits clinicians to review and trend items such as laboratory results across various time periods, even years. This is not effectively possible with paper charts unless special requests are made, and the analysis can never be done quickly. This new capacity enhances the clinician's ability to make quicker and more accurate diagnoses.

• Improved chart review, diagnosis, and treatment capabilities off the inpatient unit. Computer terminals will be located not only in patient areas but also in the physician lounges; for those physicians associated with the hospital, connections can be made to terminals in their offices. This allows the physician to check the progress of a patient online and in real time for lab, radiology, or cardiology results or nurses notes. Because of the increased resources and speed of the analysis, the physician can prescribe treatment plans or drugs sooner. This should mean quicker recovery—a plus for the patient, the patient's insurance company, and a health care organization that is reimbursed on a case rate or low per diem.

• Increased legibility owing to online documentation

• Improved patient satisfaction as patients realize the benefits of the increased speed of treatment and recovery from their illness or trauma

• Accelerated speed of documentation in the chart. Clinical documentation is always better the sooner it is recorded. Locating a terminal at the bedside, in the physician lounge, and in the physician's office should shorten the time frame for recording the documentation. Swifter documentation leads to better documentation, which leads to better clinical analysis. This ultimately leads to better coding and reimbursement.

• Increase quality of care because nursing and other clinical personnel are spending less time on administrative or clerical matters and more time at the patient's bedside, administering care

In summary, the value of clinical systems is still virtually untapped. But at RHMC and many other health care organizations, using computers for documenting, analyzing, diagnosing, and researching the patient's condition is at the starting line. It should revolutionize the practice of medical care.

Impact of the Internet

Health care IT offers greater promise in the future than has been experienced in the past. There are opportunities for unprecedented progress in patient care applications that should have positive implications for financial performance of the health care organization. In addition, there are nonfinance applications that can have positive benefits. For example, three years ago RHMC developed a Website for community access to information about RHMC's patient services, with hot links to dozens of consumer, clinical, and professional health-related Websites.

The RHMC site receives more than two hundred hits a day, surely creating a close bond with consumers in its community.

In addition, RHMC has planned some major Internet applications for the next two years:

- *Internet access for physicians.* Physicians can access the Internet from the lounge or medical library for medical research. This is a burgeoning area of interest for physicians and allows them to find information of any type that can aid in diagnosis and treatment issues. Further in the future, the physician will have this access at the patient's bedside and in the outpatient treatment areas.

- *Online patient records.* In the near future, the most effective placement and use of computerized patient records will be on the Internet. This allows clinicians to access CPR information from any computer terminal with Web capability, throughout the world (provided the clinician has the proper security code; see HIPAA requirement). RHMC consistently monitors the development of CPRs. As the development gets closer to usable reality, RHMC is waiting for CPRs systems to become more stable and usable. When the time comes, it plans to invest in the technology in a big way.

- *Management use of the Internet.* Offering selected key users (managers and directors) access to the World Wide Web means they can research new revenue-generating ideas and regulatory issues. It has already been shown to be a big asset in reducing the time spent in these areas and has enhanced the manager's ability to keep current in leading-edge change in his or her area of expertise.

- *Intranets.* Creating an intranet means a department or division like human resources or nursing can save money and increase access to policy and procedure manuals. An intranet works like a normal Web browser but without using an external modem. Instead, using a big computer server and the organization's local area network, manuals of information are now easy to use. Staff looking for information can easily access it using the Find key, without having to slog through books of several thousand pages.

In summary, the uses for IT in health care have only just begun to have a dramatic impact on patient care and finances. The future for technology in health care is limitless. Like most other health care organizations, RHMC is running as fast as it can so as not to be left behind.

Budget Presentation to the Board Finance Committee

After all the work of the previous five months, RHMC's administration presents its proposed 2002 budget to the finance committee of the board for committee

TABLE 10.2. RHMC CASH INFLOWS AND OUTFLOWS BASED ON 2002 BUDGET (IN THOUSANDS OF DOLLARS).

	2001 Projected	2002 Budget
Cash inflows		
Operating margin	$3,100	$2,920
Add back: depreciation	10,500	11,500
Total cash inflows	13,600	14,420
Cash outflows		
Capital expenditures	10,000	11,500
Principal payments on outstanding debt	13,500	3,600
Total cash outflows	13,500	15,100
Net cash inflows (outflows)	$100	$(680)

approval. Upon approval by the finance committee, it is sent to the full board of directors for final approval. This is usually a formality, as the full board has generally ceded responsibility for detailed review and debate to the finance committee. Still, an occasional controversy may occur, perhaps around the level of budgeted capital expenditure in relation to net income. For example, the administration may propose spending more money for capital acquisition and replacements than is available from cash inflow (see Table 10.2).

It is possible that the finance committee could decide to approve this scenario because it has been presented as a one-time problem. This could be the result of a major shift or reduction in third-party reimbursement, such as the Medicare BBA or an incursion of managed care into the organization's region. Yet the full board may be unsympathetic to the argument that administration should dip into its rainy-day funds. It could therefore decide not to approve the upcoming budget and instead return it to the administration with instructions to rethink the cash flow results so that there is no cash flow loss (that is, reduce planned capital spending).

In this case, RHMC's board has already discussed the issue and decided that if there is a proposed cash flow loss because of HIPAA issues or dramatic change in the reimbursement system, the board will allow it. So the presentation by administration proceeds. At RHMC, a twenty-three-page document is presented over a two-hour time frame. It is important to note that this document was sent out to the finance committee members one week before the meeting so that the members could review it in detail before the actual meeting. Table 10.3 is a (columnar)

TABLE 10.3. RHMC 2002 PROPOSED BUDGET, REPRESENTATION OF TABLE OF CONTENTS.

Reports	Page Number in Document Given to Board	Table, Figure, or Exhibit Number in This Chapter
CEO's memorandum to the board	1–2	Exhibit 10.2
Executive summary	3	
Statement of revenues and expenses	4	Table 10.4
Ratio analysis and key success factors	5	Table 10.5
Key volume assumptions and gross revenue percentage	6	Table 10.6
Analysis of revenue and contractual allowances	7	Table 10.7
Salary expense and FTE summary	8	Table 10.8
Salary reconciliation	9	Exhibit 10.3
Employee benefits	10	
Financial effect of debt issues	11	
Capital budget	12–16	
Cash budget	17	Table 10.2
Updated strategic financial plan information	18–19	
Graphs of financial and statistical trends		
Admissions	20	
Patient days and outpatient visits	21	
Total expenses and expense per adjusted admission	22	
Gross revenues, net revenues, and total expenses	23	Figure 10.4

representation of the table of contents. The presentation includes chart, graphs, tables, and variance analyses to enhance the committee's understanding of the budget.

There is an interesting feature to the structure of this budget. Several of the budget document pages are designed to look exactly like the pages presented to the finance committee in its monthly financial statements. This is a great time saver to the finance staff. In prior years, the finance staff had to scurry around throughout the year to extrapolate budgeted volumes or ratio analysis data that had not been specifically reported during the budget process. Several years ago, the RHMC finance administrator redesigned both the monthly financial statement and the annual budget report to align the outputs. All parties were pleased with the outcome of the alignment. It resulted in elimination of many obsolete analyses and inclusion of pages that matched the monthly financial report, such as the ratio analysis and key success factors (page 5 of the budget report, according to the table of contents in Table 10.3) and key volume assumptions and gross revenue percentages (page 6).

The CEO's memorandum to the board is designed to put the entire budget into perspective, coming from the individual with primary organizational responsibility for success or failure. In effect, this final budget product is the financial representation of the CEO's goal and vision for the organization. Therefore this memo is a personal message from the CEO to the board, which is responsible for approving the vision. For the year 2002 budget, the CEO's vision and the board's vision are somewhat at odds because the operating margin does not meet the board's 4 percent target. In this case, the CEO's memo becomes an essential tool for formally describing the reasons for divergence. Exhibit 10.2 shows how personal and direct this memo can be.

Following the CEO's memorandum is the final proposed statement of revenues and expenses, shown in Table 10.4.

We have already seen the development of these budgeted revenues and expenses. But the board gets to see only this final version. Ratio analysis (in the table of contents represented by Table 10.5, the page number is 5) and key volume assumptions (page 6) are then provided to place the budgeted bottom line in context. Additionally, there are explanations of variance as represented by the analysis of revenues and contractual allowances (page 7), salary expense and FTE summary (page 8), salary reconciliation (page 9), employee benefits (page 10), and interest expenses (the debt issues, page 11). There are also graphs that show selected financial and statistical trend results over the previous five or six years.

Table 10.5 places many of the expected financial results in context for the finance committee and the board. It begins with the ratios that directly relate to the organization's strategic financial plan, permitting the board members to review trends in these areas. It continues with accounts receivable information, moves to staffing information, and ends with other pertinent patient information reflecting financial outcomes. This page is set up to mimic the information presented in the financial statements every month.

In the key volume assumptions (see Table 10.6), analysis of inpatient volume begins with admissions. This is a big change from prior years, when revenues were based on per diem (or per-day) reimbursement. It meant that the health care organization was paid for each day of stay as well as all the additional diagnostic and therapeutic services rendered during inpatient stays. This was particularly important through 1983, when most third-party insurers paid the full published charges and Medicare paid its own computed actual cost for each day of stay in the hospital. Skilled nursing facilities and physician practices were treated similarly. Since then, Medicare changed its inpatient reimbursement methodology

EXHIBIT 10.2. CEO'S MEMO, OCT. 16, 2001.

October 16, 2001

To: Members of the Finance Committee
From: Richard M. Samuelson, President and Chief Executive Officer
Subject: 2002 Budget

The 2002 Budget is noteworthy for the organization. The federal government's 1997 Balanced Budget Act is beginning its fifth full year, which has produced severe consequences for the industry at large and Ridgeland Heights Medical Center in particular. Payment reductions from managed care are also continuing, but the demand for service from patients and medical staff continues unabated. Our predicament is a national and local issue as well and was anticipated to occur several years ago during discussions of prior strategic financial plans. The fact that "the sky did not fall" previously is a reflection of the growth in outpatient revenues and our ability to delay the impact of the managed care market rates (thereby generating favorable variance in contractual allowances).

The question today is, How should management and the board evaluate our budget? Clearly, the most significant trend is the sharp rise in the percentage of contractual allowances, which causes net revenues to remain relatively flat. Management suggests the board consider the following viewpoints:

- The most important consideration is that we provide quality patient care and that service shortfalls not be attributed to budget considerations. The human resource committee specifically concluded that quality should not be compromised to maintain short-term margin targets. However, on a long-term basis, both quality and financial targets must be achieved. Our ability to absorb short-term declines in operating margins is a recognized asset that the committee was willing to deploy.
- In spite of the decline in operating margins, our historical cash flow has generated a strong balance sheet, including $130 million of cash and investments through September 2001. In 2002, we will generate a negative cash flow due to projected capital expenditures exceeding our operating margin plus depreciation expenses. This one-time reduction needs to be absorbed as we restructure our services to further maximize our financial position.
- Although the 2002 budgets are submitted for approval, ideas to improve actual hospital results are being developed, including the following:
  (1) Existing program enhancement or elimination and new program development. First, analysis is being done regarding home health and skilled nursing to determine if they will continue to have a positive contribution margin. If not, other opportunities may be considered. Second, development of cardiac surgery and other new programs has not been included. Third, these projects will have short-term negative impact as they ramp up.
  (2) Cost reduction efforts are ongoing. We are exploring merging some of our outpatient clinical programs, such as home health care, to improve overall financial results. Further staff reductions may arise from a new labor productivity management program. The strategic financial plan anticipated the need for staffing cuts. Efforts to further effective use of clinical pathways and to develop best practices are necessary. This requires focused physician leadership intended to improve product standardization and utilization management.
- Putting into context the risk areas imbedded within the budget is important. Inpatient or outpatient volumes may not be achievable. Managed care contracts, which historically have been favorable, may be at or below budget in 2002. Budgeted salary reductions will be difficult and have been elusive in the past. Pharmaceutical prices and use may be problematic. Realized gains may decline due to market conditions.

In conclusion, the lack of revenue growth, in spite of volume and price increases, is the critical problem that exposes the risks identified. This requires that management remain focused on successful execution of the strategic plan to develop new or improved clinical programs, medical staff size and capability, and cost reduction efforts. The growth of our employed physician staff continues to be a centerpiece for improvement of our referral pattern. It is also essential in generating new business for the hospital. The era of declining margins makes it imperative that we maximize the returns from our core business and our investments.

TABLE 10.4. RHMC PRELIMINARY BUDGETED STATEMENT OF OPERATIONS FOR THE BUDGET YEAR TO DATE ENDING DEC. 31, 2002 (IN THOUSANDS OF DOLLARS).

	2000 Actual	2001 Budget	2001 Projected	2002 Budget	Percentage Change 2002 Budget Versus 2001 Budget	Percentage Change 2002 Budget Versus 2001 Projected
Revenues						
Inpatient revenue	$ 73,000	$ 79,000	$ 77,800	$ 87,360	−10.58	−12.29
Outpatient revenue	72,000	77,000	76,100	89,440	−16.16	−17.53
Total patient revenue	145,000	156,000	153,900	176,800	−13.33	−14.88
Less						
Contractual and other adjustments	(49,000)	(60,000)	(59,000)	(77,100)	28.50	30.68
Charity care	(2,600)	(2,700)	(2,500)	(3,000)	−11.11	−20.00
Net patient service revenue	93,400	93,300	92,400	96,700	3.64	4.65
Add						
Premium revenue	2,100	2,100	2,100	1,000	−52.38	−52.38
Investment income	6,400	5,000	6,000	6,000	−20.00	0.00
Other operating income	1,200	1,200	1,100	1,200	0.00	9.09
Total revenue	103,100	101,600	101,600	104,900	3.25	3.25
Expenses						
Salaries	36,000	35,500	36,500	37,480	5.58	2.68
Contract labor	1,000	1,400	,800	1,200	−14.29	−50.00
Fringe benefits	7,000	7,000	6,900	7,300	4.29	5.80
Total salaries and benefits	44,000	43,900	44,200	45,980	4.74	4.03
Bad debts	4,600	4,400	4,400	4,000	−9.09	−9.09
Patient care supplies	15,500	15,200	16,000	16,600	9.21	3.75
Professional and management fees Purchased services	5,400	5,600	5,600	5,600	0.00	0.00
Operation of plant (including utilities) Depreciation	11,000	11,000	10,500	11,500	4.55	9.52
Interest and financing expenses Other	3,800	3,800	4,000	4,500	−18.42	−12.50
Total expenses	97,900	97,400	98,500	101,980	4.70	3.53
Operation margin	5,200	4,200	3,100	2,920	−30.48	−5.81
Nonoperating income						
Gain/(loss) on investments	1,200	1,200	1,400	1,000	−16.67	−28.57
Total nonoperating income	1,200	1,200	1,400	1,000	−16.67	−28.57
Net income	$ 6,400	$ 5,400	$ 4,500	$ 3,920	−27.41	−12.89
4% targeted operating margin				$ 3,868		
3% targeted operating margin				$ 2,901		
2% targeted operating margin				$ 1,934		

TABLE 10.5. RHMC RATIO ANALYSIS, KEY SUCCESS FACTORS, 2002 PROPOSED BUDGET.

	2000 Actual	2001 Budget	2001 Projected	2002 Budget	Favorable/(Unfavorable) 2002 Budget Versus 2001 Projected Amount	Favorable/(Unfavorable) 2002 Budget Versus 2001 Projected Percentage
Strategic financial plan						
Operating margin	0.0%	4.1%	3.1%	2.8%	−0.3%	−8.8
Total margin	0.0%	5.3%	4.4%	3.7%	−0.7%	−15.6
Current ratio	1.27	1.33	1.35	1.28	(0.07)	−5.2
Cushion ratio	12.19	12.20	12.20	12.13	(0.08)	−0.6
Days cash on hand	525.87	510.12	501.98	485.50	(16.48)	−3.3
Average age of plant	6.55	7.24	7.35	7.85	0.50	6.8
Capital expenses as a percentage of expenses	18.8%	18.9%	18.2%	18.3%	0.00	0.9
Debt service coverage	2.28	2.16	2.04	2.04	0.00	0.1
Debt/capitalization	64.6%	62.2%	62.5%	61.8%	(0.01)	−1.1
Return on equity	7.66%	7.10%	6.80%	6.50%	(0.003)	−4.4
Return on assets	2.43%	2.10%	1.99%	1.90%	(0.00)	−4.5
Accounts receivable information						
Inpatient AR days	59.3	60.1	59.6	58	(1.60)	−2.7
Outpatient AR days	65.1	66.5	65.4	64	(1.40)	−2.1
Bad-debt expense	$4,600,000	$4,400,000	$4,400,000	$4,000,000	$(400,000)	−9.1
Net write-offs	$4,000,000	$4,300,000	$4,700,000	$4,600,000	$(100,000)	−2.1
Allowance for doubtful accounts (ADA, aka reserve for bad debts)	$5,800,000	$5,900,000	$5,600,000	$5,000,000	$(600,000)	−10.7
ADA as a percentage of AR	26.4%	26.8%	25.5%	22.7%	(0.03)	−10.7
Staffing information						
Total FTEs	980.0	1023.1	1026.0	1005.9	(20.10)	−2.0
FTEs paid per adjusted patient day	4.10	4.17	4.13	4.00	(0.13)	−3.1
Salaries, benefits, and contract labor as a percentage of net revenues and premium revenues	45.8%	47.1%	47.8%	47.5%	(0.00)	−0.6
Other patient information						
Medicare case mix index	1.32	1.33	1.34	1.34	—	0.0
All-payor case mix index	0.91	1.02	1.04	1.05	0.01	1.0
Cost per adjusted patient day	$1,122	$1,024	$1,017	$944	$(73)	−7.1
Cost per adjusted admission	$4,774	$4,200	$4,136	$3,856	$(281)	−6.8
Inpatient managed care contractual adjustments (percentage)	26.0%	29.0%	28.0%	32.0%	0.04	14.3
Outpatient managed care contractual adjustments (percentage)	20.0%	24.0%	22.0%	26.0%	0.04	18.2

TABLE 10.6. RHMC 2002 PROPOSED BUDGET, KEY VOLUME ASSUMPTIONS AND GROSS REVENUE PERCENTAGE.

	2000 Actual	2001 Budget	2001 Projected	2002 Budget	Favorable/ (Unfavorable) 2002 Budget Versus 2001 Projected Amount	2002 Budget Versus 2001 Projected Percentage
Admissions						
Adult	8,100	8,760	9,023	9,787	764	8.5
Newborn	1,950	2,145	2,165	2,382	217	10.0
Skilled nursing	800	840	850	900	50	5.9
Total admissions	10,850	11,745	12,038	13,069	1,031	8.6
Average length of stay						
Adult	3.89	4.05	4.05	4.20	0.15	3.7
Newborn	2.00	2.00	2.00	2.00	—	0.0
Skilled nursing	11.00	10.00	9.50	8.30	(1.20)	−12.6
Total length of stay	4.07	4.10	4.07	4.08	0.01	0.2
Patient days						
Adult	31,500	35,496	36,561	41,131	4,570	12.5
Newborn	3,900	4,290	4,330	4,763	433	10.0
Skilled nursing	8,800	8,400	8,075	7,470	(605)	−7.5
Total patient days	44,200	48,186	48,966	53,364	4,398	9.0
Outpatient services and visits						
Emergency visits	19,000	20,000	20,200	21,816	1,616	8.0
Outpatient surgery	4,500	5,000	5,200	5,616	416	8.0
Same-day surgery	3,700	4,000	4,500	4,860	360	8.0
Observation patients	1,950	2,000	1,890	2,041	151	8.0
Home health services	26,000	30,000	27,000	25,000	(2,000)	−7.4
All other outpatients	112,000	120,000	124,000	133,920	9,920	8.0
Total outpatient services and visits	167,150	181,000	182,790	193,253	10,463	5.7
Gross patient revenue percentage by payor						
Medicare	40.0%	39.0%	38.0%	37.5%	(0.005)	−1.3
Medicaid	4.0%	5.0%	6.0%	6.0%	—	0.0
Managed care (HMO/PPO)	26.0%	28.0%	30.0%	31.5%	0.015	5.0
All others	30.0%	28.0%	26.0%	25.0%	(0.010)	−3.8
	100.0%	100.0%	100.0%	100.0%	—	

and no longer relies on per diem costs. The Prospective Payment System (PPS) pays the organization on a per-case basis. Therefore for Medicare revenue, admission, not patient days, is now the statistic that determines net revenue.

Although many managed care companies have recently adopted per diem as the basis for reimbursement to hospitals, their per diem is on the basis of negotiations with the provider, not cost. Because managed care companies have extremely stringent utilization controls, which restrict the number of days that a patient can stay in the hospital, the number of days is limited. Hence the organization earns little if any margin from this per diem reimbursement. Therefore, although patient days are still an important statistic for determining variable costs and operating capacity, patient days no longer occupy the primary slot at the top of the key volume assumptions page.

Analysis of revenues and contractual allowances (see Table 10.7) is useful in explaining change from year to year. In particular, it allows the reviewers to see how contractual adjustment changes can positively or negatively affect net revenue. In addition, it breaks down the gross and net revenues into units (per-case, per-day) that are more easily understandable from the standpoint of financial analysis. This analysis highlights the fact that a gross revenue increase does not translate into positive net revenue results, especially in an era of declining reimbursement such as in the early twenty-first century.

The remaining analyses represent expense issues, both salary and nonsalary. There is usually little discussion on most of these items, except for staffing level and its resulting impact on salary expense. The analyses usually are able to pinpoint the issues driving staffing expense. For example, page 8 of the budget package (see Table 10.8) clearly summarizes the change in FTEs, which as we've seen in Table 7.3 of Chapter Seven has the most impact on staffing expense. In the case of RHMC, it is clear from Table 10.8 that staffing has fluctuated as the administration has attempted to rightsize it by way of productivity and volume changes throughout the years.

Meanwhile, page 9 of the budget package (see Exhibit 10.3) shows a reconciliation and explanation of how salaries increased or decreased between the current year's projected and upcoming budget year's salaries. The largest change is in the area of FTE increase or decrease, as it is again in this budget. Any policy or practice change proposed in the budget that has financial implications should be addressed in this reconciliation. Finally, merit rate increases have a carryover effect from the current year and an impact on the budget year. This last type of change would be similar if the health care organization were unionized and knew its upcoming year's negotiated wage changes.

Pages 10 (employee benefits) and 11 (financial effect of debt issues) of the finance committee budget package are summaries of specific expense items. Pages

TABLE 10.7. RHMC 2002 PROPOSED BUDGET, ANALYSIS OF REVENUE AND CONTRACTUAL ALLOWANCES.

	2000 Actual	2001 Budget	2001 Projected	2002 Budget	Favorable/ (Unfavorable)	
					2002 Budget Versus 2001 Projected Amount	2002 Budget Versus 2001 Projected Percentage
Inpatients						
Gross revenue per case						
Medicare	10,977	11,300	11,105	11,570	465	4.2
Non-Medicare	5,228	5,065	5,250	5,370	120	2.3
Total gross revenue per case	6,728	6,726	6,463	6,685	222	3.4
Gross revenue per day						
Medicare	1,505	1,502	1,478	1,506	28	1.9
Non-Medicare	1,740	1,725	1,700	1,730	30	1.8
Total gross revenue per day	1,652	1,639	1,589	1,637	48	3.0
Net revenue per case						
Medicare	4,900	4,770	4,700	4,550	(150)	−3.2
Non-Medicare	4,550	4,200	4,090	3,880	(210)	−5.1
Total net revenue per case	4,648	4,290	4,145	3,996	(149)	−3.6
Net revenue per day						
Medicare	880	850	820	790	(30)	−3.7
Non-Medicare	1,400	1,330	1,300	1,365	65	5.0
Total net revenue per day	1,141	1,046	1,019	979	(40)	−4.0
Inpatient contractual adjustment as a percentage of inpatient gross revenue						
Medicare	56.7%	58.9%	57.9%	61.0%	0.03	5.4
Non-Medicare	33.0%	38.0%	35.6%	41.2%	0.06	15.7
Total inpatient contractual percentages	41.1%	45.3%	44.2%	48.9%	0.05	10.6
Outpatient contractual adjustment as a percentage of outpatient gross revenue						
Medicare	52.3%	61.3%	59.8%	68.4%	0.09	14.4
Non-Medicare	15.0%	23.4%	22.6%	30.0%	0.07	32.7
Total outpatient contractual percentages	26.4%	33.5%	31.6%	38.0%	0.06	20.3
Bad debts and charity care as a percentage of total gross revenues						
Bad debts	2.99%	2.82%	2.86%	2.26%	(0.01)	−20.9
Charity and other free care	1.69%	1.73%	1.63%	1.70%	0.00	3.8

TABLE 10.8. RHMC 2002 PROPOSED BUDGET, STAFFING EXPENSES AND FTE ANALYSIS.

	2001 Budget	2001 Projected	2002 Budget	Favorable/(Unfavorable) 2002 Budget Versus 2001 Projected Amount	Favorable/(Unfavorable) 2002 Budget Versus 2001 Projected Percentage
Salary expenses	$35,500,000	$36,500,000	$39,000,000	$2,500,000	6.8
Total FTEs	1023.1	1026.0	1005.9	(20.10)	−2.0
FTEs per adjusted patient day	4.17	4.13	4.00	(0.13)	−3.1
Salaries, wages, and fringe benefits as a percentage of net patient service revenue	47.05%	47.84%	47.55%	−0.29%	−0.6
Nonsalary fringe benefit expenses	$7,000,000	$6,927,000	$7,270,000	$343,000	5.0

12 to 16 present an overall summary of the capital budget as well as a listing of all recommended capital items costing $25,000 or more. This detail is presented to keep the finance committee informed of items (and because the members want to see them). The committee believes that being able to review the requested items at this dollar level is consistent with its governance and approval function. RHMC's management is pleased to present the information because it shows the committee how these purchases support the organization's strategic plans.

Page 17 (see Table 10.2) is a short worksheet presentation of the organization's cash budget for the upcoming year. It is the presentation already discussed earlier in this chapter in regard to the finance committee's willingness (or unwillingness) to approve net cash outflows. In this case, management's recommendation is accepted and for the short run (that is, the year 2002) the proposed negative annual cash flow is accepted after some discussion. However, the board members challenge the administrators to attempt to beat the approved operating and capital budget. They would still like to see no negative cash flow if this can be accomplished.

The administrators accept the challenge but offer no guarantees. As with any budget or any projection, the ability to predict or foretell the future, whether in assumptions already made or an assumption not yet known, is questionable and problematic. By far, the budget assumption with the highest degree of uncertainty after volumes is managed care contractual adjustments. If none of the

EXHIBIT 10.3. RHMC 2002 PROPOSED
BUDGET SALARY RECONCILIATION.

Total full-time equivalents were budgeted at 1,023.1 in 2001. The 2002 proposal of 1,005.9 is a net decrease of 20.1 below the currently projected FTEs of 1,026.0.

RHMC's salary expense is projected to be $35.5 million in 2001 and $37.48 million in 2002, which is an increase of $1.98 million or 2.7 percent. The net increase is a result of the following changes.

2001 projected salaries	$36,500,000
Salary revisions	
Net decrease of 20.1 FTEs in 2002 (1,026.0 projected, 1,005.9 budgeted = 20.1 FTEs)	(824,100)
Increase due to staffing mix and rate changes	124,500
Wage adjustments	
2001 carryover impact of merit increases (1/2 of 4.0% increase)	730,000
2002 merit increase (1/2 of 4.0%)	749,600
2002 wage contingency	200,000
2002 proposed budget	$37,480,000

major managed care companies propose any substantial changes for the year 2002 (which is unlikely), the administration has a good chance of beating the budget.

The updated strategic financial plan information presented on pages 18 and 19 simply revise the information presented seven months earlier. This update maintains the discipline of periodically monitoring previous assumptions, summarizing actual results, explaining material variances, and reporting current projections. The explanation of variances allows the finance committee members to gain better understanding of the reasons for positive or negative differences.

Finally, the last four pages of the package present five-year trends of certain financial and statistical information in graphic form. If one picture is worth a thousand words, then these four graphs become invaluable tools in explaining the overall trends in the inputs that drive the budget dollars and the outputs from which they are derived. Page 20 graphs overall admissions for the organization, page 21 plots patient days and outpatient visits, while page 22 trends total expenses on the first Y-axis and expenses per adjusted admission (which is similar to expense per adjusted discharge) on the second Y-axis.

Page 23 (see Figure 10.4) shows the trend of gross revenues, total net revenues, and total expenses. This particular chart is a useful way to conclude the budget; in a single picture it is easy to see the relationships between these three items and whether or not they are trending in a similar manner. If they are not,

FIGURE 10.4. RHMC 2002 BUDGET, FINANCIAL TRENDS FOR THE YEARS 1998 THROUGH 2002.

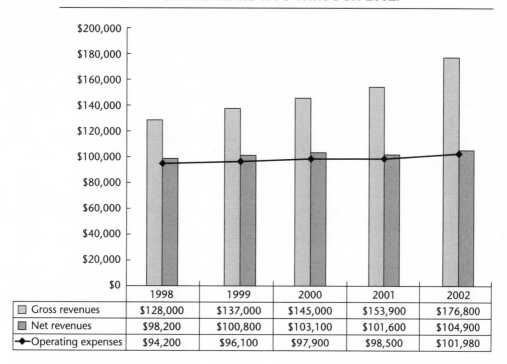

	1998	1999	2000	2001	2002
▢ Gross revenues	$128,000	$137,000	$145,000	$153,900	$176,800
▨ Net revenues	$98,200	$100,800	$103,100	$101,600	$104,900
◆ Operating expenses	$94,200	$96,100	$97,900	$98,500	$101,980

it appropriately requires the administration to explain why not. In this particular case, RHMC's trend lines move in the same direction with approximately the same slope each year. It is an accurate representation of the organization's actual financial results over the previous four years as well as the results projected for the upcoming year.

October Finance Committee Agenda Items

During the October finance committee, one of the other special agenda items was the half-yearly report on the management letter comments made by the auditors in April. However, because the auditors did not report on any internal control deficiencies in April, there are no updates to be given by management. In summary, the October finance committee is appropriately dominated by discussion and approval of the 2002 budget.

CHAPTER ELEVEN

NOVEMBER

Rick Samuelson is pensive. He shakes the feeling that a great upheaval is looming. But he is having trouble getting a clear picture in his mind of just what it might be. Just then, Sam pops his head into the CEO's office.

"Hey, Rick, what's going on?"

"Oh, hi, Sam. Come on in," says Samuelson, slightly startled by the jovial greeting.

"Rick, I was just reviewing some of our investment results from last month and thought you'd want to hear about it."

"I do. But first I'd like to share a couple of things I've just been thinking about and see what you think."

"Sure, I'd love to hear it."

"Well, you know that I've been the CEO of Ridgeland Heights for a long time. And it sure seems to be getting tougher every day. This place has so much to offer to the community. It's a place of healing. We really make people better. And we have such good people working for us. They are so committed to their jobs. But it's just getting harder and harder to maintain the high level of quality and patient satisfaction that every patient has come to expect from us."

Sam is all ears and more than happy to agree.

"I know what you mean. The payors have been taking a bite out of us for the last few years, and we're really feeling it now. The budget we just completed and got approved last month had the lowest operating margin in the last ten years. In fact, thanks to you writing your memorandum to the finance committee, they were willing to allow us to work on a lower margin target than ever before."

"That's true. And I've been thinking a lot about that. This past June, you and I had a talk about the deteriorating margin, and I remember what you said. You mentioned there were three things we could do to improve the bottom line. It was the usual things— increase revenues through higher inpatient and outpatient volumes, reduce costs through specific cost analysis and perform process improvements. But I was concerned about the reaction from our core constituents—the doctors, the staff, and the community. I was afraid they wouldn't understand the fundamental changes taking place in the financing of health care, and that they would see us as a villain in this drama."

"I know that. But it sounds like maybe you've had a change of heart."

"Yeah, I think that would be true. We continue to strive for increased volumes, but they're certainly not assured. So I want us to make a concerted and rational effort to reduce our costs. I know that you've been telling me about techniques that seem to be working at some other providers around the country. I'd like us to put some of them into place right here!"

"Well, Rick, I think that's great. I've really been hoping we could work on it. We can get started right away. The sooner we begin, the sooner we'll be able to see some positive results. And you're right. We really need to do this because even though our budget calls for a low level of profitability, even that is not assured. As you know, since we put the budget to bed we've been hit with enormous discount requests from some of the managed care companies we do the most business with. And regardless of the political party that holds office, additional Medicare cuts are probably just over the horizon. So I'm totally supportive of these initiatives."

"Well then, what are you waiting for? Stop your yapping and get started!"

The ghosts and goblins of Halloween have hardly dissipated when the month of November begins. Autumn has truly fallen upon the region, with the skies remaining increasingly gray throughout the day and the nights getting increasingly colder. Residents of the northern climes are preparing for the equivalent of the big winter hibernation as they begin preparations to hunker down against the expected turn in the weather.

Halloween is an interesting metaphor for the health care industry. Some imagine the federal government as a kind of Dracula, sucking the lifeblood out of providers through a series of small cutbacks, followed by the Big Bite of the Balanced Budget Act. Meanwhile, the Frankenstein monster of managed care has embraced and is beginning to crush the once-mighty providers, even as some of them attempt to transform themselves into the monster itself by developing their own managed care products. Still, it is much too early in the decade of 2000 to tell whether it will be the kind of eternal night that fell over the financing of the health care industry in the late 1990s, or just an aberration that will resume the 1980s' path of perpetually higher reimbursement.

Yet between shaking off some of the real and imagined monsters of Halloween and preparing to give thanks for all the good things that have taken place at the end of the month, the RHMC finance staff and managers remain hard at work. They are not worrying about what may be in the larger context of the industry so much as concerned about performing very real technical duties for their employer.

Preparation of the Budget Results and Delivery to the Department Managers

If there is one month during the year that the RHMC finance staff can sit back for a moment and take a break, it's November. Although the routine work continues as always, the budget project, which has consumed more than five months, is now relatively complete. The finance committee and the board of directors gave their approval and their blessing to the upcoming year's assumptions in October. Now the final set of assumptions, down at the department level, must be communicated. This creates an effective feedback loop, allowing managers to be cognizant of the goals and expectations placed on them.

The finance staff have certain jobs to perform before they can transmit departmental budgets back to the managers:

- Spreading the total approved financial information across certain time periods:
    Twenty-six periods of time that allow them to determine salary variances within each biweekly pay period. If an organization produces weekly paychecks, this budget spread is for fifty-two weeks.

    Twelve periods of time to determine the monthly variance for inpatient and outpatient volume statistics. This is used to determine statistical variances that often help to explain financial variance for gross revenue and expenses. The budget spread is a function of historical trends. Data are reviewed for the previous three years, by month, to develop percentages. In some cases, the financial analyst uses experience and the prior year trend to develop the volume spreads.
- Depending on the culture of the organization, some of the thirty-six months of statistical data are put through a regression analysis program to help improve the projections.

The regression analysis plots the future months' volumes based on past statistical performance. As with any projection, the results are only as good as the underlying data and the quality of assumptions. The greater the amount of historical data that can be loaded into the system, the better the possibility that the projected outcomes have validity. Therefore, for a modest cost, the results achieved from these programs can add a small amount of scientific rigor to the process.

Producing a worksheet that lists all the appropriate line items for gross revenues, contractual adjustments, salary, fringe benefits, and all other nonsalary costs is a task that spreads over the twelve monthly periods. Table 11.1 is an example of the budgeted spreadsheet produced by the finance staff for the radiology department. As you can see, the departmental line items match those in the organizationwide budget shown in Table 10.4.

These lines are a summary of a number of more detailed revenue and expense categories. For example, the patient care supplies line is an aggregation of these items:

- Bandages and dressings
- Catheters and tubing
- Disposable garments
- Drugs
- Instruments
- IV sets and supplies
- IV solutions
- Needles and syringes
- Radiology film
- Contrast media
- Processing chemicals
- Other supplies

What these items all have in common is that they vary with volume. Because they are variable expenses, they behave similarly from a budgeting perspective. This makes it easy to determine the budget spread methodology that must be employed. Because the finance staff have already spread the inpatient and outpatient volumes on the basis of historical trends, it is now simply a matter of using those budgeted monthly volume percentages to spread these variable expenses. Thus all variable nonsalary expenses are spread using the already established volumes. Similarly, nonvariable (fixed) expenses are generally spread evenly across the twelve months, one-twelfth of the total per month. Salary and fringe benefit expenses are usually spread according to the number of days in the month because salary expenses are considered fixed and payable by the calendar. Meanwhile, revenues are usually spread using the adjusted patient day methodology because revenue truly is a function of volume generation.

Budgeting and Spreading Contractual Adjustments by Department

The most difficult of the all the budget spreads is contractual adjustment by department. This is the income statement line item that gives health care organizations the most trouble. The problem stems from reimbursement methodologies that are employed by third-party payors (Medicare, Medicaid, various managed care organizations). Inpatient reimbursement methodologies can be case-based (DRGs), per diem, various percentages of charges, and regular and global capitation.

TABLE 11.1. RHMC RADIOLOGY DEPARTMENT, 2002 MONTHLY BUDGET SPREAD (IN THOUSANDS OF DOLLARS).

	Spreading Method	2002 Budget	Jan	Feb
Revenues				
Inpatient revenue	Patient days	1,984.0	164.7	146.8
Outpatient revenue	Procedures	5,657.0	486.5	413.0
Total patient revenue		7,641.0	651.2	559.8
Less				
Contractual and other adjustments	Adjusted patient days	(3,249.0)	(276.2)	(240.4)
Charity care		—	—	—
Net patient service revenue		4,392.0	375.0	319.4
Add				
Premium revenue	Carved-out member months	—		
Investment income	n/a	—		
Other operating income	Not used	—		
Total revenue		4,392.0	375.0	319.4
Expenses				
Salaries	Number of days in month	1,041.0	88.2	82.5
Contract labor	Adjusted patient days	80.0	6.8	5.9
Fringe Benefits	Even	78.0	6.6	6.2
Total salaries and benefits		1,199.0	101.6	94.6
Bad debts	n/a	—	—	—
Patient care supplies	Adjusted patient days	357.0	30.3	26.4
Professional and management fees	Even	17.0	1.4	1.3
Purchased services	Even	120.0	10.2	9.5
Operation of plant (including utilities)	Number of days in month	11.0	0.9	0.9
Depreciation	Even	—	—	—
Interest and financing expenses	Even	—	—	—
Other	Even	158.0	13.4	12.5
Total expenses		1,862.0	157.8	145.2
Operation margin		2,530.0	217.2	174.1
Patient days		1.00	0.0830	0.0740
Procedures		1.00	0.0860	0.0730
Number of days in month		1.00	0.0847	0.0792
Adjusted patient days		1.00	0.0850	0.0740
Even		1.00	0.0833	0.0833

Mar	Apr	May	Jun	Jul	Aug	Sep	Oct	Nov	Dec
160.7	156.7	158.7	158.7	182.5	180.5	160.7	184.5	158.7	170.6
446.9	463.9	463.9	446.9	509.1	486.5	458.2	480.8	469.5	531.8
607.6	620.6	622.6	605.6	691.7	667.0	618.9	665.4	628.3	702.4
(259.9)	(259.9)	(263.2)	(259.9)	(295.7)	(289.2)	(263.2)	(285.9)	(263.2)	(292.4)
—	—	—	—	—	—	—	—	—	—
347.7	360.7	359.4	345.7	396.0	377.9	355.8	379.4	365.1	410.0
347.7	360.7	359.4	345.7	396.0	377.9	355.8	379.4	365.1	410.0
88.2	85.3	88.2	85.3	88.2	88.2	85.3	88.2	85.3	88.2
6.4	6.4	6.5	6.4	7.3	7.1	6.5	7.0	6.5	7.2
6.6	6.4	6.6	6.4	6.6	6.6	6.4	6.6	6.4	6.6
101.2	98.1	101.3	98.1	102.1	101.9	98.2	101.8	98.2	102.0
—	—	—	—	—	—	—	—	—	—
28.6	28.6	28.9	28.6	32.5	31.8	28.9	31.4	28.9	32.1
1.4	1.4	1.4	1.4	1.4	1.4	1.4	1.4	1.4	1.4
10.2	9.8	10.2	9.8	10.2	10.2	9.8	10.2	9.8	10.2
0.9	0.9	0.9	0.9	0.9	0.9	0.9	0.9	0.9	0.9
—	—	—	—	—	—	—	—	—	—
—	—	—	—	—	—	—	—	—	—
13.4	13.0	13.4	13.0	13.4	13.4	13.0	13.4	13.0	13.4
155.7	151.8	156.1	151.8	160.5	159.6	152.2	159.2	152.2	160.0
192.0	208.9	203.3	193.9	235.5	218.3	203.6	220	213	249.9
0.0810	0.0790	0.0800	0.0800	0.0920	0.0910	0.0810	0.0930	0.0800	0.0860
0.0790	0.0820	0.0820	0.0790	0.0900	0.0860	0.0810	0.0850	0.0830	0.0940
0.0847	0.0820	0.0847	0.0820	0.0847	0.0847	0.0820	0.0847	0.0820	0.0847
0.0800	0.0800	0.0810	0.0800	0.0910	0.0890	0.0810	0.0880	0.0810	0.0900
0.0833	0.0833	0.0833	0.0833	0.0833	0.0833	0.0833	0.0833	0.0833	0.0833

Outpatient reimbursement methodologies can include percentage of charges, fee schedule, capitation carveout, and ambulatory payment group.

On the inpatient side, it is literally impossible to assign the actual contractual adjustment because the third-party payors did not create DRGs, per diem, and capitation with actual nursing and ancillary charges in mind. Instead, the net payments made by third parties to health care organizations, and hospitals in particular, are based on amounts that Medicare and Medicaid can impose and managed care companies can negotiate. Therefore, in assigning contractual adjustments to nursing and ancillary departments, the best method is to use reasonable statistical relationships.

As shown on Table 11.2, RHMC attempts to be as scientific as possible while working within this constraint. The real problem with the budgeted contractual adjustment is splitting the inpatient side among the various departments. In the absence of any actual information from the payors, RHMC used a percentage-of-charge methodology. This involves using the budgeted inpatient charges by department, converting them to a percentage of the total, and then calculating the contractual adjustment by department on the basis of the total budgeted contractual adjustment.

Thus, in Table 11.2, the $87.36 million of budgeted inpatient gross charges in column 1 is converted into percentage of the total in column 2. These percentages are then assigned to the $40.092 million of budgeted contractual adjustments in column 3 to calculate the inpatient contractual adjustment by department. The outpatient contractual adjustment relies less on departmental allocation because most outpatient contractual adjustments are for actual services provided. Except for capitation reimbursement, there was a direct relationship between charges and contractual adjustments. This is even true of Medicare, which now reimburses most outpatient services on the APC method or on a fee schedule. Thus, using the organization's contract payment analyzer, it was not difficult to establish the proper contractual adjustment by department.

In summary, transmission of the budget spreadsheets is important to proper functioning of all the health care organization's departments. The department managers need to know what is expected of them so that they understand the type of volume necessary if the organization is to meet its revenue and bottom-line objectives. Being able to communicate the results of the budget by late November allows the department managers enough time to prepare for the upcoming year. This could mean that the manager has to do all of the following:

- Recruit a new staff member because a new budgeted position has been approved to absorb significantly increased volume

- Plan to lay off one or more staff member because volume has been declining and fewer staff are needed to perform duties
- Prepare for acquisition of new equipment to enhance the department's ability to handle sicker patients (higher acuity) or perform more tests and therapies

Having the budget back quickly is essential to efficient and effective operation of the organization.

Issues Involving RHMC's Cost Structure

Meanwhile, as the department managers prepare for the new year, the administration is debating a problem that has become more evident over the past year or so, as the bottom line begins to shrink. There has been a lot of talk by the administration to the managers about diminishing returns. Although the best way to improve the organization's financial situation is to increase volume and net revenue, many of the efforts that have been tried thus far proved unsuccessful. In this light, managers have been asked, once again, to review the cost structure of their departments and reduce spending wherever possible, even beyond the level of the approved 2002 budget. Over the past few years, several methods have been used to deal with costs. Some of the efforts were highly successful, while some were not. The successful efforts have included these:

• Creation of organizationwide teams charged with reviewing specific issues leading to reduction of definitive costs. For example, a group was organized to review the types of glove being purchased throughout the organization. It was determined that the same type was being purchased from three manufacturers. The group's analysis concluded that all the manufacturers' quality is comparable and there will be no resistance from the nursing, clinical, or physician staff to making a change. Thus a three-month trial period was established to use a single glove manufacturer's product. Because the trial was successful, a change to a single manufacturer was made—at total organizational savings of *$50,000 a year!* This arose from additional volume discounts and the ability to negotiate aggressively. This was just one item of potential savings.

• Creation of a formalized "suggestion box," whereby each employee was required to submit at least two cost reduction suggestions over a one-month time frame. This method assumes that employees working at the detailed level (nurses, technicians, therapists, clerical staff) have a much better idea of the waste that is taking place and improvements that are possible if it is addressed. RHMC's one thousand employees offered almost two thousand suggestions. An organization-

TABLE 11.2. RHMC MONTHLY SPREAD OF BUDGETED CONTRACTUAL ADJUSTMENT, FOR THE BUDGET YEAR ENDING DEC. 31, 2002 (IN THOUSANDS OF DOLLARS).

Department	Inpatient		
	Gross Revenue	Gross Revenue as a Percentage of Total	Computed Contractual Adjustment
			$40,092
2 East (medical/surgical nursing floor)	$3,400	3.89%	$1,560
2 Southwest (medical/surgical nursing floor)	2,170	2.48%	996
3 Northwest (medical/surgical nursing floor)	5,000	5.72%	2,295
Labor, delivery, and postpartum (LDRP)	7,350	8.41%	3,373
Pediatrics	800	0.92%	367
Critical care step-down unit	5,220	5.98%	2,396
Critical care unit (CCU)	3,870	4.43%	1,776
Skilled nursing facility (SNF)	2,680	3.07%	1,230
Psychiatric unit	4,720	5.40%	2,166
Surgical suites (operating rooms)	7,880	9.02%	3,616
Postanesthesia care unit (PACU)	1,270	1.45%	583
Same-day surgery	0	0.00%	0
Outpatient procedures and treatment center	0	0.00%	0
Anesthesia	1,470	1.68%	675
Emergency department	2,770	3.17%	1,271
Renal dialysis	320	0.37%	147
Home health services	0	0.00%	0
Eye center	0	0.00%	0
Respiratory care	3,000	3.43%	1,377
Fertility center	0	0.00%	0
Physical therapy	1,550	1.77%	711
Occupational therapy	750	0.86%	344
Cardiology	1,400	1.60%	643
Cardiac rehabilitation	0	0.00%	0
Cardiac catheterization	1,320	1.51%	606
Radiology	2,210	2.53%	1,014
CT scan	1,610	1.84%	739
Ultrasound	260	0.30%	119
Magnetic resonance imaging (MRI)	560	0.64%	257
Laboratory	8,700	9.96%	3,993
Pharmacy	10,340	11.84%	4,745
Nuclear medicine	1,000	1.14%	459
Central supply	5,740	6.57%	2,634
Total	$87,360	100.00%	$40,092

Gross Revenue	Outpatient		Total	
	Gross Revenue as a Percentage of Total	Computed Contractual Adjustment	Gross Revenue as a Percentage of Total	Computed Contractual Adjustment
		$37,008		$77,100
$800	0.89%	$331	$4,200	$1,891
300	0.34%	124	2,470	1,120
600	0.67%	248	5,600	2,543
400	0.45%	166	7,750	3,539
100	0.11%	41	409	
400	0.45%	166	5,620	2,561
200	0.22%	83	4,070	1,859
0	0.00%	0	2,680	1,230
0	0.00%	0	4,720	2,166
13,240	14.80%	5,478	21,120	9,095
2,000	2.24%	828	3,270	1,410
4,000	4.47%	1,655	4,000	1,655
5,000	5.59%	2,069	5,000	2,069
3,000	3.35%	1,241	4,470	1,916
6,200	6.93%	2,565	8,970	3,837
3,500	3.91%	1,448	3,820	1,595
4,500	5.03%	1,862	4,500	1,862
400	0.45%	166	400	166
1,200	1.34%	497	4,200	1,873
3,500	3.91%	1,448	3,500	1,448
3,400	3.80%	1,407	4,950	2,118
400	0.45%	166	1,150	510
2,700	3.02%	1,117	4,100	1,760
500	0.56%	207	500	207
1,700	1.90%	703	3,020	1,309
5,400	6.04%	2,234	7,610	3,249
5,000	5.59%	2,069	6,610	2,808
1,500	1.68%	621	1,760	740
3,500	3.91%	1,448	4,060	1,705
7,000	7.83%	2,896	15,700	6,889
6,000	6.71%	2,483	16,340	7,228
2,400	2.68%	993	3,400	1,452
600	0.67%	248	6,340	2,883
$89,440	100.00%	$37,008	$176,800	$77,100

wide, manager-led committee was established to review the ideas and bring the most promising ones forward for swift implementation. There were many detailed steps taken to move from idea to implementation, but the result was a $4 million cost savings. These savings were particularly valuable because they positively affected not just the year of implementation but all future years.

Meanwhile, unsuccessful efforts have usually all had the same elements:

- No well-defined goal
- No department manager involvement in establishing the goal
- No staff involvement in establishing the goal
- No accountability
- No follow-up by administration

RHMC's administration was aware of the successes and the failures. In addition to these five reasons for failure, some other distinguishing characteristics were lack of appropriate staffing, lack of political will, distraction, differing priorities, and outright resistance to change. The administrators knew they needed to enhance cost-reduction efforts and were determined to achieve a lower level of unit cost while going beyond previous successes.

The first step RHMC took to determine its current cost structure was to attempt to understand it in a macro sense. In other words, before looking at the components of cost (the micro level), it looked at its global cost structure to determine if, in fact, it was out of line with the rest of the industry. To do this, RHMC had to benchmark costs against those of peers. Benchmarking is a standard of excellence, achievement, and the like against which similar things can be measured or judged. Therefore, it had to obtain benchmarking data on overall costs for health care organizations. Because RHMC was no longer only a hospital, it felt it needed to benchmark against organizations like itself, those having a hospital-based program such as psychiatric services, an SNF unit, or a full-scale home health agency. Furthermore, it was interested in organizations that were managing a physician practice as well.

To obtain benchmarking data on overall hospital cost, RHMC reviewed information on the available benchmarking services. Although every industry in America has some, RHMC was interested only in those representing the health care industry. The review turned up a number of companies performing just this sort of service; many of them were dedicated solely to the health care industry. The review identified some health care benchmarking companies that specialized in only the financial aspects of the industry, others that specialized in only clinical aspects, and others that performed in both segments.

Other distinguishing characteristics separated the various benchmarking companies specializing in health care:

- The number of health care organizations that are participating in the review (this has a significant impact on the sample size)
- Whether the benchmarking company is obtaining its data from health care organizations (which gives access to a greater amount of data at the micro level)
- Whether the information is being obtained from governmental sources at the federal or state level (which means more assumptions are being made in attempting to standardize the cost information)
- The quality and extent to which the benchmarking companies have supplied the organization's financial analyst with explanations on how to aggregate the departmental data

On this last point, the degree to which explanations are available heavily weighs on the quality of the outcomes reported for all the peer organizations being benchmarked. It also helps or hinders the financial analyst's ability to convince department managers that the quality of the data is good. Good data allow the manager to concentrate on the results of the benchmark study rather than on the quality of the data itself.

After selecting two types of benchmark company to work with, RHMC discovered some interesting findings. The most intriguing to the administrators was that the organization had a high expense base, according to both sources. This was further validated by a third benchmarking outcome; expense in this case was measured as a function of a unit of measure. The two most frequently used units of measure for expenses are patient days or patient discharges, adjusted for outpatient volume. These are commonly called expense per adjusted discharge (EPAD) or expense per adjusted patient day (EPAPD). (As an aside, the words *cost* and *expense* are used interchangeably. Further, use of discharges or admissions has almost no impact on the final calculation because in any given period—month, year—there should never be a material difference.)

Figure 11.1 is a graph of RHMC's EPAD over the previous four years. Even more interesting than the slope of the line, which is not decreasing but should be, is the position of RHMC's line compared to the median EPAD of the benchmark peer group. An organization can easily delude itself into thinking that it is cost-efficient and even getting better if all that is available as a guide is analysis of its own results. Only by looking at other organizations and finding out which are using best practices can a valid comparison be drawn.

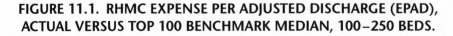

FIGURE 11.1. RHMC EXPENSE PER ADJUSTED DISCHARGE (EPAD), ACTUAL VERSUS TOP 100 BENCHMARK MEDIAN, 100–250 BEDS.

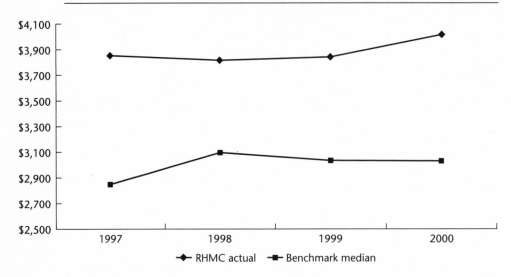

Every health care organization can set the benchmark target as desired. Some may aspire to be the best, thereby setting the target at or above the 90th percentile. Other organizations may be satisfied to be at the 50th percentile, or the median level for the benchmark group. This usually depends on the organization's culture and leadership. It may also be a function of the level of competition in the area and whether or not there is a pressing need to set a high target.

RHMC is feeling the need to improve cost structure given the negative reimbursement change it is experiencing. The cost graph in Figure 11.1 is convincing enough for the administration to begin a series of evaluation steps that it expects to conclude in serious improvement in cost structure. This will come in conjunction with the new budget year and be led by all the division heads, each of whom is responsible for a department where additional cost reduction can be made.

How to Improve the Organization's Cost Structure

There are several ways to improve the cost structure of the health care organization:

- Enhance communication with physicians
- Standardize the organization's supplies

- Reduce utilization of services and supplies
- Obtain best pricing for supplies and products
- Establish and implement optimum productivity and staffing levels

Enhance Communication with Physicians

In all hospitals, physicians control most of the cost of supplies. They place orders for pharmaceutical and medical supplies to be used for patients. They often do not know the cost of supplies because it has never been shared with them. They will usually make rational and reasonable choices in use of supplies so long as they have an understanding of the issues. Thus, it is important to create formal and informal communication channels with physicians.

There are several ways to establish a communication channel. One is for the health care organization to publish its charge master, with the actual cost of each item prominent, in places such as the physician's lounge. This allows the physician to review the cost of an item before writing an order, especially if there is a less expensive alternative available. A better way is to require the physician to order her own supply and ancillary service online. In this case, the organization can list the cost of each requested order on a monitor, along with the charge. When the physician places the order, an alert pops up showing possible alternatives that are clinically appropriate. This point-of-service alert offers the greatest opportunity for changing the physician's ordering pattern. The biggest problem is that in most health care organization the physician does not enter her own orders either because she does not want to or the organization believes she does not want to. This is an area ripe for change. There are numerous benefits to having the physician entering her own order and using the computer for more than just looking up the location of a patient. Future issues of this sort are explored further in Chapter Twelve.

Standardize the Organization's Supplies

The concept of standardizing supplies is once again wrapped around physician ordering patterns. Physicians often practice medicine the way they were taught in medical school and in their residency programs. They are often taught only one way of performing their duties. The interesting aspect of this educational feature is that the teaching of medicine varies with the school. In fact, there are many ways to practice good medicine. Some of them are less expensive than others, yet the clinical outcomes are usually similar.

Thus physicians from the same hospital often want to practice medicine the way they were taught, even if it means a variety of practice and ordering patterns abound at the health care organization where they are currently working. This is particularly true for surgeons who become attached to the instruments of specific manufacturers that were used in the residency program they attended. Because the look, feel, and function of each manufacturer's surgical instrument differ, the surgeon often bonds with that manufacturer's instruments for life. The problem for the health care organization is that this creates a group of nonstandard surgical supplies that may be quite expensive.

For example, consider that the major supply item for hip replacement surgery is the artificial hip. At RHMC, there were actually seven artificial hips ordered by the organization's nine orthopedic surgeons who perform this procedure. Ordering from seven manufacturers does not allow the organization to partake of discounts for volume buying, and it necessitates an inflated level of inventory to keep a complete set of hips for each size from all seven manufacturers. This nonstandardization is quite obviously inefficient and costly to RHMC. Yet none of the surgeons wants to give up the product on which he has trained and performed all of these surgeries throughout his career.

What to do? It is another case of an irresistible object meeting an immovable force. What gives? A couple of potential solutions may be considered. The first involves a mandate from the administration that standardization must take place in the interest of cost reduction. The timing of a mandate of this sort is always interesting. It could come when the organization is already hemorrhaging red ink, in which case the surgeons may recognize the financial need; this allows them to acquiesce without controversy, banding together to help the organization survive. Or the mandate could come while the organization is still financially sound and the standardization could help them stay that way.

Still, the financially sound organization faces a problem convincing surgeons to abandon their comfort zone. To do so successfully, the organization should facilitate a group meeting with the physicians, led by the clinical chair of the surgery service. The chair should explain the financial problems caused by multiple vendors and the need to economize because of reduction in reimbursement. It is extremely important that the physicians be allowed to determine which one or two vendors should remain. Administratively imposed decisions in this regard would be suspect and challenged by the physicians.

If the first solution is politically untenable, a second solution involves a compromise whereby all the physicians agree to help the organization negotiate for the best price on artificial hips without changing vendors. They do this by letting each of the seven salespeople know they are seriously considering changing their hip preference unless a significant discount is offered to the health care organization. This discount should produce the price that would be available if the organization used only one type of artificial hip. Each vendor must get the same message, and any vendor that does not comply should be dropped by the surgeon and the organization. This solution allows the organization to obtain significant pricing concessions, though lack of standardization means that the inventory is still too large. Even so, it is better than nothing and keeps the physicians relatively happy about not having to change hip vendors.

Standardization throughout the organization holds great potential for savings. In many cases, it involves little pain to most of the users of supplies. It allows the organization to reduce inventory of high-priced supplies and deal with fewer vendors, thereby creating efficiency for the material management (purchasing) department. To achieve effective standardization, however, a lot of work is required by the clinical users and the purchasing agents:

- Evaluation of opportunities for standardization
- Determination of which vendor's product they want to standardize
- Organization of a clinical trial or test of the product in those areas that will be using it
- Evaluation of the results of the trial
- Implementation of the standardization

Reduce Utilization of Services and Supplies

This is another way to achieve significant cost reduction in a hospital. The organization can perform analyses to help it understand the types of supplies and services that are being overused and who is placing orders to do so. Rational improvement cannot be made without the data. This is especially true because the primary group that orders supplies is the physicians, and they demand data when their efforts are being reviewed. To summarize the steps that should be taken to effectively analyze, develop, and implement improvement in supply utilization (using the organization's decision support system, or an outside agency specializing in clinical decision support):

1. Segregate the inpatient discharges by DRGs
2. Further segregate the inpatient discharges by ICD.9 diagnosis level
3. Determine the supplies being used at the ICD.9 level
4. Analyze use by the organization's physicians against outside benchmarks
5. Identify best-practice treatment protocols
6. Use these protocols (either internal or external) as standards of practice
7. Measure individual physician variance
8. Determine the reasons for variance
9. Develop an action plan to achieve change

TABLE 11.3. RHMC UTILIZATION ANALYSIS OF DRG 89, PNEUMONIA, SUBSET: NO SUBSTANTIAL CCS OR MODERATE CCS.

	Average Dollars					Number of Cases	Grand Total
	Price	Frequency	Distri-bution	Other	Unit Total		
DRG subset							
1. No substantial CCs or moderate CCs	1,900	200	1,400	1,500	5,000	150	750,000
2. Major CCs	1,800	1,300	4,000	2,000	9,100	20	182,000
3. All other	100	(1,000)	(20)	400	(520)	10	(5,200)
Total DRG 89	1,789	256	1,610	1,494	5,149	180	926,800

10. Implement change in practice
11. Monitor the results of the change
12. Provide feedback of the monitoring results to the appropriate parties

These steps are critical to a successful conclusion. Some interesting findings may be uncovered using these techniques. Also, use of benchmarks is essential to a successful outcome.

Consider a case study from RHMC. A national clinical benchmarking firm was retained to review the utilization levels of a specific number of DRGs. They were reviewing the differences between RHMC's actual utilization and the available benchmark group utilization. The DRGs were selected according to the high number of cases seen at the organization. One selected was DRG 89, a medical DRG consisting of simple pneumonia and pleurisy, age greater than seventeen with at least one comorbidity or complication (CC) if present. (CC generally means that the patient is sicker and requires more care than a patient without CC.) The benchmarking firm first sorted all of RHMC's DRG 89 pneumonia cases into their ICD-9 components, because usage at the level of diagnosis code represents a much more homogenous mix than aggregated at the DRG level (see Table 11.3).

The variance analysis was then sorted by price, frequency, distribution, and other factors. Positive price variance means that RHMC's unit cost of products is higher than the benchmark. The frequency variance measures how often each patient is receiving a particular type of service or supply; for example, in the case of a complete blood count lab test this category would measure whether the test was ordered and performed more (or less) for RHMC's actual patients than for the benchmark group. The distribution variance represents the number of pa-

FIGURE 11.2. RHMC ANALYSIS OF CT SCANS, DRG 89, NO SUBSTANTIAL CCS OR MODERATE CCS, FOR THE TWELVE MONTHS ENDED DEC. 21, 2000.

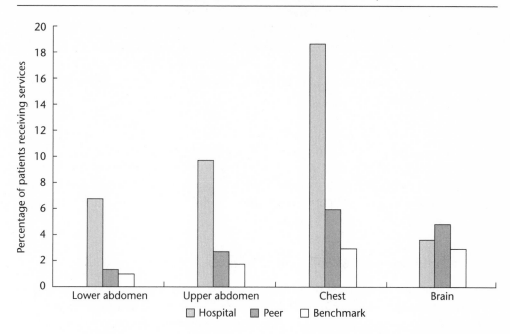

tients within the diagnosis code who are getting the service. In other words, it indicates the percentage of the total patients in DRG 89 receiving antibiotics at RHMC compared to the percentage for the benchmark group.

When stratified, it is clear from the "unit total" variance and the number of cases that further analysis is warranted for the subset of "no substantial CCs or moderate CCs." Next, using that subset as the new variable, they determined variances between RHMC and peer and benchmarking groups for major ancillary services (laboratory, radiology, cardiology, pharmacy). They also reported variance in the average length of stay.

This review immediately highlighted one interesting variance in the radiology (or imaging) service. The CT scan service appeared to be costing the organization much more money than what was reported by the peer and benchmarking group. Upon further review, it was noted that although the figures for patients receiving services were 3 percent for the benchmark group and for the peer group 6 percent, RHMC's utilization rate was over 18.7 percent, six times that of the benchmark group (see Figure 11.2).

Upon learning of this, RHMC performed further analysis. It was discovered that a long-standing practice at the organization was for the radiologists who read the routine chest X ray to "recommend" a CT scan for many patients, in the case of a negative finding, as a precaution for the patient. Because of this recommendation from the radiologist, the attending physician had to order the test, from a medicolegal standpoint. Now that the organization had the national data, it questioned the radiologists about this recommendation. Although surprised by the data, the radiologists did not hesitate to change their recommendation methodology on the spot.

A cost saving and a revenue enhancement accrued from just this one change. First, the variable cost of the CT scan was saved. Second, because there was a waiting list for the organization's CT service, they were able to replace the unnecessary and generally unreimbursed tests with reimbursed outpatient services. The quality of the data and the depth of the analysis impressed the physicians. They became more than willing to listen to the results of subsequent review because of the outcomes for pneumonia.

Obtain Best Pricing for Supplies and Products

Obtaining best pricing is the most mundane of the cost-saving ideas. It is time-tested and easy to achieve. There is little magic to doing so for the supplies and products being acquired by a health care organization. One of the primary methods to achieving best product pricing is to understand and practice the fine art of negotiation. But there may be some problems with this approach if used alone.

First, the negotiator, often the purchasing agent, may not have enough experience or training to negotiate the best available price from the salesperson. Second, the negotiator may not have any leverage to command the best price (this is true in the artificial hip example). If physicians tell the salesperson that they have no intention of switching to another hip regardless of what they are told by the health care organization, the purchasing agent will never be able to obtain a good price from the salesperson. Third, and most important, the health care organization may not be big enough to command the best prices from the manufacturer or distributor of the product. The best prices are usually given to those purchasers who order the greatest quantity of goods. Most stand-alone health care organizations do not look or act like a major purchaser.

Thus it is important to look like a much bigger purchaser than is really the case. To do this, various health care providers band together to form a purchasing alliance. Three of the biggest current alliances (also known as group purchasing organizations, or GPOs) belong to Amerinet, Voluntary Hospitals of America (VHA), and Premier.

For the price of membership, health care providers are permitted to participate in supply and service contracts. The GPO has already negotiated the prices for the goods. In most cases, the health care provider merely has to agree to purchase a minimum number to get pricing at a cost far less than would have been available had it negotiated as a freestanding entity. This is possible because the GPO comes to a negotiating table with tremendous purchasing clout: the ability to deliver millions of dollars of sales to the manufacturer or distributor of supplies.

In any case, the GPO member is often assured of obtaining the best price (or close to the best) for much of the clinical and nonclinical goods required in running an efficient organization. This is a primary tenet in managing supplies in a health care organization. Other materials management concepts are discussed later in this chapter.

Establish and Implement Optimum Productivity and Staffing Levels

Productivity management is a technique established and used for many years in other industries. Health care was late to adopt many of the techniques because until recently cost management was not a top priority. As stated earlier in the book, prior to 1983 Medicare reimbursed the hospital segment of the industry according to cost; the system rewarded higher costs. Labor costs represent the highest portion in the health care industry. Because there was actually a disincentive to reducing costs prior to 1983, most health care companies did not practice labor productivity management.

Subsequent to 1983, these incentives changed. For inpatient care, Medicare's decision to pay a specific rate according to diagnosis, regardless of the patient's length of stay or resources consumed, led administration to take some notice of cost. Still, many organizations had a small number of Medicare patients and a reasonable percentage of charge-based payors. They were therefore insulated from most financial disasters throughout the 1980s. But the rapid rise of managed care plans in the 1990s around the country made almost no health care organization immune from cost pressure. Organizations started to recognize a need for cost reduction and identified labor as the most likely area to attack.

A typical method for identifying optimum labor and productivity levels is as follows:

1. Develop a list of the tasks performed by each employee.
2. Determine the amount of time it took the staff to do each task.
3. Determine the appropriate unit of service to be used by which to multiply the task.
4. Do the multiplication to determine the amount of total staff time needed according to the projected volume.

5. Compare the staff needed (from the calculation) to the actual staffing.
6. Reassign the staff that made up the excess if actual staffing exceeded the calculation; maintain the status quo if the calculation exceeded actual staffing.

Many organizations either performed these steps on their own or engaged consulting firms to do so. When RHMC did so, the results were mixed. Some departments were able to determine they had been performing tasks that were non-value-added. When this was discovered, the tasks were often eliminated, thereby freeing up staff time. In the best case, staff could then be used to treat patients who were waiting for revenue-producing care. In the worst case, staffing was downsized, through attrition, relocation, or position elimination. Over a short period of time (six months), in a small number of departments (twelve) and with a moderate number of staff members (four hundred), RHMC was able to reduce its staff by twelve members, or 3 percent.

This is not an overwhelming reduction; however, it was achieved and taught the organization's administration and managers two valuable lessons. First, understanding the actual task and job assignment improves the relationship between manager and staff. It allows a dialogue based on objective data. It enables rational discussion. For example, if the staff feel overworked, the manager and staff can review the task list and determine whether there are any additional non-value-added tasks that can be eliminated without sacrificing core values.

Second, it is important to monitor ongoing productivity. Once the tasks are known and the unit-of-service standards are set, the organization needs to maintain a system whereby variance is monitored by pay period. This encourages vigilance on these important costs.

Thus understanding, measuring, and managing labor costs is critical to maintaining a health care organization's cost structure. The level of labor and nonlabor costs plays a great role in whether the organization remains financially viable or struggles to survive. Cost management is crucial in an era when volume is stagnant or slightly declining and reimbursement rate is declining. RHMC has chosen to place great emphasis in these areas and has been successful using such techniques.

Materials Management in Health Care

Integral to the concept of cost management is the field of materials management, or supply chain management. Materials management in health care is generally defined as managing supplies and goods (clinical and nonclinical) used by staff to perform their duties. In theory, materials management is the responsibility of every employee and nonemployed physician in the health care facility. In practice, the materials management function is performed by these staff members:

- Purchasing staff, who negotiate and contract with outside suppliers and distributors
- Receiving staff, who accept and log in all the supplies offloaded at the receiving dock
- Central supply staff, who maintain the organization's inventory and distribute it to all the users around the facility

The staff working in these materials management areas are aware of the magnitude of their job. At RHMC, for example, they are responsible for acquiring $16.6 million in patient care supplies as budgeted for 2000. That's 16 percent of RHMC's total expenditures, which is comparable to many health care organizations around the country.

There are a couple of basic tenets that good materials managers follow to maximize return for their employers.

Obtain Best Pricing

The first is to obtain best pricing for goods and supplies. This was discussed at length in the previous section. The primary method is to contain the cost of goods, but it is not the only one.

Develop Close Relations

The second tenet is to develop close relations with distributors. Distributors are the middlemen in the supply chain. One of their basic functions is to consolidate the medical and surgical supplies of many manufacturers and resell them to health care providers for a small mark-up. The distributor/consolidator simplifies the procurement process through this one-stop shopping approach. Distributors that do a good job of performing their tasks are often taken for granted by the materials manager. But it is important for the materials manager to develop close relations with distributors, for a number of reasons.

Over the past couple of years, the number of major distributors has decreased as that segment of the industry experienced significant alliances and combinations. The materials manager is responsible for ensuring that the goods needed by clinical and nonclinical users are available when required. The distributors control the availability, receiving schedule, and pricing for these goods. Although the materials manager has a choice of distributors, this choice is dwindling. Good management technique obligates the materials manager to maintain close and effective relations with the one or two distributors that supply a majority of the organization's goods.

Adopt Just-in-Time Inventory Management

Just-in-time (JIT) inventory management has become extremely important over the past ten years as health care providers adopted techniques pioneered in the automotive industry. Prior to adoption, the health care provider maintained an entire inventory within the four walls of the facility. The provider therefore bore the risk for the holding cost of all the goods being warehoused in the facility as well as an increased chance for obsolescence and shrinkage (theft).

JIT allows the health care organization to significantly downsize its storeroom or warehouse. This produces significant savings to the organization. It can use an onsite, vacated, or downsized storeroom for a more productive or revenue-producing activity, or it can vacate warehouse space that may be leased outside the four walls, thereby saving significant rent expense.

JIT shifts the risk of these holding costs and shrinkage back onto the supplier or the distributor. These companies now become responsible for warehousing the products and shipping them to the organization expeditiously. JIT increases the frequency of delivery to the organization, often from once a week to three to five times per week. It becomes imperative that the supplier's truck appear at the provider's receiving dock at the time that it is expected each day. Otherwise, patient tests or surgeries may have to be postponed. Consequently, there are caveats to using a JIT method. The supplier or distributor must be extremely reliable in its delivery schedule. And the supplier or distributor must also have a reliable pipeline to obtain or manufacture the goods.

Because the holding costs and risk of shrinkage have been shifted back to the distributor or supplier, that business generally charges a slightly higher rate for this service and the risk it entails.

Create In-Service Training

Creating and maintaining an in-service program for the organization's entire management group is fundamental to running the materials management program efficiently. It allows the materials manager to communicate and educate managers and their staff on major internal and external issues surrounding their role in materials management issues:

- Understanding the materials management and central supply process
- Instructing managers on the proper procedures for requesting a purchase order number, which, when assigned, is a legal contract obligating the organization to pay the supply ordered
- Whether the manager should attempt to do his own negotiating with vendors or refer the salespeople to the organization's purchasing agent

- How to deal with a salesperson who has been known to break the organization's rules about the steps to be taken before contacting a specific department manager

This type of in-service helps the organization maintain a good materials management system.

Adopt Consignment

Adopt consignment as a business model. In most cases, a health care organization acquires goods by purchasing them from a distributor or supplier. The goods are ordered by the health care provider, sent by the supplier, received by the provider, billed by the supplier, paid by the provider, stored for a short time in the user's department, and then finally consumed. Under the consignment method, the methodology changes because the provider acquires the goods for use, but payment is made only if used. If it is not used, the item can be returned to the supplier. Consignment is most often used for relatively expensive, specialized equipment usually consumed in the surgical suite (operating room).

Consignment is an economical model that benefits the organization positively, through access to a variety of high-cost equipment without the monetary outlay usually associated with acquisition. There is no significant downside to the provider, so it is likely to grow in popularity.

Implement E-Commerce

Since the late 1990s and the advent of widescale use of the Internet, a number of distributors, suppliers, manufacturers, and purchasing organizations have been busy developing tools and techniques to significantly improve the efficiency and effectiveness of health care supply chain management. Companies on the Web (such as neoforma.com and medibuy.com) have been created to help with the following tasks:

- Ordering goods (hospital department manager)
- Processing the order (purchasing department)
- Pricing the order according to prescribed details in the computer program
- Transmitting the order from the hospital to the distributor
- Sending the order from the distributor back to the hospital
- Tracking the order
- Receiving the order at the hospital dock
- Transporting the order to the appropriate department
- Invoicing the hospital (distributor)
- Paying the distributor (hospital)

These are just some of the big process areas that e-commerce can help stream-line. E-commerce is already quite a bit down the road in achieving many of these goals. An interesting aspect of health care e-commerce is that today distributors and GPOs want to be sure they have a role to play in the Web-enabled future. For that reason, it was the large distributors and GPOs that developed and now own Websites (such as the two just mentioned). There will be much greater use of this type of Website in the near future as further refinements are adopted.

It is clear that sound materials management policies and practices within a health care organization can have a positive impact on facility cost management. It is an area that merits highlighting whenever the concept of cost reduction is proposed.

Benefits of Tax Status to the Health Care Organization

Back in Chapter Two, the issue of not-for-profit versus for-profit health care was briefly touched on. Throughout the book, the not-for-profit model has been con-tinuously emphasized because RHMC (like more than 80 percent of hospitals or health systems) operates under this Internal Revenue Code designation. There are several positive financial implications associated with this designation, and one large drawback. Here is a summary of the various financial benefits associ-ated with the two designations:

Not-for-Profit

- Exempt from federal income tax on profits
- Exempt from state income tax on profits
- Exempt from property taxes (in most cases)
- Exempt from state and local sales taxes (not exempt from excise taxes)
- Able to issue bond debt (income from which is tax-exempt to the purchaser of the debt) to raise capital

For-Profit

- Able to issue stock to raise capital
- Able to offer stock options to recruit and retain staff at various levels
- Limited obligation to provide indigent or uncompensated care

If we were just counting the number of benefits in this listing, it would appear that the not-for-profit entity has an advantage. After all, it benefits from consid-erable operating cost savings throughout the year, which translates into a greatly

TABLE 11.4. OPERATING TAX BENEFITS FOR RHMC AS A REPRESENTATIVE NOT-FOR-PROFIT HEALTH CARE ORGANIZATION.

		Total Potential Tax Liability Savings
2002 projected net income	$ 3,920,000	
Federal corporate tax rate	34.00%	
Potential federal income taxes	$ 1,332,800	$ 1,332,800
State corporate tax rate	10.00%	
Potential state income taxes	$ 392,000	392,000
Potentially taxable property at estimated appraised value	$200,000,000	
Approximate property tax rate	2.50%	
Potential property taxes	$ 5,000,000	5,000,000
Value of goods to be purchased including supplies and capital equipment	$ 30,000,000	
State and local sales tax	8.00%	
Potential sales taxes	$ 2,400,000	2,400,000
Amount of tax-exempt bond debt issued	$150,000,000	
Average difference between taxable and nontaxable interest rates	1.20%	
Actual annual interest expense savings	$ 1,800,000	1,800,000
Total potential and actual annual operating expense tax savings due to not-for-profit status		$10,924,800

improved bottom line. Using RHMC's 2002 budget as an example, Table 11.4 shows that the organization benefits by saving $10,924,800 in taxes. That is an enormous benefit to the nonprofit organization.

The government has granted this benefit because, historically, not-for-profit health care organizations have taken care of the poor, needy, and indigent who needed health care. These health care organizations did not discriminate against anyone who presented in an emergent care situation; they would often provide care even in an urgent or elective situation. Much of this has changed over the years as the government imposed greater and greater requirements on health care providers, both voluntarily (if the organization accepted 1948 Hill-Burton grants) and involuntarily (the COBRA and EMTALA regulations of 1988).

A requirement for providing services to the indigent was imposed in the late 1940s with the passage in Congress of the Hill-Burton Act. This act allowed the government to grant or lend money to health care organizations for the express purpose of building or renovating their facilities. Aside from the fact that this legislation was the first time the federal government had really opened the spigot for a great flow of funds to the health care industry, the act required the recipient organization to ensure that a minimum number of dollars was spent on care for the indigent. It generally amounted to 10 percent of the amount borrowed each year over a twenty-year period. This was the equivalent of a 200 percent return on the borrowed funds in aid to community residents who could not afford this health care.

Although the reporting requirements were onerous, the actual requirements to treat indigent patients were not a problem for most nonprofit institutions. This, after all, was part of their mission. Keep in mind that this program was begun almost twenty years before Medicare and Medicaid, to spur the growth of health care facility availability for the soldiers returning from World War II and their families. There were also almost no for-profit health care facilities in the country at that time. It allowed the nonprofit organizations to share in the largesse of the government.

The advent of Medicare and Medicaid in 1966 considerably changed the equation. There was now far greater coverage for the poor, the elderly, and the impoverished elderly. Although these programs did not cover all the needy, initially the pool shrank. Depending on the location of the health care provider, there could be a large or small number of the indigent requiring care. Residents whose annual income falls below the government's federal poverty guidelines often populate inner cities and rural areas; higher-earning individuals are often located in suburbs. Thus, there are varied opportunities for not-for-profit health care organizations to give free or low-priced service to residents of a community.

There is an interesting counterpoint to the concept of providing community services. The late 1960s saw the first great wave of for-profit health care spring up. Hospital Corporation of America incorporated at this time, with a mission to maximize shareholder wealth. This was in stark contrast to the not-for-profit mission to provide health care to all members in the community who needed it. For-profit health care organizations are not obligated to seek out indigents within their community. Their mission therefore differs from that of the not-for-profit health care organization.

In many communities where for-profit organizations set up their operations, they sought out the best-paying patients. This is known as "skimming." To maximize profits, they specifically attempted to avoid providing services to less-than-full-paying patients except where it was required by law. This occasionally led to another practice, "dumping," which is defined as discharging or transporting patients without insurance to their home or to county facilities before any treatment has been rendered.

To some extent, the desire by certain health care providers not to treat patients who could be a financial drain led to a new law to combat dumping. The

Consolidated Omnibus Budget Reconciliation Act of 1988 set up requirements that all health care facilities, for-profit or nor-for-profit, must treat and stabilize any patient who presents for care in a health care organization's emergency department. Thus, in the case of skimming and dumping, thanks to COBRA there is no longer any advantage or disadvantage to the health care provider on the basis of tax status.

Preparation and Implications of the Annual IRS 990 Report

Not-for-profit, tax-exempt status confers certain responsibilities. One is submission of an annual corporate tax return. The IRS 990 is similar in many respects to a for-profit tax return. It requests information on the organization's income and expenses just as for other corporations. But unlike these other organizations, there is no tax assessment on any revenue exceeding total expenses. This is true for the operating margin as well as any total margin (which includes income on investment). Although the IRS 990 is initially due in March, RHMC took advantage of allowable extensions until November.

Part III, Statement of Program Service Accomplishments, of the IRS 990 encourages the nonprofit organization to highlight its community service activities of the tax year. Hospitals have developed community service benefit reports that summarize their large and small contributions made to the community: annual health screenings and immunization clinics, community health programs such as first aid classes, school health fairs, CPR classes, stress management and nutrition programs, prenatal care programs, support groups, sponsorship, and so on.

The community service benefits report was developed and promoted by the Catholic Health Association as a way to advocate the social value of its mission of caring and healing. During the 1980s, many of the ideas and features of the report were adopted by other not-for-profit health care organizations as a defined method to report their contributions to the community. Table 11.5 is a summary of the community service report included in Ridgeland's IRS 990.

The report is separated into several categories:

- Value of traditional charity provided to the community, the cost of providing free or discounted care to patients in accordance with the organization's policies
- Unpaid costs of public programs, representing the net loss (or cost) of providing care to patients insured by government programs such as Medicare or Medicaid

TABLE 11.5. RHMC 2000 COMMUNITY SERVICE REPORT, SUMMARY OF QUANTIFIABLE BENEFITS.

	Persons Served	Total Expenses	Offsetting Revenues	Net Community Benefits	Percentage of Hospital Expenses	Percentage of Hospital Revenues
Traditional charity care	506	$567,000	$0	$567,000	0.58	0.39
Unpaid costs of public programs						
Medicare	80,000	40,000,000	30,000,000	10,000,000	10.21	6.90
Medicaid	1,500	1,400,000	800,000	600,000	0.61	0.41
Subtotal unpaid cost of public programs	81,500	41,400,000	30,800,000	10,600,000	10.83	7.31
Community services						
Nonbilled services						
Community health education and outreach	24,000	330,000	90,000	240,000	0.25	0.17
Patient education on disease prevention	2,000	40,000	10,000	30,000	0.03	0.02
Other nonbilled services	8,000	30,000	0	30,000	0.03	0.02
Subtotal community services	34,000	400,000	100,000	300,000	0.31	0.21
Medical education						
Physicians, nurses, technicians, other	0	0	0	0		
Scholarships, funding for health professionals	0	0	0	0		
Other medical education	0	0	0	0		
Subtotal medical education	0	0	0	0		
Subsidized health services						
Emergency and trauma care	0	0	0	0		
Neonatal intensive care	0	0	0	0		
Freestanding community clinics	5,200	400,000	0	400,000	0.41	0.28
Collaborative efforts in preventive medicine	0	0	0	0		
Other subsidized health services	0	0	0	0	0.00	0.00
Subtotal subsidized health services	5,200	400,000	0	400,000	0.41	0.28
Research	0	0	0	0		
Cash and in-kind donations	0	45,000	0	45,000	0.05	0.03
Grand total	121,206	$42,812,000	$30,900,000	$11,912,000	12.17	8.22

- Nonbilled community services, the organization's cost of offering community health education and outreach services
- Medical education, the net cost to the organization of teaching and education for health professionals
- Subsidized health services, the organization's cost of providing specialized or free health services to the community
- Research, usually limited to an academic medical center
- Cash and in-kind donations, reportable when the organization donates cash, goods, or services for community services

RHMC adopted this reporting practice several years ago because of its highly structured definitions. It affords a defensible reporting mechanism and a framework for year-to-year comparison. The administration uses this report in an effort to understand and budget for community service benefits.

It is important for a tax-exempt organization to be clear, concise, and complete in describing tax-exempt achievements because the description is likely to be reviewed by community and noncommunity members interested in the sources and uses of the organization's funds.

There are some specific rules regarding public access to the IRS 990. The document is available through the IRS or through the tax-exempt organization to anyone requesting public inspection or a copy. If requested through the organization, all parts of the return and all required schedules and attachments— other than the schedule of contributors to the organization—must be made available during regular business hours at the organization's principal business office and at each of its regional or district offices having three or more employees (Section M. Public Inspection of Completed Exempt Organization Returns and Approved Exemption Applications, Returns for Organizations Exempt from Income Tax Under Section 501(c)(3) of the Internal Revenue Code, Department of Treasury, Internal Revenue Service, General Instructions for Form 990 and Form 9990-EZ). Failure of the organization to properly respond to requests will result in a significant fine.

The not-for-profit 990 tax return has one particular piece of information that is often scrutinized by certain segments of the public more than any other. Schedule A of the 990 requires the organization to report the names, occupations, and salaries of the five highest-paid employees who are not officers of the corporation. On another page, the salaries of any paid officers of the corporation are reported. Therefore salaries of the organization's top officials are likely to appear on one or the other page. Additionally, compensation of the five highest-paid independent contractors for professional services is required on Schedule A. The organization's auditors, lawyers, and consultants often dominate these lines. Many local newspapers around the country have regular features reporting these wages and contract services at not-for-profit corporations.

Thus the IRS 990 report has many uses, both for the organization and for the public. As with any tax return, it is imperative to make the required information timely and accurate, following the rules and regulations set down by the government. In the case of the 990, it is also important to understand the potential implications of the need to report the salaries of the highest-paid employees and service providers. The RHMC finance staff and managers responsible for preparing and submitting these tax returns are aware of the rules for reporting and filling requests for information. In fact, they use outside tax experts to review their preparation each year before the filing date to ensure that they have made no errors. This also attests that they have complied with any new rules effective with the tax year in question.

CHAPTER TWELVE

DECEMBER

Self-doubt dominates Sam's dreams. He is worried. He is trying to move along a clearly marked road, his destination shining in the distance. But he is mired in mud, unable to make any progress. And he does not know why.

"Come on, come on, let's go," he tells himself. "I can do this. I can get there! What do I need to do to break out of this rut and get going?"

Just then a booming voice echoes through his thoughts: "And just where is it you think you're going?" the Voice asks.

"Whaddya mean, where am I going?" the incredulous Sam replies. "Obviously, I'm heading out there. It's my destination, my goal."

Now it's the Voice's turn to act incredulous. "Oh really, Sam? And just what does that destination represent to you?"

"Huh?"

"Come on, Sam, don't be so obtuse. You can see the beacon out there on the horizon, and you can even see what looks like a path. But if you look closer, you'll notice that there are some gaps along that paved road. In fact, you're standing in one of those gaps right now, a patch of mud so deep it'll take you quite a bit of hard thinking to get out of it."

"Well, I still don't know what you're talking about. Me, obtuse? I don't think so. Never was, never will be."

"Oh, really?" says the Voice. "If you're so smart, then you tell me where you're heading, and why."

"Well, of course I know where I'm heading. Out there is stability, for me and this crazy industry I'm in. We're going through some pretty unstable times at the moment in the financing of health care. There are a lot of these reimbursement cutbacks destabilizing delivery of patient care. There's also a big problem for many families that stand to lose their take-home pay if someone is laid off because of these cutbacks. So yeah, I'm worried. Wouldn't you be?"

"Now that you ask, yeah, I guess I would be. But anyway, now that you've been able to pinpoint the problem, the next question is, What are you going to do to work out a solution so that you can begin the move forward again?"

"Oh, man, you're one big pain. Questions, questions. I answer one, but is it good enough for you? No! Right away you hit me with another big one. I'll tell you, no rest for the weary."

"Hey, hey, nice try, but I can see right through you. Stop avoiding the question. What are you going to do about the financial instability in the industry?"

"Me? Why me? Why do I have to be the one to do anything about the financial instability in the industry? Who am I? I'm no politician. I can't make the managed care

*companies pay providers any more money. I can't make the feds increase their reimburse-
ments to the industry to reflect an appropriate return on investment. Not only do they
think we already make too much money, they claim they really don't have the money
to fully fund the industry even if they want to. Their funding source is eventually going
broke. Also, politicians always take the expedient way out. They don't lead; they react.
They're afraid to alienate any constituency that votes, so they refuse to make a decision
that would put the right kind of incentive in place, that would begin to minimize
Medicare trust fund disbursements."*

"Oh, really? Tell me more."

*"Well, it doesn't seem like anybody's dealing with the conflict between patients
who are demanding more services and payors who are demanding less payment. The
patients want to get better but want someone else to pay. The payors want to limit benefits so they don't have to pay. They need to raise their premiums to produce a bottom-
line margin for their own health plans or insurance companies, but until recently they've
been stymied. After all, the employers feel like they've maxed out on medical insurance
premiums," is Sam's stream-of-consciousness reply.*

"And your point is?"

*"We need to rationalize the financing of care. We need someone to make the hard
decisions. If there's too much capacity in the health care delivery system, contributing to
too much fixed cost, someone needs the authority to close it down. If too many providers
are in a certain geographical area, a facilitectomy needs to be performed! If there aren't
enough facilities in certain areas, like rural settings, then a facility graft should be made."*

*"Come on, Sam, grow up," says the Voice. "You know a proposal of that kind is a
nonstarter. First, no politician is going to take you up on it; it's political suicide. Second,
in some cases, it's been tried. Some of what you suggest is in the hands of state-run
certificate-of-need boards. Third, it sounds like another government boondoggle, letting
an authority make a decision that's better left to the free market."*

*"Blah, blah, blah. Hey, Voice, you sound just like every one else who puts up obstacles
because it's easier to maintain a bad status quo than to work out a better future. What
you just said is nonsense. Most certificate-of-need boards were disbanded by their states
because of ineffectiveness, and they didn't have the authority to delete facilities. They
could only decide whether or not to add health care facilities and services, and usually
only within certain provider types, which sure made for severe unfairness. They might
have to approve addition of an MRI service for a hospital, but they might not be able to
stop a physician's office from adding one. Pretty dopey stuff. So it's certainly a bad
model to use.*

*"As far as your comment about government boondoggles and letting the free mar-
ket prevail," Sam huffs onward, "that's problematic. This country has over forty million
underinsured or uninsured citizens, which is about 15 percent of the population. Who's
speaking for them? Certainly not the free-market thinkers. And what about the population that's aging? Right now, Medicare covers only one hundred skilled nursing home
days, and in many cases that leaves a string of poor, uninsured older people with very
few options. Medicaid has become the payor of last resort—and it's already government
funding. If we leave government to always be the final payor of services, then maybe we
need to have it participate in the initial discussion of a solution."*

*"Sam, Sam, Sam. Boy, sometimes you're such a bleeding heart. How can govern-
ment be the solution when it's so often the problem? Don't you remember when the*

president tried to do this in 1993 and 1994? It failed miserably. Nobody wanted it. Health planning was set back for years because of it."

"Aha," Sam thinks, out of hearing of the Voice inside his head. "I've got him now."

"Oh, yeah?" he retorts smartly. "Well, that's where you're wrong, buster. The 1993 initiative failed for three reasons. One, the process was handled very badly. The lesson learned was to be less arrogant and get more constituencies involved. Second, the opposition mounted a brilliant campaign. The people responsible for providing commercial health insurance had a heavy self-interest in seeing the proposals defeated. They convinced a number of legislators through scare advertising that government-run health care would be as inefficient as the post office. They also convinced many people that there were no problems in health care finance. Their motto was 'If it ain't broke, don't fix it.' But you and I know it's broke, structurally and financially. Third, the proponents were ahead of their time. It was obvious to many of us in the industry that there was a health care-financing problem already in the early 1990s, but it wasn't obvious to the legislators."

"So what, Sam? That's still a lot of rehash. Anyway, this is getting tiresome. You're living in the past. I don't see any of that mud loosening up. I still don't see you moving ahead. You seem to have analyzed a lot of the problem. You still haven't told me what feasible ideas you have to help solve the financing instability problem, and when— or if—you propose to present them."

"OK, already. Maybe there are a few things I can do. I'm nothing but a small cog in a small wheel, but at the moment, what I can do is continue doing the best job possible for RHMC. That means continuing to maximize the revenues, staying within all the laws, and helping the clinical and nonclinical department managers contain their costs through assistance with reporting and benchmarking, so we can maintain management accountability.

"But the other thing I can do is help get out the message about health care financial management and health care financing. They're the two sides of the same coin. It's a fact that you can't be the best health care financial manager without having a solid understanding of health care financing issues. And if you have a truly good understanding of the financing issues, it's hard to ignore them and try to improve it because of the significant impact they have on each facility's bottom line."

"So what are you going to do?"

"I suppose I could write a book that blends theory with practice, anecdote with history, and narrative with exposition. It should be something that helps in understanding the day-to-day functioning of health care managers and their staff. The real efforts it takes to keep a health care organization running as smoothly as possible in this difficult day and age. My hope would be that it allows readers to gain understanding, and that as a result one reader, or a bunch of them, can take the next steps to improve financing of the health care delivery system in the future. None of us is going to solve this alone. It will take a concerted effort by a strong group committed to an overall solution, not just Medicare and Medicaid. Everything and everyone."

With that, Sam is startled out of his dream. As he regains consciousness, he feels his sore feet loosen up as he jumps out of bed to get to his word processor.

December. Thanksgiving gone. Christmas and New Year's Day to come once
again, and quickly. The air is brisk as it skims across the Great Plains and
the Canadian frontier, heading east to a rendezvous with the denizens of northern Illinois. The winter coats are out, and the first dusting of snow has already
been felt in the region. The winter doldrums are beginning to set in.

Getting Ready for Year-End Reporting . . . Again

Come early December, the finance staff are engaged in the routine business of
preparing the November financial statement and taking the first steps in getting
ready for year-end reporting. During the November closing of the books, the staff
take extra time to analyze and evaluate the balance sheet and income statement
accounts. They are searching for unexplainable variance.

Any variance has to be understood and appropriately adjusted before the
close of the year, and it is always better to make these adjustments in November
rather than December. December adjustments are more obvious to the primary
readers of the financial statements—the CEO and the board—because they have
become conditioned to inquire about significant December line item changes. It
is best to have no adjustments made by the auditors, but it is also preferable to
have no major internal adjustments in December, if they can be avoided. It's
much better to make the adjustment in November.

Open Heart Surgery Pro Forma

Meanwhile, RHMC administration has continued to analyze the future of the organization. The administrators have determined that the time has come to fill a
major hole in product offerings. As a medium-sized community hospital, RHMC
does not perform cardiovascular (open heart) surgery. When this procedure was
first developed in the 1960s, it was performed only by surgeons at major academic (teaching) medical centers that had been involved in the initial trials or by
surgeons who had subsequently trained or assisted with the original ones.

Over the years, many surgeons have been trained on this procedure. In addition, the steps required to perform these procedures have become well known,
and in the 1980s some community hospitals began offering CV surgery. The mor-
tality rate at many a hospital was now equivalent to that at the teaching hospitals,
which encouraged some other community hospitals to offer the service. In the
late 1990s, it was important, in a competitive service area, for some community

hospitals to provide this service to its patients. It indicated to patients and their physicians that the organization practiced serious medicine, surpassing other community hospitals that did not offer the service, and placing one's organization on par with some academic programs.

RHMC administration decided it was time to attempt to implement one of the main tactics in its strategic plan. They knew that to continue to compete for patients in the core and secondary service areas, they must develop a cardiac surgery program. Heart disease is and has been the number one killer of Americans for many years. Heart disease, which leads to death, also may occasion the need for significant inpatient and outpatient services. For RHMC to access more of these patients for treatment, an open heart surgery program was required.

To determine the financial implications of such a program, the finance division was asked to develop a financial pro forma. Unlike the pro forma developed for the MRI that we saw in Chapter One, which was relative easy because it involved only one department (radiology) and involved only one set of volume assumptions, the open heart surgery program involves many more departments and personnel. This creates a number of additional variables, thus increasing the complexity of the analysis, which increases to some extent the risk that assumptions are unsound.

Development of Volume and Revenue

The first step in developing an open heart surgery pro forma, as with almost every other pro forma, is to determine the volume of services that can be provided. In this case, there are two prevalent procedure types. A coronary artery bypass graft (CABG, often pronounced "cabbage") is generally the procedure referred to when people talk about open heart surgery. Percutaneous transluminal coronary angioplasty (PTCA) is a procedure that cleans out plaque that has formed on the vessels leading to the heart, also through invasive surgery.

Tables 12.1 and 12.2 show the detailed and summary volume projections, which are based on usage rate within the organization's service area as well as the actual volume of cardiac catheterization procedures currently performed at RHMC. The best way to initially determine if they can achieve a CABG volume of two hundred per year (a number generally agreed to be a minimum for competence in the industry) is to review the current volume that it is generating. After that review, the medical center should look at volume in the surrounding community. Thus, the medical center's plan is to convert 100 percent of its current catheterization patients who have been transferred to other facilities into its own CABG patients. This, however, gives only 120 potential patients a year. So administration then reviewed the patient origin data of all CABG patients within its surrounding

TABLE 12.1. RHMC CARDIAC SURGERY PROGRAM, PROJECTED CARDIAC PROCEDURES, GROSS REVENUES AND NET REIMBURSEMENT, YEARS 1–5.

DRG No.	Projected Procedures	Year 1	Year 2
103 Heart transplant		0	0
104 Cardiac valve proc w/cardiac cath		7	7
105 Cardiac valve proc w/o cardiac cath		8	8
106 Coronary bypass w/cardiac cath		30	55
107 Coronary bypass w/o cardiac cath		30	55
108 Other cardiothoracic procedures		0	4
110 Major cardiovascular procs w/cardiac cath		0	14
111 Major cardiovascular procs w/o cardiac cath		0	4
112 Percutaneous cardiovascular procedures		85	100
116 Other perm cardiac pacemakers implant or PTCA w/ stent		0	0
Total cardiac procedures		160	247
Total CABG and valve procedures		75	125
Total PTCAs		85	100
Total other procedures		0	22
Total cardiac procedures		160	247

DRG No.	Unit Gross and Net Revenue by DRG	Year 1	Year 2
103 Heart transplant		0	0
104 Cardiac valve proc w/cardiac cath		80,000	80,000
105 Cardiac valve proc w/o cardiac cath		74,000	74,000
106 Coronary bypass w/cardiac cath		74,000	74,000
107 Coronary bypass w/o cardiac cath		65,000	65,000
108 Other cardiothoracic procedures		65,000	65,000
110 Major cardiovascular procs w/cardiac cath		67,000	67,000
111 Major cardiovascular procs w/o cardiac cath		67,000	67,000
112 Percutaneous cardiovascular procedures		33,000	33,000
116 Other perm cardiac pacemakers implant or PTCA w/ stent		33,000	33,000

DRG No.	Total Gross and Net Revenue by DRG	Year 1	Year 2
103 Heart transplant		0	0
104 Cardiac valve proc w/cardiac cath		560,000	560,000
105 Cardiac valve proc w/o cardiac cath		592,000	592,000
106 Coronary bypass w/cardiac cath		2,220,000	4,070,000
107 Coronary bypass w/o cardiac cath		1,950,000	3,575,000
108 Other cardiothoracic procedures		0	260,000
110 Major cardiovascular procs w/cardiac cath		0	938,000
111 Major cardiovascular procs w/o cardiac cath		0	268,000
112 Percutaneous cardiovascular procedures		2,805,000	3,300,000
116 Other perm cardiac pacemakers implant or PTCA w/stent		0	0
Total cardiac procedures		8,127,000	13,563,000
Total CABG and valve procedures		5,322,000	8,797,000
Total PTCAs		2,805,000	3,300,000
Total other procedures		0	1,466,000
Total cardiac procedures		8,127,000	13,563,000

Payor Mix		DRG no. 106	
Blue Cross		2	1.57%
HMO		23	18.11%
HMO Sen		28	22.05%
Medicare		55	43.31%
Medicaid		2	1.57%
PPO		17	13.39%
Total		127	100.00%

Year 3	Year 4	Year 5
0	0	0
20	20	20
20	20	20
80	80	80
80	80	80
4	4	4
14	14	14
4	4	4
100	100	100
0	0	0
322	322	322
200	200	200
100	100	100
22	22	22
322	322	322

Year 3	Year 4	Medicare Year 5	Contractual Reimburse	Percentage
0	0	0	0	
80,000	80,000	80,000	31,823	60.22%
74,000	74,000	74,000	24,345	67.10%
74,000	74,000	74,000	24,156	67.36%
65,000	65,000	65,000	17,687	72.79%
65,000	65,000	65,000	17,687	72.79%
67,000	67,000	67,000	18,080	73.01%
67,000	67,000	67,000	18,080	73.01%
33,000	33,000	33,000	9,106	72.41%
33,000	33,000	33,000	10,498	68.19%

Year 3	Year 4	Managed Care Year 5	Contractual Reimburse	Percentage
0	0	0		
1,600,000	1,600,000	1,600,000	21,824	72.72%
1,480,000	1,480,000	1,480,000	17,526	76.32%
5,920,000	5,920,000	5,920,000	20,782	71.92%
5,200,000	5,200,000	5,200,000	17,795	72.62%
260,000	260,000	260,000		
938,000	938,000	938,000		
268,000	268,000	268,000		
3,300,000	3,300,000	3,300,000	7,660	76.79%
0	0	0		
18,966,000	18,966,000	18,966,000		
14,200,000	14,200,000	14,200,000		
3,300,000	3,300,000	3,300,000		
1,466,000	1,466,000	1,466,000		
18,966,000	18,966,000	18,966,000		

DRG no. 107	
2	2.56%
50	64.10%
14	17.95%
4	5.13%
2	2.56%
6	7.69%
78	100.00%

TABLE 12.2. RHMC CARDIAC SURGERY PROGRAM, SUMMARY OF ASSUMPTIONS, DECEMBER 2001.

Capital Costs

Equipment
Renovations
   Total capital costs

	Year 1	Year 2
Volumes		
CABG and valve procedures	75	125
PTCA and other valve procedures	85	122
Total volumes	160	247
Total volumes per day at 260	0.62	0.95
Charge per test		
CABG and valve procedures	70,960	70,376
PTCA and other valve procedures	33,000	39,066
Gross revenues		
CABG and valve procedures	5,322,000	8,797,000
PTCA and other valve procedures	2,805,000	4,766,000
Total revenues	$8,127,000	$13,563,000
Payor mix		
Medicare	40.00%	40.00%
Managed care	55.00%	55.00%
All other	5.00%	5.00%
Total payor mix	100.00%	100.00%
Contractual allowances		
CABG and valve procedures		
Medicare	72.80%	72.80%
Managed care	72.60%	72.60%
All other	20.00%	20.00%
PTCA and other valve procedures		
Medicare	72.00%	72.00%
Managed care	77.00%	77.00%
All other	20.00%	20.00%

Notes: Volume and service mix are based on research from current RHMC cath lab volumes and external sources.

Payor mix is based on Smith Memorial Hospital actual data for DRGs 106 and 107.

Gross revenue is based on full-year operations for DRGs 106 and 107. All other DRGs are estimated from 106 and 107.

Contractual allowances are based on Medicare and managed care approximate rates from other regional hospitals.

Gross charges are projected to increase at 0 percent per year.

Variable expenses are projected to increase by an inflationary rate of 5 percent per year.

Equipment is depreciated over eight years.

Spinoff revenues and expenses are provided at a 5 percent increase over the 2000 actual cardiovascular service line.

			CV Program
			$1,092,553
			$ 5,000
			$1,097,553
Year 3	Year 4	Year 5	Total
200	200	200	800
122	122	122	573
322	322	322	1373
1.24	1.24	1.24	1.06
71,000	71,000	71,000	
39,066	39,066	39,066	
14,200,000	14,200,000	14,200,000	56,719,000
4,766,000	4,766,000	4,766,000	21,869,000
$18,966,000	$18,966,000	$18,966,000	78,588,000
40.00%	40.00%	40.00%	
55.00%	55.00%	55.00%	
5.00%	5.00%	5.00%	
100.00%	100.00%	100.00%	
72.80%	72.80%	72.80%	
72.60%	72.60%	72.60%	
20.00%	20.00%	20.00%	
72.00%	72.00%	72.00%	
77.00%	77.00%	77.00%	
20.00%	20.00%	20.00%	

community, which is available from a state database, to determine which other hospital's volume it could divert. This is called a market-based solution.

After determining the volumes, the financial analyst estimates the gross revenues chargeable for the service based on the current market rate. In addition to gross revenue, RHMC needs to estimate the mix of payors that will represent the CABG and PTCA patients. It does this on the basis of surveys of area hospitals willing to share such data. It can also validate these data by reviewing the payor mix of its catheterization patients. RHMC needs to perform this estimate to project its net revenue, which depends on the contractual rates that can be negotiated with third-party managed care payors as well as acceptance of the rates paid by Medicare and Medicaid for these services. Finally, to complete net revenue projections, the medical center must estimate contractual rates. This also uses information from other area hospitals, and in some cases a best guess from the medical center's managed care negotiator.

The Importance of Financial Analyst Objectivity. To reiterate a comment from the pro forma development in Chapter One, the absolute toughest assumption in any pro forma is volume projection. However, the second toughest is often the net revenue rate assumptions because of the significant possibility of being too optimistic.

It is important to be conservative when estimating both volume and net revenue. In this industry, as well as most others, optimistic pro forma projection has often given way to greenlighting a project that subsequently fails because of problems within these two areas. Nobody, particularly the financial analyst, wants a finger pointed because of overly optimistic projections. The finance pro forma developer must use great judgment in critically evaluating the numbers presented from the operations representative. Keep in mind that the latter individual has a bias toward getting a project approved, since this affords growth in that area of responsibility.

The finance representative should never have such a bias. She must remain independent and objective at all times. If the pro forma shows a very good internal rate of return, then it is obvious to all reviewers that the project will be approved on its merits. Do not help the result by improving these critical pro forma elements just because it seems like a good project to do, or because the operations representative is pushing to do so. Also, the pro forma finance representative developer should not become a champion of the project. That is the role of the operations or business development representative. Always stay objective.

Development of Expenses. After completing the volume assumptions, projection of expenses can begin. Like revenues, expenses are both fixed and dependent on the volume projection. Because most project expenses are variable (that is, they vary with volume), it is important to have the volume assumption completed before an estimate of staffing and supplies can begin. Table 12.3 is the CV surgery projected income statement (pro forma). In addition to its summary of gross and net revenues, it shows expenses by specific category.

Staffing Expenses. A key expense assumption is estimating the number and type of staff required to perform the services. In the case of the open heart surgery program, several types of employee required: specialized operating room nurses and technicians; intensive care unit nurses; additional cardiac catheterization nurses and technicians; and cardiology, respiratory therapy, and cardiac rehabilitation technicians. In this case, RHMC estimates it needs a total of 16.7 additional FTEs in the first year of the program, rising to 23.5 FTEs in the fifth year.

Fringe Benefits. RHMC is consistent in its use of a 30 percent fringe benefit rate on all of pro formas (the derivation of this rate was explained in detail in Chapter One), and in this pro forma the center continues to do so.

Variable Start-Up Staffing Expense. As with most new programs, there are expenses incurred to start up before any revenue is generated. These start-up costs are usually related to training the new program staff, whether new employees from the outside or retraining existing staff from other departments. This training is obviously important because the staff must be ready to perform competently on the day that the service opens to the public.

In the case of the open heart surgery program, training is extensive for all levels of staff involved. Most new staff receive eight weeks of intensive training, both in the classroom and on the job, at other hospitals that are already performing the service. In addition, currently employed staff receive the necessary training to treat and service new patients. The cost of their training, as well as the cost of replacement staff paid while others are training outside the unit, is included in start-up cost.

Variable Expenses. To determine variable expenses for the new service, which involves several hospital departments, it is essential to be able to estimate two items with the greatest possible precision. They are the volume (units of service) of the new services to be rendered (which we know is already available because of the work performed to determine revenue) and the cost per unit of service.

Determining the cost per unit of service does not have to be an onerous task. If the organization has developed a cost accounting system, then it should not be difficult to use the cost already established for each individual service code

TABLE 12.3. RHMC CARDIAC SURGERY PROGRAM, INCOME STATEMENT PRO FORMA, DECEMBER 2001.

	Year 1	Year 2
Revenues		
Gross revenues	$8,127,000	$13,563,000
Less contractual allowances	5,751,656	9,600,616
Net revenue before spinoff	2,375,344	3,962,384
Marginal spinoff revenue	207,500	311,250
Total net revenues	2,582,844	4,273,634
Expenses		
Staffing	1,008,296	1,156,089
Fringes at 30%	302,489	346,827
Total staffing and benefits	1,310,785	1,502,916
Variable startup staffing costs	131,532	
Variable expenses		
Laboratory	75,337	120,587
Radiology	31,912	52,027
Pharmacy and IVs	51,293	82,539
Other ancillaries	19,814	31,725
Supplies, RHMC direct variable	683,519	1,004,343
Marginal spinoff cost	112,500	168,750
Total variable expenses	974,375	1,459,970
Fixed expenses		
Franchise fee—teaching hospital	250,000	175,000
Contract labor, perfusionists	18,750	31,250
MD house coverage	327,840	340,954
Medical director fee	25,000	25,000
Education	44,480	13,480
Maintenance costs	64,154	64,154
Marketing	250,000	200,000
Equipment depreciation	140,319	140,319
Building renovation depreciation	0	625
Total nonstaffing expenses	1,120,543	990,782
Total expenses	3,537,235	3,953,668
Contribution to overhead	($ 954,391)	$ 319,967
Internal rate of return		

Year 3	Year 4	Year 5	Total
$18,966,000	$18,966,000	$18,966,000	$78,588,000
13,385,201	13,385,201	13,385,201	55,507,874
5,580,799	5,580,799	5,580,799	23,080,126
415,000	415,000	415,000	1,763,750
5,995,799	5,995,799	5,995,799	24,843,876
1,285,934	1,336,223	1,388,524	$ 6,175,066
385,780	400,867	416,557	$ 1,852,520
1,671,714	1,737,090	1,805,081	$ 8,027,586
174,419	174,419	174,419	$719,182
78,924	78,924	78,924	$320,711
121,082	121,082	121,082	$497,078
45,928	45,928	45,928	$189,322
1,627,793	1,627,793	1,627,793	$ 6,571,240
225,000	225,000	225,000	$956,250
2,273,146	2,273,146	2,273,146	$ 9,253,783
100,000	100,000	100,000	$725,000
50,000	50,000	50,000	$200,000
354,592	368,775	383,526	$ 1,775,687
25,000	25,000	25,000	$125,000
13,480	13,480	13,480	$98,400
64,154	64,154	64,154	$320,770
100,000	100,000	100,000	$750,000
140,319	140,319	140,319	$701,596
625	625	625	$2,500
848,170	862,354	877,105	$ 4,698,953
4,793,030	4,872,590	4,955,332	21,980,322
$ 1,202,769	$ 1,123,209	$ 1,040,467	$ 2,732,022
			28.08%

(procedure code). These procedure code costs should then be applied against the projected volume to determine the variable expenses of the new service. If the organization has not developed a cost accounting system, it can still use the simple, though less-sophisticated, method of the ratio of cost to charges, available to all health care organizations that file a Medicare cost report. The RCC was reviewed in detail in Chapter Four.

Fixed Expenses. The fixed expenses are generally specific to the program, and of course, by definition, they do not vary with volume. In this case, there are three key fixed expenses:

1. A franchise fee
2. A cost for twenty-four-hour physician coverage of the cardiology patients in the hospital
3. Marketing costs

Regarding the first fixed expense, because RHMC is a community hospital and does not have prior experience or expertise in open heart surgery, it has decided to affiliate with a respected academic medical center just on the fringe of the RHMC service area, to make the requisite experience and expertise available. The academic medical center decided to charge RHMC a franchise fee for its services, including onsite and offsite training of RHMC staff, any and all required technical assistance, and use of its CV surgeons.

Second, again because RHMC is itself not a teaching hospital, it does not have interns and residents to cover inpatients through the day and night. The RHMC administration decided that to promote and market its new service to primary care and specialist physicians (especially cardiologists) in its service area and beyond, it must offer this twenty-four-hour onsite coverage by hiring its own set of physicians to cover the inpatients. This coverage allows referring cardiologists to increase their comfort level that their patients have adequate care available, especially at night.

As for marketing costs, we see in the projected income statement that this program should earn net revenues of almost $25 million over the first five-year period. The administration has determined that it is worth $750,000 over that same time period to bring this new program to the attention of its prospective customers, primarily the referring physicians (primary care physicians and area cardiologists). There will be a small amount of marketing directed to the consumer, but this is considered only a secondary consideration because most patients in the early years of the twenty-first century will still be unable to self-refer for nonprimary services.

Financial Conclusion: Open Heart Surgery Program

The contribution margin, or contribution to overhead, over the five-year period is a positive $2,732,022, including depreciation charges. On its face, this appears to be a good return. But this does not tell the whole story. As was explained in Chapter One, many health care organizations use either the net present value calculation or the internal rate of return. RHMC prefers the percentage methodology inherent in the internal rate of return. The 28.08 percent internal rate of return on initial investment for the open heart surgery program justifies the administration in taking this program and its $1,092,553 initial investment to the December finance committee and the board of directors.

It is important to note that the finance division did more than just present the models in Tables 12.1, 12.2, and 12.3. Staff also built sensitivity models that assign more optimistic and more pessimistic volumes to assess the impact of other possible scenarios. The finance committee requires this sensitivity because members are aware that a pro forma is only as good as the volume assumptions made.

December Finance Committee Special Agenda Items

In addition to the CV surgery program that the administration presents in December to the finance committee and in the regularly scheduled monthly financial statements and accounts receivable report, there are two more routine reports to be presented: a review of the organization's insurance coverage, and a request for approval of the external auditors and their fees for the following year.

Review Malpractice Insurance Coverage

An important feature and function of RHMC's cost structure and risk management program, professional liability insurance (or malpractice insurance, as it is commonly known) is reviewed with the finance committee once a year. The committee is concerned about the level of coverage as well as the premium costs. Exhibit 12.1 shows the report presented to the committee. As with most insurance, the cost of coverage decreases on each layer above the primary or first layer because there is less chance for a claim being made against these additional layers. RHMC was fortunate to have experienced a reduction of premiums in 1998 and 1999 as a result of a small number of claims being filed. In addition, there were even fewer payments, or losses, against claims made. Still, it is incumbent on the organization to guard itself against potential claims of poor treatment or poor outcomes. It is within the fiduciary responsibility of the finance committee members

EXHIBIT 12.1. RHMC PROFESSIONAL LIABILITY SELF-INSURANCE STATUS PREMIUM UPDATE, DECEMBER 2001.

RHMC's self-insurance administrator has estimated the premiums required to maintain our coverage for professional liability over the period through December 2002. The coverage will be identical in amount and structure to that which was in effect in 2001. An optional third layer of excess coverage was added effective January 1, 1999.

	Per-Occurrence Limit	Aggregate Limit	Funding
First layer	$ 1,000,000	None	Primary trust
Second layer	$10,000,000	$20,000,000	Excess trust
Third layer	$10,000,000	$10,000,000	Excess coverage

The schedule below indicates the premiums that have been paid for the policy years beginning in 1997:

	1998	1999	2000	2001	2002
First layer	$450,000	$400,000	$600,000	$ 650,000	$ 680,000
Second layer	250,000	250,000	280,000	300,000	310,000
Third layer	—	100,000	95,000	90,000	90,000
Total	$700,000	$750,000	$975,000	$1,040,000	$1,080,000
Budget	$900,000	$800,000	$900,000	$1,000,000	$1,100,000

to be apprised of and understand the significance of the level of malpractice coverage. They are comfortable with the current level and understand the need to pay self-insurance premiums.

Review and Approve Auditors and Their Fees for the Current Year

The final action that is taken by the finance committee this year is approval of the auditors, along with their proposed fees. The audit partner and the manager of the CPA firm that RHMC has been using for a number of years have been invited to present a proposal indicating the scope of the audit, a high-level discussion of how they plan to conduct the audit, and the various responsibilities of the client. They present the arrangement letter spelling out, in detail, the responsibilities of both the audit firm and RHMC. It also spells out any additional services that the organization has commissioned the auditors to perform and the fees for those services. The arrangement letters are standard and have evolved over time as the auditors defended themselves and their firms in court, particularly in cases where the auditor's client went bankrupt, leaving a line of creditors looking for some recourse.

The audit partner spends some time pointing out current items of interest in the industry (hot topics!) and commenting on any topics the finance committee members might want to know more about. The finance committee at RHMC is charged with selecting an audit firm each year. It is important for the members to feel comfortable with their choice because the auditors are passing judgment on the quality of the work of the finance managers. They want a professional and unbiased opinion of the financial statements and of the financial managers and staff. It is an important decision that is made easier if an ongoing relationship has been established over the years.

The committee reviews the audit fees for consistency. The members are interested in any rate of increase over the prior year. In addition, the committee periodically requests that management perform a comparison of pricing with other audit firms in the region to determine if they are being charged more than their peers. Although the committee values a long-standing relationship, members do not want to overpay for it. Thus it is in the best interest of the current audit firm to stay competitive because they know it will be checked.

Finance Committee Annual Achievements

The December finance committee meeting concludes its members' work for the year. They have had a productive year, reviewing management's work across most aspects of health care financial management. In doing so, they touched on certain topics:

- Monthly financial statement reporting and analysis, particularly the variances between actual results and approved budget
- Special review regarding the ongoing payment changes wrought by Medicare and Medicaid through the BBA, subsequent give-back provisions of the BBRA and BIPA, and reductions continuing to be evident with managed care plans
- Accounts receivable issues and analysis
- Bond debt status
- Health and malpractice insurance analysis
- Approval of the auditors, their fees, and the annual audit and auditors' management letter
- Pension status and actuary's report
- Materials management analysis
- Information systems plans, particularly concerning HIPAA implementation and the new systems needed by the organization
- Approval of the five-year strategic financial plan linked to the organization's strategic plan early in the year
- Approval of the annual budget for the coming year

Throughout the year, as part of their monthly review of the financial statements, they also were apprised of the income earned on investments. The negative market conditions of the previous two years have not been pleasant for the committee members. However, their review was cursory because a separate investment committee was primarily involved with investment opportunities and results. Although investment policies and practices are beyond the scope of this book, in the second half of the 1990s all of this was extremely important in producing overall positive results for health care organizations, especially with significant reductions in reimbursement by all the major payors. Still, RHMC managed to avoid the negative investment results of 2000 and 2001 that had proven so onerous to other organizations, thanks to some judicious market timing and "going to cash."

Although the committee is somewhat disappointed in the overall operating margin results, management's ongoing education of the members regarding payment reduction and ongoing concerns about cost management have given the members a better appreciation of the challenges confronting health care organizations. They are in a better position to assess the year just past and the years to follow. They are concerned about the financial integrity of the organization and worried about how to maintain and even improve the high level of patient care that currently exists. There have been discussions regarding the future of RHMC's financial position as well as that of the industry in general. It takes on a crystal ball feel, but it is a necessary step and a required management technique for future planning.

Looking into the Future of Health Care Finance

The future of health care financial management and health care financing is anyone's guess. It could take any of a hundred paths, twisting and winding, approaching forks in the road not currently evident to planners. Decisions could be made by government employees or politicians, seeking to save the Medicare trust fund for future beneficiaries, who may or may not achieve intended consequences. Decisions could also be made by the executives at managed care plans seeking to increase their profits at the expense of patients or providers by limiting their exposures on medical loss ratios. Decisions could also be made by employers around the country, some of whom have grown tired of subsidizing medical insurance for their employees.

Several of these paths could be taken simultaneously, as seems to be the case now, at the beginning of a new century. Or they could diverge. Clues abound everywhere about the possible futures of health care finance. There are comprehensive industry models as well as segment models. RHMC and its administration are concerned about the financial implications of future trends. They would be delighted to recognize any particular emerging trend and be one of the first to implement services that would improve revenue. They would also be amenable to applying any new ideas that produce efficiency without compromising patient care or patient satisfaction.

For this discussion, it is best to look at the trends for the industry as a whole, for the payors, and for the providers. Over the course of this book, we have seen many concepts used in financial and general operations. We have seen many theories turned into practice and used to maximize the clinical, operational, and financial outcomes for RHMC. It is time to do some crystal ball gazing and see how some of the current trends might reach into the future.

General Macro Health Care Trends

Two trends appear to be emerging faster and with more power (as they did at the time of the first edition of this book in 1999).

First, cutting-edge research and development in gene therapy has already produced some startlingly positive results in a few diseases, with the promise of landmark breakthrough in other diseases in the very near future.

Second, the growing value of drug therapy in curing or containing illness is already helping to produce some dramatic quality-of-life improvements in the lives of patients with certain diseases.

Here are some fascinating details regarding these two trends.

Genomic Medicine and Gene Therapy. Most likely, gene therapy will be the primary medical treatment of the twenty-first century and have a profound effect on delivery of medical care. The human genome is the set of genetic instructions carried within a single cell of an organism. Gene therapies will be the outgrowth of the Human Genome Project, funded by the federal government to find all human genes, and Celera Genomics, a private company that gave the government quite a bit of competition. In February 2001, scientists from the government and Celera, in a joint statement, announced they had located 95 percent of the sequencing of human genetic information with accuracy greater than 99 percent. Interestingly, the announcement also revealed that humans are 99.9 percent genetically identical (Olivier and others, 2001).

Additionally, according to an article in the *Chicago Tribune,* the most sweeping, near-term benefit of knowing our genes is likely to be a major improvement in health that could supersede the tremendous advances made by vaccines and antibiotics. The article quotes a physician as saying "even thought we like to think we're fairly sophisticated in medicine, we don't cure disease. We make it more bearable, or we prolong people's lives. Genomic medicine is different. It is the fact that you're getting at the root cause of the disease and you have rational new ways of treating it." In fact, another physician who is working on gene repair and gene therapy is quoted as saying "We can envision a hospital some day that is strictly a gene-therapy hospital" (Kotulak, 1999, p. 1).

Time magazine devoted forty-five pages of its special January 11, 1999, edition to genetics. Titled "The Future of Medicine: How Genetic Engineering Will Change Us in the Next Century," it offers in-depth coverage of the history of modern genetic research, the current climate, and some of the medical advances that should be available in the near future. Among the possible developments on the horizon:

- Replacing defective cells to generate healthy tissue in combating Alzheimer's disease, heart disease, and diabetes
- Developing fruits and vegetables to deliver drugs that stave off infectious diseases or treat various chronic conditions rather than relying on injection to do so
- Developing better vaccines to coax the body to churn out killer T-cells, which strike at offending microbes with great specificity
- Lengthening the tip of certain chromosomes that might control the aging process (if this is determined to be correct, it is theoretically possible to rejuvenate a part of any organ with a simple injection)

There are great social and ethical issues at work here, and much bioethical debate is currently under way. The private sector is heavily involved in its own human genome research, and some companies have already developed practical solutions to dealing with some diseases.

In a related development, President Bush is now urging Congress to pass legislation that would outlaw discrimination on the grounds of genetic testing. In his weekly radio address on June 23, 2001, the president said, "By better understanding the genetic codes in each human being, scientists may one day be able to cure and prevent many diseases. As with any other power, this knowledge of the codes of life has the potential to be abused."

Because new genetic research should make it possible to identify an individual's lifetime risk of cancer, heart attack, and other diseases, the average American is already worried that this information could be used to discriminate in hiring, promotion, or insurance. Employers and insurers could potentially save millions of dollars if they used predictive genetics to identify in advance, *and then reject,* applicants who are predisposed to develop chronic disease. Fear of discrimination could discourage people from seeking useful information about their genetic makeup.

In any event, the genie is out of the bottle. Rampant development of these therapies is likely to be the number one health care story in the next century.

Drug Therapy. Drug therapy is an extension of much of the gene therapy that was done throughout the 1990s. Wonder drugs that significantly improve the health of patients with specific conditions are beginning to come to market—with enormous price tags attached. Many of these new drugs will reduce a patient's pain or create a cure to long-standing illness. The wonder drugs continue to come to market, often with assistance from the same genetic research that is powering genomic medicine. The new science of pharmacogenetics marries the discoveries of the Human Genome Project to technologies like DNA chips and traditional medicine (Begley, 2001). This allows patients to use drugs that have been designed specifically for a rare disease that they may be carrying. This is a great advance for them, allowing them to live a longer and more productive life.

Still, there is a great up-front cost for these advances. In the case of personalized medicine, the big drug makers are unlikely to produce a big profit-generating drug if each one is individually tailored to specific patient needs. But as stated in the *Newsweek* article, "if pharmacogenetics comes through, a simple $500 test will decode your genome, so every doctor you consult can check whether your genes make you a good candidate for a particular therapy. And then, rather than making you sick, your genes will ride to the rescue" (Begley, 2001, p. 69).

Meanwhile, the hospital and physician side of the industry and the insurance companies will be tested in their resolve to use and reimburse these new therapies. Pharmaceutical expenses represent a high percentage of dollar increase in coming years. It is not expected to get better as efficacious miracle drugs make their way through the FDA's testing process and become available for prescription use. So providers and insurers are already gearing up for seemingly inevitable cost increases related to these new drug therapies. It remains to be seen if these high-cost drugs eventually lower the overall cost of health care throughout the nation.

National Health Care Expenditure Projection. In the first chapter of this book, it was shown that the United States spent more than $1.2 trillion on health care in 1999, the last year for which data were available. This accounted for 13.0 percent of the country's GDP. Yet in information published on the government's Website, it is estimated that health care spending will increase to $2.64 trillion, or 16.6 percent of the GDP, by the year 2010, an increase of more than 100 percent over an eleven-year period. This is a huge dollar increase, backed up by an enormous movement of additional funds being spent on the nation's sick care and well care.

According to the summary of the study shown in Table 12.4, the areas with the greatest expenditure increase between 1999 and 2010 are drugs (a whopping 267.5 percent) and other personal health care (231.6 percent). As was just recounted, the reasons for drug increases should be no surprise. A major part of the increase in other personal health care expenditures is related to alternative medicine, which has also been discussed previously.

Meanwhile, hospitals (84.3 percent) and nursing homes (103.8 percent) expect much smaller increases, in large part because the federal and state governments are continuing to ratchet down these institutional payments, and because of ongoing, tough, and tedious managed care negotiations. Perhaps the biggest surprise is that home health care (162.8 percent) is not hit harder. This is because the need for these services is projected to continue increasing greatly even while the unit payments are being severely reduced.

No matter how this pie is sliced, $2.6 trillion is a gigantic pile of money that is going to be paid to health care industry providers. In no way is this an industry in decline. Not only does the gross number increase, the GDP percentage does also. In the near future, this industry will continue to play a large part in the financial wealth of the nation, as it has always played the key role in its health.

Industry Payor Trends

Along with the general health care trends, it is important to concentrate on the trends playing out in the payor community.

Medicare. The major player in the payor community is Medicare. In its current form, it is the largest payor of health care services. As a government agency, it is subject to politics in a significant way. In 2001, the future of the Medicare program is once again being debated at the highest levels of government.

Prior to 2001, the last time the government attempted to do some heavy lifting over the future of Medicare was in 1998, when President Clinton appointed the National Bipartisan Commission on the Future of Medicare to debate and present a proposal. The commission met from early 1998 to March 1999, to determine how to keep the Medicare trust fund from going bankrupt in 2008.

Of major interest is what would happen to health care expenditures after the then-current projections were evaluated. Medicare has to share in the brunt of the expenses. The commission was charged with recommending changes to the current program. The members were concerned that between 2011 and 2030, seventy-seven million baby boomers will turn sixty-five, and there will be fewer

TABLE 12.4. NATIONAL HEALTH EXPENDITURE AMOUNTS, 1999 ACTUAL AND 2010 PROJECTED, SELECTED YEARS (IN MILLIONS OF DOLLARS).

	1999 Actual	2003 Projected	2007 Projected	2010 Projected	Percentage Change 2010 Projected Versus 1999 Actual
Payors					
Out-of-pocket payments	186.5	257.8	336.1	404.0	116.6
Third-party payments (insurance)	475.6	682.4	895.3	1,054.4	121.7
Medicare	213.6	276.6	330.2	441.4	106.6
Medicaid	187.6	252.2	350.5	446.0	137.7
Other government	147.3	197.4	274.3	291.6	98.0
Total	1,210.6	1,666.4	2,186.4	2,637.4	117.9
Providers					
Hospital care	390.9	504.8	626.7	720.5	84.3
Physician services	269.4	363.3	463.5	545.9	102.6
Dental services	56.0	74.3	93.2	108.9	94.5
Other professional services	37.9	54.3	73.5	89.5	136.1
Nursing home care	90.0	119.1	153.6	183.4	103.8
Home health care	33.1	51.4	71.2	87.0	162.8
Prescription drugs	99.6	175.8	272.4	366.0	267.5
Durable medical equipment	18.1	22.9	28.4	33.4	84.5
Other nondurable medical products	29.5	37.3	44.1	49.1	66.4
Other personal health care	33.2	50.8	79.0	110.1	231.6
Program administration, public and private	72.0	101.5	133.4	164.2	128.1
Government public health activities	41.1	58.3	80.5	100.4	144.3
Research and construction	39.8	52.6	66.9	79.0	98.5
Total	1,210.6	1,666.4	2,186.4	2,637.4	117.9
U.S. population	277.8	287.0	296.1	302.9	9.0
Per capita spending	4,357.8	5,806.3	7,384.0	8,707.2	99.8
Percentage change from 1999		33.2	69.4	99.8	

Sources: National Health Expenditures Projections (http://www.hcfa.gov/stats/NHE-Proj/tables/t01.htm); National Health Expenditures Projections (http://www.hcfa.gov/stats/NHE-Proj/tables/t02.htm); National Health Expenditures Projections (http://www.hcfa.gov/stats/NHE-Proj/tables/t03.htm).

workers per retiree to fund the Medicare program. So their goals for twenty-first century Medicare was for the program to be

1. Responsive to the needs of the beneficiaries
2. Cost-effective, for both the beneficiary and the taxpayer
3. Available to younger workers, who expect a financially viable program when they retire
4. Fair to providers (Medicare Commission, 1999)

Exhibit 12.2 is a summary of the proposed changes. Its cochairmen, Sen. John Breaux (D-La.) and Rep. William Thomas (R-Calif.), issued the proposal as a final draft on March 15, 1999. It recommends major changes in the method by which Medicare pays for services. Although there were some new features proposed by the chairmen and it was supported by a vote of ten to seven, it lacked the crucial eleven-vote supermajority needed to formally adopt the proposal and move it on to the Congress. In fact, President Clinton came out against the proposal just before the vote, praising the commission for its work but saying that "it falls short in several respects" and that he would develop his own plan (McGinley, 1999).

As we know from Chapter Four, as currently formulated Medicare pays providers, such as hospitals, physicians, nursing homes, and home health agencies, for services rendered under specific payment guidelines. Under the proposed bipartisan commission guidelines, Medicare would subsidize patients' purchase of health care coverage from managed care plans that bid to participate in the program. Called "premium support," this proposal is similar to the plan currently offered to federal employees under the Federal Employees Health Benefits Program (FEHBP). Medicare beneficiaries would be given a voucher worth a specific amount of money from which they can purchase a basic package of benefits. Any voucher dollars left over are used to increase benefits beyond the basic package; or the Medicare beneficiaries can pay extra, out-of-pocket premiums for additional coverage.

The commission's other major proposal was to include pharmacy benefits for specific sets of individuals or plans, as outlined in Exhibit 12.2. This proposal was extremely delicate, but because it does not endorse comprehensive pharmacy benefits, President Clinton rejected it. Half the commission was adamant that the drug benefit be included out of fairness because Medicare HMO beneficiaries currently receive drug benefits. But heavy lobbying by the pharmaceutical industry since the inception of Medicare has kept this benefit out of the hands of most Medicare beneficiaries (Lagnado, McGinley, and Tanouye, 1999). Still, legislative threats to impose the equivalent of price controls on the pharmaceutical industry allowed the commission to agree to this partial, yet rejected, concession.

The bipartisan commission's recommendations, had they been adopted, would have changed the Medicare program dramatically (including raising the age of eligibility from sixty-five to sixty-seven). Although federal employees currently use this premium support system, it is unclear how it would fare with Medicare recipients. In any event, this type of radical change was sure to create upheaval in delivering medical care to the elderly. There was no assurance that the change would have been positive or negative. HCFA actuaries released a report during the last week of February 1999 indicating that the premium support proposal should save at least $75 billion over a ten-year period.

Still, it was not clear that the proposal would save enough money to keep the Medicare program solvent through the year 2030. So why are we looking at a "rejected" program in this book? Because politics is a fickle field, and a bill rejected one year may well have a way of making it back in another year. In fact, in this case the election of George Bush to the presidency in 2001 has seen the bipartisan commission's proposal reemerge, under the leadership of Senator Breaux, who still very much believes in the features outlined in the proposal.

What has also changed is the financial climate. When the commission was initially debating the future of the Medicare program and the Medicare Part A trust fund, the fund appeared to be solvent only through 2008. What was not factored in was the significant positive impact of the 1997 BBA on the solvency of the Part A trust fund. In fact, the latest information available from the 2001 annual report of the board of trustees of the Federal Hospital Insurance trust fund shows that the Part A trust should remain solvent until the year 2029. This takes some pressure off the program.

Still, there are many possible paths and futures for health care financing. It could embrace interesting and alternative futures. These various proposals continue to make the future of health care financial management quite entertaining.

Managed Care. As we already saw in Figure 4.7, more than eighty million Americans, or 30.1 percent of the population, are enrolled in managed care programs. Most of these members are enrolled through their employers. Still, according to the latest government statistics, 14.5 percent of Medicare 1997 patients, or 5.6 million (14.5 percent times 37.66 million); and 54 percent of 1998 Medicaid patients, or 21.95 million (54 percent times 40.66 million), are enrolled in managed care programs where the program contracts directly with the HMO to pay the appropriate annual premium (National Center for Health Statistics, 2000).

Managed care emerged quickly in the 1990s to supersede the old indemnity health insurance polices that paid providers the charges that were billed to insurance companies. When the ultimate payors—the employers—tired of premiums rising at an ever-increasing level, they moved most of their plans to managed care. Throughout the 1990s, managed care plans controlled employers' premium

EXHIBIT 12.2.   NATIONAL BIPARTISAN COMMISSION ON THE FUTURE OF MEDICARE, SUMMARY OF BREAUX-THOMAS PROPOSAL, MAR. 15, 1999.

Medicare Board
The board would provide information to beneficiaries, negotiate with plans, compute payments to plans (including risk, geographic, and other adjustments), and compute beneficiaries' premiums (collected via Social Security system as with Part B premiums now). Board approval would be required for plan service areas and benefit package designs.

Benefits
The standard benefits package specified in law would consist of all services covered under the existing Medicare statute (Medicare-covered services). Plans could establish their own rules as to how the benefits would be provided. Board approval would be required for all benefit design offerings, and the board would allow variation only within a limited range as the risk adjusters were proven over time.

Prescription Drugs
Private plans.   All private plans would be required to offer a high option that included at least the standard benefits package plus coverage for prescription drugs. The minimum drug benefit for high-option plans would be based on an actuarial valuation, with standards and examples set by the board.

Low-income.   The proposal would immediately extend coverage of prescription drugs to qualifying beneficiaries under 135 percent of poverty under Medicaid with full federal funding of the additional cost. That coverage could be provided through high-option plans when the premium support system was implemented. (A special premium support schedule could be used to combine premium and drug subsidies for low-income beneficiaries.)

Fee-for-service.   The Health Care Financing Administration (HCFA) would be allowed to contract with or enter joint marketing arrangements with private insurers offering prescription drug benefits. That would allow a public-private high-option plan or plans, with HCFA providing coverage for Medicare-covered services and its private partner(s) providing coverage for drugs. HCFA's share of the premium in a public-private high-option plan would simply be the premium for its standard-option plan. In the long run, HCFA would be allowed to transition the government-run fee-for-service plan to a more privately managed basis overall, possibly with different alternatives available regionally.

Medigap.   The National Association of Insurance Commissioners would develop new model plans immediately under a federal directive. All plans would include basic coverage for prescription drugs. One plan would be drug-only. Plans would vary regarding the degree Medicare coinsurance was covered.

Premium Formula Basics
Beneficiaries would pay 12 percent of the premium for the standard benefits package on average, pay no premium for plans less than about 85 percent of the national weighted average, and pay all of the additional premium for plan premiums above the national weighted average. (An example of this type of premium schedule was included in the estimate from February 17, 1999.)

Although all plans would be available on the national premium schedule, only the cost of standard benefits (Medicare-covered services) would count toward computing the national weighted average premium. Plans with only a high option would be required to separate out the cost of extra benefits in their submission to the board for that purpose. If early versions of the risk adjuster would otherwise fail to prevent excessive premium differences between high- and standard-option plans, the board's actuaries could require that differences in premiums reflect the difference in value of benefits offered for private plans with multiple benefit options.

In areas where only the government-run fee-for-service plan operated, the beneficiary obligation would be limited to the lower of 12 percent of the fee-for-service premium or 12 percent of the national weighted average premium.

Fee-for-Service Benefits
The government-run fee-for-service plan would have a $400 combined deductible, indexed to the growth in Medicare costs. Ten percent coinsurance would be charged for home health, laboratory services, and certain other services not currently subject to coinsurance. No coinsurance would be charged for inpatient hospital stays and preventive care.

Management of the Government-Run Fee-for-Service Plan
All plans, private and government-run fee-for-service, would compete in the premium support system; all plans would have premiums and would be available on the national schedule. The fee-for-service plan would have a premium like any other plan; it would adjust its premium in subsequent years based on its cost experience.

The proposal recommends that efforts to contain costs in the fee-for-service plan continue. Toward that end, HCFA would be allowed to pursue competitive purchasing strategies in areas where its payments were not appropriate. The estimate assumes that the growth of fee-for-service spending would be moderated somewhat by a combination of HCFA and congressional efforts. Without such ongoing savings, the fee-for-service plan could gradually lose its competitive position with private plans.

Special Payments (Education, Disproportionate Share, Rural Subsidies)
Under the proposal, federal support for direct medical education (DME) would be carved out of Medicare. DME funding would continue through either a mandatory entitlement or a multiyear discretionary appropriation program separate from Medicare. Depending on the nature of the replacement program for DME, the federal budget as a whole might not be affected by the carve-out. The proposal would also recommend exploring funding disproportionate share hospitals (DSH) and indirect medical education (IME) outside of the Medicare program and financing those items through a mandatory or multiyear discretionary appropriation program. Any special payments remaining in Medicare would not be included in premiums for the government-run fee-for-service plan or private plans.

Retirement Age
The normal age of eligibility would be gradually raised from sixty-five to sixty-seven to conform with that of Social Security. Congress would develop an exemption process for affected beneficiaries with special needs, such as those unable to work and otherwise get health coverage. Eligibility requirements under that exemption process would not necessarily be the same as the requirements for eligibility based on disability for those under sixty-five, although the waiting period for eligibility based on disability could also be waived or shortened for those affected by the change.

Long-Term Care
The proposal indicates that long-term care issues should be separated from Medicare (an acute-care program). The proposal would require a study of various long-term care issues. The cost estimate does not include any impact on the budget from long-term care items.

Financing
The proposal would implement a combined trust fund, with guaranteed general revenue funding to grow at the same rate as overall program costs if it otherwise would exceed 40 percent of the program's cost (without further congressional approval). The initial balance in the combined fund would equal the balance in the Part A and Part B funds at the time of enactment.

Source: National Bipartisan Commission on the Future of Medicare. (www.medicare.commission.gov/ medicare/btp31599.html)

increases through utilization controls and heavy emphasis on payment limitations to providers.

By the end of the century, managed care plans' control on both areas was under severe attack. The government has been attempting to pass patient protection legislation since 1997, and although it has not yet been achieved (through 2001), there is a good possibility that it will succeed soon. This legislation removes some of the utilization controls that the health plans have been using primarily to limit specialist referrals, often for highly expensive tests. In addition, employers have been hearing a loud-and-clear call from their employees that they want more choice in provider selection than has been available through the basic managed care health plan. This has led to new point-of-service (POS) offerings in many plans that allow the member to receive service from providers outside the plan's panel with very little financial disincentive. This freedom of choice, however, carries a price with it.

Inevitably, the industry is starting to see the return of health care inflation that outstrips the inflation inherent in the rest of the economy. Since 1999, employers have been feeling the pinch as managed care plans proposed 6 to 12 percent premium increases (Walker, 1999). At the same time, it has been reported that the percentage of U.S. workers enrolled in restrictive managed health care plans fell for the first time in 1998, according to a survey suggesting that the managed care strategy has run its course. The report found that 47 percent of employees covered by U.S. companies were members of either an HMO or a POS plan, down from 50 percent in 1997. Meanwhile enrollment in the less-restrictive PPOs climbed from 35 percent to 40 percent (Winslow, 1999). This is an indication that the restrictive managed care plan premise of "less access, less cost" was no longer acceptable.

These upward trends in cost are a function of several phenomena:

- Plans with less restriction and more choice
- The upward surge of pharmaceutical costs, which are borne in large part by the health plan
- The increase in the health plan's medical-loss ratio, which itself has been driven by lower-than-required premium increases over the past several years

Although the short-term future of managed care is probably secure, its long-term future is questionable. Medicare's plan to offer premium support payments to patients, as well as Medicaid's drive to enroll as many eligible members as possible, may well reinvigorate the plans. To be successful, though, the plans have to convince a skeptical public that they care as much about quality (or more) as they do about cost. Otherwise, these profit-driven plans may be replaced by nonprofit, community-based plans controlled by hospital and physician providers that can demonstrate quality above cost. Or employers may well decide they do not need an intermediary adding a 20 to 25 percent cost factor to the premium. They may choose to contract directly with providers (Relman, 1998). Any one of these propositions is possible.

Industry Segment Trends

The previous macro and payor trends have a direct impact on the various segments of the health care industry.

Hospitals. In 1975, there were approximately 1.5 million hospital beds in America. By 1999, this number had shrunk to just over 1.0 million, a reduction of about 33 percent in just twenty years (National Center for Health Statistics, 2000). In addition, the total number of hospitals had decreased from 7,156 to 6,201 in the same time period (and down to 5,890 not long thereafter) (American Hospital Association, 2000). If the bed count reduction is extrapolated out, there should be no need for any more hospital beds by the year 2038. But the demise of the American hospital is not likely to come that soon, and possibly not forever.

Here's a riddle concerning the future of hospitals and hospital care. If the health care community is going to practice Star Trek medicine in the future, with medical tricorders and magic pills developed through the use of gene therapy that do away with the need for surgery, why does the *Starship Enterprise* have a sick bay? It may have to do not only with the technical competence and proficiency of the nurses, doctors, and technicians that treat the patient; it may also involve the compassionate care given by these same individuals. Patients have come to prize the high-tech and high-touch environment of hospital care.

There is good reason to believe that hospitals will have to reinvent themselves in the current century to offer improvements in many areas and remain a viable delivery system. There is also ample evidence to believe that they can do so. Improvements might include the following:

• *Patient-friendlier processes,* from the registration function to the clinical climate, followed by discharge planning and billing requirements. Many hospitals have already begun to adopt systems to deal with these issues. Heavy reliance preregistration and point-of-service registration processes has been adopted at many facilities. Most new hospitals are built with private rooms only; semiprivate rooms and wards are a thing of the past in many communities. Similarly, most renovation projects on the patient floor adopt the private room concept. Many hospitals have also adopted highly structured discharge planning techniques that emphasize patient and family education and a variety of posthospital options. This is often called continuum of care, and it improves the awareness of patients and their caregivers.

• *Development of additional revenue sources.* For hospitals to prosper and thrive in the future, they have to tap into new health care services that may not exist today. One obvious developing area is the gene therapy clinic, but it is still too early. However, there are a number of areas where hospitals could increase their inpatient and outpatient revenues. Some of these outpatient care areas are alternative medicine centers, midlife women's centers, and digestive disorder centers, along with stroke centers, frail elderly units, and cardiac crisis centers. To survive in the future, hospitals must develop these new revenue sources or steal market share from competitor organizations that are also trying to do the same.

• *Cost reduction from improved clinical decision support systems.* There is an enormous opportunity in most hospitals to improve the cost structure through utilization and consumption controls, along with standardization of protocols and supplies. This was covered in some detail in Chapter Eleven. Hospitals of the future have to stop talking and start doing. The best chance these providers have to accomplish this task is through clinical decision support systems that include the hospital's unit costs and volumes segregated by physician and clinical coding (such as ICD-9 and CPT-4 codes). This could and should be incorporated into clinical (critical) pathway development and monitoring. These systems exist now. Successful providers will take a leadership position and enlist their physicians in changing their ordering patterns to reduce costs while maintaining or improving quality.* Using clinical decision support tools is one of the best opportunities for health care systems of the future to position themselves as low-cost, efficient, patient-friendly providers.

• *Develop the concept of a virtual hospital or a hospital without walls.* This entity may include only a small physical structure for major surgery and critical care beds. All other activities would take place at a cluster of widely separated (or neighboring) facilities (for example, imaging center, same-day surgery center, and ambulatory center) for activities that cannot be accomplished over the phone or

---

*According to an article in the February 1999 issue of *Healthcare Financial Management,* "information systems can help build critical pathways, measure variations in patterns of care, perform comparative performance assessments, and offer analytical services, such as quality and utilization outcome comparative data for special units or services. Other capabilities include order entry, laboratory test results posting, alerts and reminders, and giving clinicians with access to diagnostic algorithms, treatment standards, and educational services. The computerized electronic medical record enables providers to improve data accessibility and accuracy, give on-line reporting capabilities, reduce duplication, and improve productivity, while reducing errors and cutting labor and office supply costs" (Rosenstein, 1999, p. 52).

through telemedicine. There would also be a communications center to facilitate electronic monitoring of chronic patients and telemedicine capabilities.

Physician Practice Management. Physicians, of course, will continue to practice medicine, and their practices will evolve with the coming wave of pharmaceutical and gene therapies. How they run their offices is another matter entirely. There has been a major revolution in how a physician runs an office over the past five to seven years. Physician practice management companies, the high-flyers of the second half of the 1990s, have fallen out of favor. Recall the discussion of MedPartners and PhyCor in Chapter Nine. There is dramatic rethinking of what it takes to successfully operate a physician practice in the near and far future.

A clue is offered in a report published by the Medical Group Management Association (MGMA), "Performances and Practices of Successful Medical Groups." This is a benchmarking study that profiles groups showing superior performance in profitability and operating costs; production, capacity, and staffing; and accounts receivable and collections. As summarized in a *Modern Healthcare* article, highly successful physician groups manage their practices with seven common techniques:

1. Using detailed cost accounting
2. Knowing the true cost of delivering care
3. Employing zero-based budgeting
4. Applying physician incentive compensation
5. Using effective managed care contracting
6. Employing effective coding techniques
7. Improving service delivery (Jaklevic, 1999)

Physician practice is one of many areas where good past practices will work well in the future. All the items in this list are nothing more than good management practice. Any physician who wants to manage using good practices can do so, easily. The challenge on the physician side of the industry is to effect a major change in the thinking of physicians who simply do not believe they need to change. In the future, because of the major reimbursement changes for physicians over the past ten years, behavior that follows the payment rules will lead to good financial results. If this happens, the industry could experience dramatic cost savings as physicians strive to maintain or enhance the bottom line through cost-effective management.

Skilled Nursing Facilities. SNFs will either be financially profitable or a major cost drain in the future. It depends on whether the SNF is freestanding or hospital-based. Under the new prospective payment system (PPS) of reimbursement for SNFs, a single national rate will be in effect for Medicare patients by the year 2002. This payment rate, which is variable and dependent on patient severity, should increase the revenues of many low-cost, freestanding SNFs while drastically cutting the revenues of higher-cost hospital-based units.

The reason for this is simple. Until 1998, skilled nursing facilities were reimbursed on their cost (with a reasonable cost limit). Thus hospitals received higher reimbursement because of their higher cost basis, usually associated with personnel-related and overhead costs. Conversely, the freestanding facilities were paid lower rates as a result of their lower costs. When the government decided to level the playing field and pay one rate regardless of ownership, not surprisingly it chose the lower rate. This will probably cause many hospital-based units to close over the next three years, as the full impact of the PPS becomes onerous in 2002.

The remaining SNFs stand to be highly successful. The aging of the population requires eldercare on a much more intense scale than at present. The baby boomer generation is approaching old age, and many of those already elderly are getting older. The frail elderly, usually defined as individuals eighty-five and older, are increasing in number. Their needs are greater; the SNF operators that figure out the proper formula of care should profit, probably through facility consolidation. They should be capable of financially successful operation that does not sacrifice high-quality care.

Home Health Agency Services. Home health agencies (HHAs), by contrast, may continue to suffer greatly at the hands of government rate makers. New prospective payment rates have been developed and in place since October 1, 2000. These rates have a chance to slightly improve the financial condition of home health agencies, which were devastated in the first two years of the Balanced Budget Act.

Home health care is an important cog in the continuum of care in the industry. The dramatic reduction of providers in the late 1990s, along with the reduction of SNFs, could leave a gaping hole that will be difficult to fill. Thus it was no surprise that when it became obvious to policy makers that access to care was threatened, the government stepped in and restored the home health rates to a rational level. Providers and patients already left in the dust will be nothing more than a memory.

Health Care IT Trends

Information system advances hold out a great opportunity for improving quality and efficiency at health care organizations. Because the clinician knows more about the patient and his or her medical, social, and economic history than anyone, capture of this knowledge in an electronic medical record that can store, retrieve, and display this information in a user-friendly and timely manner is coming soon. Information of this type will permit the clinician to develop a treatment plan sooner because he will be able to make a correct diagnosis quicker. In fact, in the future, the computers will be assisting the clinician in patient diagnosis. Medical databases are being developed that can assess the probability of a diagnosis according to the input of symptoms and complaints presented by the patient. The databases will be updated constantly in real time with the latest clinical findings as published in clinical journals from around the world. Once the diagnosis is made, these databases will also recommend the most efficacious treatment pattern. Clearly, a targeted approach to treating a properly diagnosed illness has a better chance of clinical success with a lower cost for achieving it.

These databases are just one of many improvements that IT holds out. Each year in February, the magazine *Healthcare Informatics* looks at the nine hottest trends. In the February 2001 issue, the hot trends are listed as application service providers, data security, integration, supply chain management, workflow automation, wireless, customer relation management, convergence, and disease management. Typically, the trends are chosen on the basis of at least one of three critical components to health care delivery: lowering overall costs, offering a competitive advantage, or improving patient care.

These are some important areas of concentration at this moment in time. Yet as the past is prelude, these hot items will pass, to be replaced with the next big thing. Still, IT in the future of health care will play a key role in helping organizations achieve goals, mundane or lofty. When it comes to technology, there are few limits on the improvement that can be made to the care of the patient at a reasonable cost.

Future Conclusions

All this prognosticating about the future holds big promises and big threats. As the health care industry continues to prepare for its unknown future, it faces a daunting financing challenge. The industry needs to decide if it truly believes that projected expenditure levels can be sustained. Also, will the country continue to allow a disproportionate amount of its wealth to be used for health care in the manner it has in the past? The industry is going to have to face public schizophrenia and political posturing as it winds its way down the path to an unknown tomorrow. The one constant we are assured of is that there will always be change.

A study commissioned by the League of Women Voters with the Henry J. Kaiser Family Foundation shows just how great a task this will be. The study found these results:

- Americans love Medicare, and they say they're willing to do whatever is necessary to keep it, but they are loath to raise payroll or personal contributions.
- Americans say people should be responsible for themselves as much as possible, but they think that the government should cover long-term nursing home care so they won't have to use personal savings.
- Americans know that Medicare is in serious trouble, but their major proposal for fixing it is to eliminate waste and fraud.
- Americans don't want to cut payments to doctors and hospitals because they are afraid that if payments are reduced, fewer payors will take Medicare patients.
- Americans think that raising the Medicare eligibility age from sixty-five to sixty-seven is a bad idea that would push large numbers of people into the ranks of the uninsured (Quinn, 1999, p. 3).

In the end, health care finance professionals have to understand all the factors that affect the finances of the industry. Whether they are managers, accountants, financial analysts, payroll or accounts payable specialists, materials management buyers, receivers or distributors, registrars, billers, collectors, or ombudsmen, they all have a common goal: to support patient caregivers in every way possible. This usually means using their expertise to maximize revenues or minimize costs, to produce the highest possible operating and net margins so that the health care organization they represent can continue to buy the latest medical equipment and hire the best-qualified personnel to provide the best in patient care. This may be why *CFO* magazine published an article titled "Critical Condition—Why Healthcare CFOs Have the Toughest Finance Jobs in America." The article quotes a number of health care CFOs. As one says: "The whole industry is in turmoil, and I don't think any of us know where this is going. We have a lot of options and I'm not sure any one is the right one, but decisions have to get made. It's not just a business; there are enormous social considerations. Every day we have to consider that the consequences of not doing a good job are just terrible. We take it very, very seriously" (McCafferty, 1999, p. 71).

◆ ◆ ◆

They take it seriously at Ridgeland Heights Medical Center, with an occasional sip of goofball humor thrown in on the side. Finally, the finance management and staff are happy to conclude another successful year of doing their jobs to the best of their ability. Then the clock strikes midnight on December 31, 2001. As the second hand rolls over into a new year, many of them are hopeful that a new era may dawn for health care finance . . . or is it just a dream?

"Dad, are you finally done?" asks an overly tired Susie.

"Well, honey, I guess I'm done with this book," says a greatly relieved Sam. "But I don't think I'm done getting out the message of how important the things that we do in health care finance are. I suppose I'll keep doing something of this sort for a while. You know I enjoy doing it, so I'll just stay with it."

"Yeah, Dad, that's great. But remember, I just heard you tell this whole story over the last year. I'd really rather go out and kick the soccer ball around with you."

"You're right," her proud dad beams at the active little girl. "Let's go."

REFERENCES

Advisory Board. *The New Competitive Standard for Hospitals.* Washington, D.C.: Advisory Board, 1996.

American Hospital Association. *Estimated Useful Lives of Depreciable Hospital Assets.* Chicago: American Hospital Association, 1988.

American Hospital Association. *AHA Annual Survey Database, Fiscal Year 1999.* Chicago: American Hospital Association, 2000.

American Institute of Certified Public Accountants. *Audit and Accounting Guide for Health Care Organizations.* New York: American Institute of Certified Public Accountants, 1992, 1996.

Begley, S. "Made-to-Order Medicine." *Newsweek,* June 25, 2001, pp. 65–69.

Berger, S., and Ciotti, V. G. "HIS Consultants: When Are They Necessary and Why?" *Healthcare Financial Management,* June 1993, pp. 45–49.

Berman, H. J., Weeks, L. E., and Kukla, S. F. *The Financial Management of Hospitals.* (6th ed.) Ann Arbor, Mich.: Health Administration Press, 1986.

Bohlmann, R. C. "Hospital-Affiliated Practices Reduce 'Red Ink.'" *Medical Group Management Journal,* Nov.-Dec. 1998.

Cleverly, W. O. *Essentials of Healthcare Finance.* (4th ed.) Gaithersburg, Md.: Aspen, 1997.

Cleverly, W. O. *Almanac of Hospital Financial and Operating Indicators, 1998–1999.* Columbus, Ohio: Center for Healthcare Industry Performance Studies, 1998.

Cleverly, W. O., Knott, P. J., and Dye, C. F. *The 1997–1998 Physician Practice Acquisition Resource Book.* Columbus, Ohio: Center for Healthcare Industry Performance Studies, 1998.

Conn, J. "Remote Control: Security and Stability Concerns Make Physicians Leery of ASP Technology." *Modern Physician,* Jan. 29, 2001, p. 24.

Cook, B. "Judgment Day: MedPartners' Pullout Raises Questions About the Future of PPMs." *Modern Physician,* Dec. 1998, p. 2.

Cowling, P. *Certification Examination Preparation: CORE Manual.* Westchester, Ill.: Healthcare Financial Management Association, 1998.

Eisenberg, D. M., and others. "Unconventional Medicine in the United States." *New England Journal of Medicine,* 1993, *328*(4), 246.

First Consulting Group. *Report on the Impacts of the HIPAA Final Privacy Rule on Hospitals.* Chicago: American Hospital Association, 2001.

"Fortune 500 Largest U.S. Corporations." *Fortune,* Apr. 16, 2001, p. F19.

Gapenski, L. C. *Financial Analysis and Decision Making for Healthcare Organizations: A Guide for the Healthcare Professional.* Chicago: Irwin, 1996.

Gardner, J. "Budget Battle Looms: Clinton Uses Fraud Fines, User Fees to Pay for Programs." *Modern Healthcare,* Feb. 9, 1998.

Gibson, R. P., Berger, S., and Ciotti, V. G. "Selecting an Information System Without an RFP." *Healthcare Financial Management,* June 1992.

Heimoff, S. "Round and Round and Round and Round: PPMs Regroup and Retool to Try to Stay Alive." *Modern Physician,* Jan. 2000.

Horngren, C. T., and Foster, G. *Cost Accounting: A Managerial Emphasis.* (6th ed.) Upper Saddle River, N.J.: Prentice Hall, 1987.

Ingenix. *Almanac of Hospital Financial and Operating Indicators: A Comprehensive Benchmark of the Nation's Hospitals.* Ingenix, 2001.

Irving Levin Associates. *Physician Medical Group Acquisitions Report.* (5th ed.) New Canaan, Conn.: Irving Levin Associates, 2000.

Jaklevic, M. C. "Practices with the Best Practices." *Modern Healthcare,* Feb. 8, 1999.

Jaklevic, M. C. "Still Struggling: Not-for-Profit Hospitals Post Small Increases in Margins, New Study Shows." *Modern Healthcare,* Apr. 23, 2001.

Kaufman, K., and Hall, M. *The Capital Management of Healthcare Organizations.* Ann Arbor, Mich.: Health Administration Press, 1990.

Kaufman, K., and Hall, M. *The Financially Competitive Healthcare Organization: The Executive's Guide to Strategic Financial Planning and Management.* Chicago: Probus, 1994.

Kotulak, R. "Genetics Reshaping Medicine: The Future Is Now for Powerful New Tool." *Chicago Tribune,* Feb. 21, 1999.

Lagnado, L. "Hospitals Profit by 'Upcoding' Illnesses." *Wall Street Journal,* Apr. 17, 1997, p. B1.

Lagnado, L., McGinley, L., and Tanouye, E. "Dose of Reality: Idea of Having Medicare Pay for Elderly's Drugs Is Roiling the Industry." *Wall Street Journal,* Feb. 19, 1999, p. 1.

McCafferty, J. "Critical Condition: Why Health Care CFOs Have the Toughest Finance Jobs in America." *CFO,* Jan. 1999.

McGinley, L. "Medicare Overhaul Shifts to Capitol Hill: National Commission Fails to Endorse a Proposal; Clinton Criticizes It Too." *Wall Street Journal,* Mar. 17, 1999.

Medicare Commission. "Medicare Commission Continues Analyses, Details Criteria for Medicare for Next Millennium." (Press release.) Medicare Commission, Jan. 5, 1999. (http://medicare.commission.gov/medicare/med1599-2.html)

Micheletti, J. *Understanding and Managing Under APCs.* Marblehead, Mass.: Opus Communications, 2001.

National Center for Health Statistics. *Health, United States, 1996–1997, and Industry Chartbook.* Hyattsville, Md.: National Center for Health Statistics, 1997.

National Center for Health Statistics. *Health, United States, 2000, with Adolescent Health Chartbook.* Hyattsville, Md.: National Center for Health Statistics, 2000.

Ngeo, C. "Trouble at Home." *Modern Healthcare,* July 27, 1998, p. 40.

Olivier, M., and others. "A High-Resolution Radiation Hybrid Map of the Human Genome Draft Sequence." *Science,* Feb. 16, 2001, pp. 1298–1302.

Pallarito, K. "Auditing the Auditors." *Modern Healthcare,* Sept. 21, 1998.

Pearman, W. A., and Starr, P. *Medicare: A Handbook on the History and Issues of Health Care Services for the Elderly.* New York: Garland, 1988.

Quinn, J. B. "Public Is in Medicare Dream World." *Chicago Tribune,* Feb. 28, 1999.

Relman, A. "The Decline and Fall of Managed Care." *Hospitals and Health Networks,* July 5, 1998.

Rosenstein, A. "Inpatient Clinical Decision-Support Systems: Determining the ROI." *Healthcare Financial Management,* Feb. 1999, p. 52.

Tschida, M. "Breakaway: Systems Divest the Practices They Had." *Modern Physician,* Apr. 2000.

Versel, N. "Dying Breath: Phycor Sees Losses Mount, Considers Bankruptcy." *Modern Physician,* May 2001.

Walker, T. "Experts Predict 6% to 12% Premium Increase in 1999: Employer and Employees to Pick Up the Monetary Slack After Healthcare Cost Hikes in Recent Years. *Managed Healthcare,* Jan. 1999, p. 17.

Weissenstein, E. "A One-Year Dip, Medicare Inpatient Spending to Resume Climb in '99." *Modern Healthcare,* Feb. 2, 1998.

Winslow, R. "Measure of HMO Membership Falls for First Time." *Wall Street Journal,* Jan. 16, 1999.

Worley, R., and Ciotti, V. "Selecting Practice Management Information Systems." *MGM Journal,* May-June 1997.

INDEX